Anatomy

2014–2015

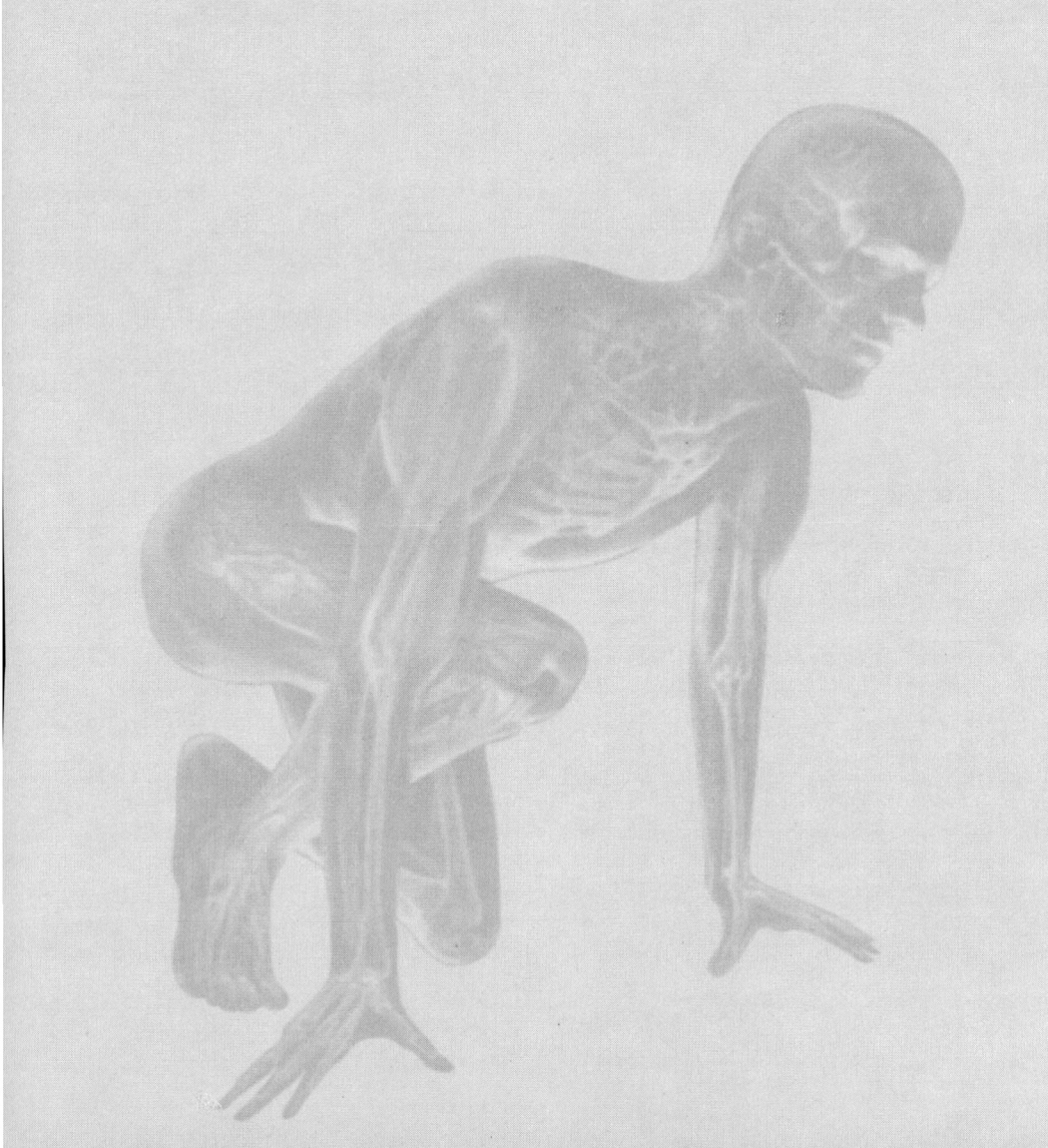

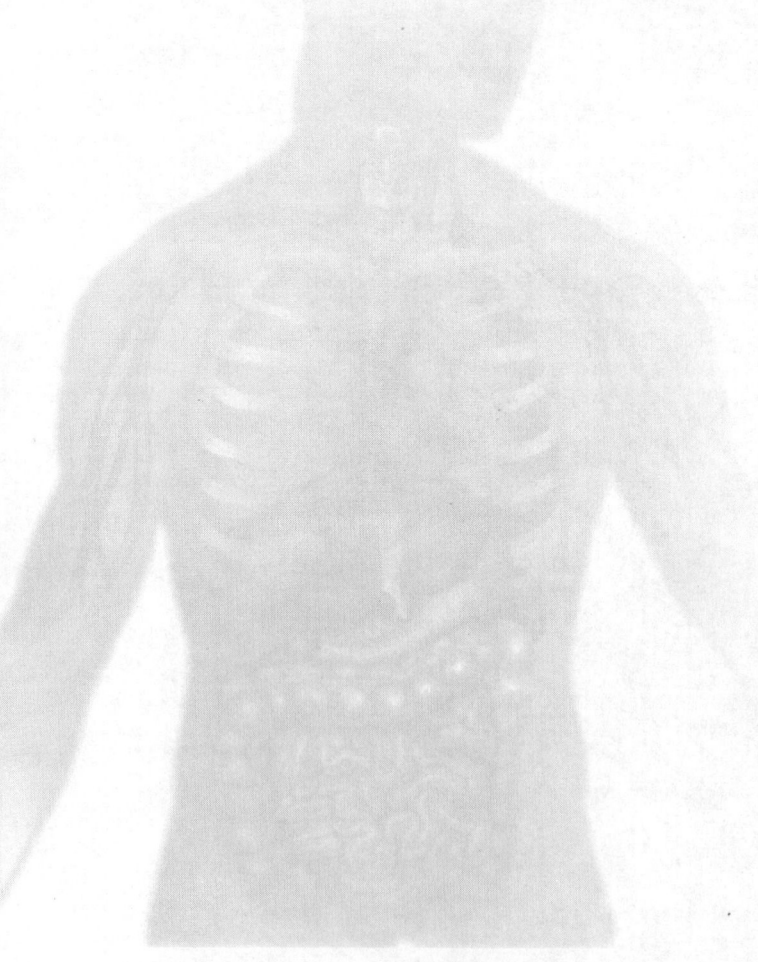

Quick Review *in*

Anatomy

2014–2015

Prof Ghulam Hassan

Ex-Professor and Head
Government Medical College, Srinagar, SKIMS Medical College, Srinagar
and Al Qassim University, Kingdom of Saudi Arabia

Ashfaq Ul Hassan

Lecturer, SKIMS Medical College, Srinagar

Shifan Khanday

Resident, SKIMS Medical College, Srinagar
Lecturer, Dubai Medical College for Girls, Dubai, UAE

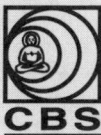

CBS

CBS Publishers & Distributors Pvt Ltd

New Delhi • Bengaluru • Chennai • Kochi • Mumbai • Pune
Hyderabad • Kolkata • Nagpur • Patna • Vijayawada

Quick Review in
Anatomy
2014–2015

ISBN: 978-81-239-2445-8

Copyright © Authors and Publishers

First Edition: 2014

Published by Satish Kumar Jain for

CBS Publishers & Distributors Pvt Ltd
4819/XI Prahlad Street, 24 Ansari Road, Daryaganj, New Delhi 110 002, India.
Ph: 23289259, 23266861, 23266867   Fax: 011-23243014   Website: www.cbspd.com
e-mail: delhi@cbspd.com; cbspubs@airteimail.in.

Corporate Office: 204 FIE, Industrial Area, Patparganj, Delhi 110 092
Ph: 4934 4934   Fax: 4934 4935   e-mail: publishing@cbspd.com; publicity@cbspd.com

Branches

- **Bengaluru:** Seema House 2975, 17th Cross, K.R. Road, Banasankari 2nd Stage, Bengaluru 560 070, Karnataka
  Ph: +91-80-26771678/79   Fax: +91-80-26771680   e-mail: bangalore@cbspd.com
- **Chennai:** 20, West Park Road, Shenoy Nagar, Chennai 600 030, Tamil Nadu
  Ph: +91-44-26260666, 26208620   Fax: +91-44-42032115   e-mail: chennai@cbspd.com
- **Kochi:** 36/14 Kalluvilakam, Lissie Hospital Road, Kochi 682 018, Kerala
  Ph: +91-484-4059061-65   Fax: +91-484-4059065   e-mail: kochi@cbspd.com
- **Mumbai:** 83-C, Dr E Moses Road, Worli, Mumbai-400018, Maharashtra
  Ph: +91-22-24902340/41   Fax: +91-22-24902342   e-mail: mumbai@cbspd.com
- **Pune:** Bhuruk Prestige, Sr. No. 52/12/2+1+3/2 Narhe, Haveli (Near Katraj-Dehu Road Bypass), Pune 411 041, Maharashtra
  Ph: +91-20-64704058, 64704059, 32392277 Fax: +91-20-24300160 .   e-mail: pune@cbspd.com

Representatives

- **Hyderabad** 0-9885175004
- **Nagpur** 0-9021734563
- **Kolkata** 0-9831437309, 0-9051152362
- **Patna** 0-9334159340
- **Vijayawada** 0-9000660880

Printed at Magic International, Pvt. Ltd., Greater Noida

Preface

Thanks to Almighty for guidance in life and blessings to Prophet Mohammed [PBUH].

We provide this book for the benefit of quick revision of anatomy for students of PG preparation as well as first MBBS students who at the end of their studies do not find ample time for quick revision.

The book contains all the important points and topics and clinically relevant points on applied anatomy along with the latest MCQs, newly framed and taken from DNB, AIIMS, PGI, State level examinations.

We hope this book will give maximum benefit to the students.

Prof G. Hassan
Dr Ashfaq Ul Hassan
Dr Shifan Khanday

Preface

Acknowledgments

Prof Showqat Zargar MD DM, Director, SKIMS/Principal, SKIMS Medical College, Srinagar

Prof Khaleel Baba, Dean, SKIMS, Soura

Prof Nisar Chaudhary, Professor of Surgery, SKIMS, Soura

Prof Khursheed, Ex-Dean, SKIMS, Soura

Prof A Halim, Ex-Professor and Head, Anatomy, King George Medical College, Lucknow

Prof Muzzamil, Ex-Professor, Anatomy, Aligarh Muslim University

Prof RN Bargotra, Ex-Professor and Head, Anatomy, GMC, Jammu

Prof Sunnanda, Professor and Head, Anatomy, GMC, Jammu

Prof Shaheen Shadad, Professor and Head, Anatomy, GMC, Srinagar

Prof Mohammed Shafi, Ex-Professor and Head, GMC, Srinagar

Dr Ghulam Mohd Bhat, Associate Professor, Anatomy, GMC, Srinagar

Dr Bashir Ahmed, Assistant Professor, Anatomy, GMC, Srinagar

Dr Mohammed Saleem, Assistant Professor, Anatomy, GMC, Srinagar

Contents

1

Upper Limb

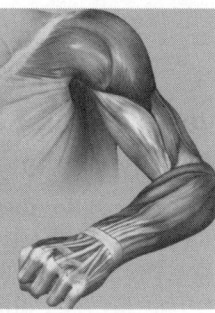

AXILLA

Axilla is a space between the upper part of the arm and the upper part of the side of the thoracic wall. **It resembles a "four sided pyramid"**.

Boundaries of Axilla

Anterior wall	• Pectoralis major • Pectoralis minor • Subclavius and clavipectoral fascia
Posterior wall	• Subscapularis • Latissimus dorsi • Teres major
Medial wall	• Upper four ribs • Side of the thorax • Serratus anterior
Lateral wall	• Upper part of shaft of humerus • Biceps brachii • Coracobrachialis
Apex	• Bounded by the middle third of clavicle—outer border of 1st rib • Upper border of scapula
Floor/Base	• Axillary fascia

Contents of Axilla

• Axillary artery
• Axillary vein
• Axillary lymph nodes
• Axillary fat
• Infraclavicular part of brachial plexus

- Long thoracic nerve
- Intercostobrachial nerve

Vessels of Upper Limb
Axillary artery

It begins at the **outer border of the 1st rib** as a continuation of the **subclavian artery** and **ends at the lower border of the teres major by becoming the brachial artery**. The pectoralis minor muscle divides the artery into three parts.
- The 1st part above it,
- The second part behind it and
- The third part below it.

Ist part:	gives (1) **Superior thoracic artery**
2nd part:	gives (2) **Thoracoacromial and lateral thoracic arteries**
3rd part:	gives (3) **Anterior circumflex humeral, posterior circumflex humeral and subscapular arteries**

Brachial artery

Extends from lower border of **teres major** muscle to elbow just **medial to tendon of biceps**. The pulsations of brachial artery are **auscultated for blood pressure measurement**.

Branches of brachial artery

- Muscular branches.
- **Profunda brachii artery with its branches:** *Anterior descending, posterior descending and ascending branch*
- Superior ulnar collateral
- Inferior ulnar collateral
- Nutrient artery to humerus
- **Terminal branches:** Ulnar and radial.

Branches of ulnar artery

- Muscular branches
- Anterior ulnar recurrent
- Posterior ulnar recurrent
- Palmar and dorsal carpal branches
- Common interosseous artery

Branches of radial artery

- Muscular branches
- Radial recurrent
- Palmar carpal branch
- Superficial palmar branch

Axillary vein

Begins at the **lower border of teres major as the continuation of the basilic vein and ends at the outer border of the first rib by becoming the subclavian vein**. It lies on the medial side of the axillary artery.

Axillary lymph nodes

These are arranged in five main groups

- **Anterior or pectoral group:** Lie along the lower border of pectoralis major and sends efferents to apical nodes.
- **Posterior or subscapular nodes:** Lie along subscapular vessels and they also send efferents to apical nodes.
- **Lateral nodes:** Lie along the axillary vein and drain into apical nodes.
- **Apical nodes:** Lie behind the clavicle at the apex of axilla. The efferents either pass to the lower group of the deep cervical lymph nodes or directly reach the subclavian lymph trunk.
- **Central nodes:** Lie along the base of the axilla and drain into the apical nodes.

BREAST

- **Apocrine gland/modified sweat gland**
- **Well developed in females**
- **Rudimentary in males**

Extent

- Vertically from the **second or third to the sixth rib**
- From the **sternal edge, medially, almost to the midaxillary line** laterally in the transverse plane.
- The superolateral quadrant is prolonged towards the axilla along the inferolateral edge of pectoralis major, from which it projects a little, and may extend through an opening in the deep fascia **(foramen of Langer)** up to the apex of the axilla **(axillary tail of Spence).**
- The breast lies upon the **deep pectoral fascia, which in turn overlies pectoralis major and serratus anterior**. Between the breast and the deep fascia is loose connective tissue in the **'submammary space'**.

- The **nipple** projects from the centre of the breast anteriorly. It lies at the fourth intercostal space in most young women.
- The **areola** is a darkly pigmented area of skin, which circles the base of the nipple
- **Montgomery's tubercles are sebaceous glands underlying the areolar skin which enlarge during pregnancy and lactation.**

Important Points

✓ *Retraction of nipple* is due to fibrous contraction of lactiferous ducts in breast cancer.

✓ Invasion of retrommary space by cancer cells can cause fixity of breast to pectoral fascia by cancer cells.

✓ Contraction of ligaments of Cooper by cancer cell infiltration can cause dimpling of skin.

Arteries

The breasts are supplied by:

- Branches of the **internal thoracic artery** (2nd–6th intercostal arteries).
- Branches of the **axillary artery:** Namely the **superior thoracic, the pectoral branches of the thoracoacromial artery, the lateral thoracic and the subscapular arteries.**
- The **second perforating artery** is usually the largest, and supplies the upper region of the breast, and the nipple, areola and adjacent breast tissue.

Veins

There is a circular venous plexus around the areola. From this, and from the glandular tissue, blood drains in veins which accompany the corresponding arteries that supply the breast.

Lymphatic Drainage

Superficial lymphatics

Drain skin over breast except nipple and areola. They pass to axillary, internal mammary, supraclavicular lymph nodes.

Deep lymphatics

Drain parenchyma of the breast plus nipple and areola. They pass to axillary, posterior intercostal nodes.

Axillary nodes (chief nodes) receive more than 75% of the lymph from the breast. They are:

- Pectoral (anterior)
- Subscapular (posterior)

- Central and
- Apical.

Surgically, the nodes are described in relation to pectoralis minor.

- Those lying below pectoralis minor are the low nodes **(level 1)**,
- Those behind the muscle are the middle group **(level 2)**,
- While the nodes between the upper border of pectoralis minor and the lower border of the clavicle are the upper or apical nodes **(level 3).**

The subareolar plexus of Sappey **is a collection of large lymph vessels situated under the areola and is not to be considered as a collecting zone of lymph and it communicates with the lymphatics of the breast tissue.**

Lake of Stiles

Plexus of lymph situated on anterior sheath (deep fascia) of pectoralis major is called Lake of Stiles. It receives lymphatic communications from subareolar plexus of Sappey.

The internal mammary nodes receive lymph from both the medial and lateral portions of the breast. Lymph enters the thorax along the anterior perforating branches of the internal mammary artery and along the lateral perforating branches of the intercostal vessels. Most of the lymph goes to the internal mammary chain, but a small amount may pass to the posterior intercostal nodes along the heads of the ribs.

- Breast is a **frequent site of carcinoma.**
- Approximately 60% of them occurring in **upper lateral quadrant.**
- Cancer cells may infiltrate the **suspensory ligaments**. The breast then becomes fixed. Contraction of the ligaments can cause puckering of the skin.
- Infiltration of lactiferous ducts and their consequent fibrosis can cause **retraction of the nipple.**
- Because of communications of the superficial lymphatics of the breast across the midline, **cancer may spread from one breast to the other, and to the opposite axillary nodes as well.**
- Entrance of cancer cells into the blood vessels accounts for **metastasis in the distant bones.**

Nerve Supply

The breast is innervated by anterior and lateral branches of the **fourth to sixth intercostal nerves**

Brachial Plexus

- The anterior/ventral primary rami of **C5, 6, 7, 8 and T1** take part in its formation.
- Often C4 also takes part and it is then called **prefixed.**
- Often T2 also takes part and is called **postfixed.**
- The parts are **roots, trunks, divisions and cords**.

1

Upper Limb

> – C5 and C6 unite to form upper trunk.
> – C7 remains as such and forms middle trunk.
> – C8 and T1 unite to form lower trunk.

- Each trunk divides into an **anterior and posterior division**.

> – All posterior divisions meet and form **posterior cord**.
> – The anterior divisions of upper and middle trunks unite to form **lateral cord**.
> – The anterior division of the lower trunk only forms the **medial cord**.

- The roots lie in the neck between scalenus anterior and medius.
- The trunks lie in the lower part of the posterior triangle.
- The divisions lie behind the middle third of clavicle.
- The cords lie in the axilla.

Nerves from roots
- Dorsal scapular nerve (nerve to rhomboids) C5
- Nerve to serratus anterior C5, 6, 7

Nerves from medial cord
- Medial pectoral nerve C8, T1
- Medial cutaneous nerve of arm T1, T2
- Medial cutaneous nerve of forearm C8, T1
- Medial root of median nerve C8, T1
- Ulnar nerve C7, C8, T1

Nerves from lateral cord
- Lateral pectoral nerve C5, C6, C7
- Lateral root of median nerve C5, C6, C7
- Musculocutaneous nerve C5, C6, C7

Nerves from posterior cord
- Axillary nerve C5, C6
- Radial nerve C5, C6, C7, C8, T1
- Nerve to latissimus dorsi C6, C7, C8
- Upper and lower subscapular nerve C5, C6

Erb's Point

Union of six nerves, namely C5, C6, suprascapular nerve, nerve to subclavius, anterior and posterior division. Damage to it results in Erb's paralysis.

Erb's Palsy

Lesion of upper trunk of brachial plexus (C5, C6) caused by forceful downward traction of shoulder with lateral displacement of head to the other side (Policeman's tip).

The deformity causes:
- Hanging of arm by the side
- Extension of elbow
- Pronation of forearm
- Flexion of wrist.

Klumpke's Palsy

Lesion of lower trunk of brachial plexus (C8,T1) caused by forceful upward traction of the arm.

The deformity causes:
- Claw hand
- Sensory loss on ulnar side of forearm
- Horner's syndrome

Crutch Palsy

Damage of brachial plexus in the axilla from pressure of the crutch as a result of damage of radial nerve.

Saturday Night Palsy

Due to prolonged pressure on radial nerve in the spiral groove of humerus, there is radial nerve palsy after consuming liquor on weekends (especially Saturdays) when patient falls asleep with his arm hanging over back of chair. In the morning he suffers from radial nerve damage particularly wrist drop.

Winging of Scapula

Is excessive prominence of medial border of scapula due to paralysis of long thoracic nerve of bell.

NERVES

Radial Nerve

It is a branch of posterior cord of brachial plexus.

Root value is: C5, C6, C7, C8, and T1.

It is commonly injured in fracture shaft of humerus, intramuscular injections in arm.

It supplies:
- **Triceps**
- **Anconeus**
- **Brachioradialis**
- **Lateral part of brachialis**

- Brachioradialis
- Extensor carpi radialis longus

Cutaneous Branches

- Lower lateral cutaneous nerve of arm
- Posterior cutaneous nerve of arm
- Posterior cutaneous nerve of forearm

Lesion in Spiral Groove Causes

✓ Wrist drop
✓ Loss of supination
✓ Triceps is spared

Lesion Below Elbow Causes

✓ Wrist drop
✓ Loss of supination
✓ Sensory loss on lateral part of dorsum of hand.

Musculocutaneous Nerve

It is a branch of lateral cord of brachial plexus.

Root value is: C5, C6, C7

It supplies:
- Biceps
- Brachialis
- Coracobrachialis

Cutaneous Branches

Lateral cutaneous nerve of forearm

Lesion Causes

✓ Loss of flexion of elbow
✓ Weak supination
✓ Loss of biceps jerk

Median Nerve

It is a branch of medial and lateral cord of brachial plexus.

Root value is: C5, C6, C7, C8, T1.

It supplies:
- Pronator teres in arm

In forearm to:
- Flexor carpi radialis
- Palmaris longus
- Flexor digitorum superficalis

Damage in Wrist Causes
- Paralysis of thenar muscles and lumbricals 1 and 2
- Loss of opposition of thumb
- Ape thumb deformity
- Sensory loss over thumb, adjacent 3½ fingers and radial 2/3rd of palm.

Carpal Tunnel Syndrome
Compression of median nerve as it passes deep to the flexor retinaculum.

Ulnar Nerve
It is a branch of medial cord of brachial plexus.
Root value is: C8, T1.
It supplies:
- Flexor carpi ulnaris and medial half of flexor digitorum profundus in forearm
In hand:
- *Hypothenar muscles:* Palmaris brevis, abductor digiti minimi, flexor digiti minimi, opponens digiti minimi
- Medial two lumbricals
- Palmar and dorsal interossei
- Adductor pollicis

Damage in Wrist Causes
- Paralysis of all intrinsic muscles of hand (except those supplied by median nerve)
- Claw hand
- Loss of adduction of fingers
- Loss of adduction of thumb
- Wasting of hypothenar muscles
- Sensory loss over dorsal aspect of distal and middle phalanges of these fingers.

Structures under Cover of Deltoid
- Bony prominences, namely upper end of the humerus with greater and lesser tubercles, bicipital groove, upper part of shaft and surgical neck of humerus, coracoid process of scapula.
- Origin of muscles like coracobrachialis, short head of biceps, long head of biceps and long head of triceps.

1

Upper Limb

- Insertion of the muscles, namely pectoralis minor, subscapularis, supraspinatus, infraspinatus, teres minor, pectoralis major, teres major and latissimus dorsi.
- Anterior and posterior circumflex humeral vessels.
- Axillary nerve
- Shoulder joint
- Subacromial and subdeltoid bursae.

Rotator Cuff/Musculotendinous Cuff

Comprises four tendons of the muscles which are arising from the scapula and get inserted into either the greater or lesser tubercle of the humerus. They are at the place of the insertion fuse with the capsule of the shoulder joint and strengthen it.

They include:
- Subscapularis
- Supraspinatus
- Infraspinatus
- Teres minor

SPACES

Quadrangular space is bounded
Above: By subscapularis and teres minor
Below: By teres major
Medially: By long head of triceps
Laterally: By surgical neck of humerus
Through this passes axillary nerve and posterior circumflex humeral vessels.

Upper triangular space is bounded
Above: By teres minor
Below: By teres major
Laterally: By long head of triceps
Through this space passes circumflex scapular vessels.

Lower triangular space is bounded
Above: By teres major
Below: By long head of triceps
Laterally: By humerus
Through this space passes radial nerve and profunda brachii artery.

Important Anatomical Changes Taking Place at the Level of Insertion of Coracobrachialis Muscle

- The shaft of humerus above this level is circular and below triangular.
- Corresponds to insertion of deltoid laterally.
- Marks the beginning of origin of brachialis and medial head of triceps.
- The medial and lateral intermuscular septa start becoming more prominent.
- The basilic vein pierces the deep fascia.
- Median nerve crosses the brachial artery from lateral to medial side.
- The medial cutaneous nerve of arm and forearm pierce the deep fascia here.
- The medial intermuscular septum is pierced here by ulnar nerve and superior ulnar collateral artery.
- The lateral intermuscular septum is pierced at this level by radial nerve and radial collateral branch of the profunda brachii artery.
- The nutrient artery to humerus passes into the bone.

Lateral intermuscular septum extends from the lateral lip of the intertubercular sulcus of the humerus along the lateral supracondylar ridge to the lateral epicondyle. It is perforated by the radial nerve and the radial collateral branch of the profunda brachii artery.

The thicker medial intermuscular septum extends from the medial lip of the inter-tubercular groove of the humerus along the medial supracondylar ridge to the medial epicondyle and blends with the tendon of coracobrachialis. It is perforated by posterior branch of inferior collateral artery, and ulnar nerve.

The medial and lateral intermuscular septa divide the upper arm into anterior and posterior compartments.

The muscles of anterior compartment are coracobrachialis, biceps brachii and brachialis.

The muscles of Posterior compartment are triceps and anconeus.

Cutaneous Nerve Supply of the Axilla and Upper Arm

- Supraclavicular on the lateral side of the shoulder C3, C4
- Intercostobrachial on the medial side of axilla T2
- Upper lateral cutaneous nerve of arm (axillary)
- Lower lateral cutaneous nerve of arm (radial)
- Medial cutaneous nerve of arm T1, T2 (medial cord)
- Posterior cutaneous nerve of arm (radial)

1

Upper Limb

Muscles of the Front of the Upper Arm

Muscle	Origin	Insertion	Action
Biceps brachii	Long head from supraglenoid tubercle of humerus Short head from coracoid process	Main tendon into posterior part of radial tuberosity. The bicipital aponeurosis into deep fascia	Supinator and flexor of elbow. Long head maintains the head of humerus in proper position
Brachialis	From front of the lower shaft of the humerus	Tuberosity of ulna	Primary flexor of elbow
Coracobrachialis	Coracoid process	In the middle part of the medial margin of the humerus	Flexes and adducts the arm

Muscles of the Back of the Upper Arm

Muscle	Origin	Insertion	Action
Triceps brachii	Long head from infraglenoid tubercle of scapula The lateral head from an area from the greater tuberosity to groove for radial nerve The medial head from posterior surface of humerus below the groove	A common tendon into the posterior part of upper surface of olecranon	Powerful extensor of elbow
Anconeus	Lateral epicondyle of humerus	Lateral border of olecranon and upper third of back of ulna	Extensor of elbow

The muscles of back of upper arm are supplied by radial nerve.

Triceps muscle can be tested by palpating its fibers during elbow extension against resistance.

Cubital Fossa

Is a triangular space which lies in front of the elbow.

Base lies above

Apex lies below

It is bounded **above** by an imaginary line between medial and lateral epicondyles of humerus.

- **Laterally**— brachioradialis muscle
- **Medially**— pronator teres muscle
- **Apex** is formed by the meeting of both the lateral and medial borders.

- **Roof** is formed by:
  - Skin
  - Superficial fascia contains cephalic vein, basilic vein, median cubital vein, medial cutaneous nerve of the arm and lateral cutaneous nerve of the forearm.
  - Deep fascia is pierced by the communication between deep veins and median cubital vein.
  - Bicipital aponeurosis.

Floor is formed by brachialis and anterior part of supinator muscle.

Contents of Cubital Fossa

- Median nerve which disappears between two heads of pronator teres.
- End of brachial artery.
- Origin of radial artery.
- Origin of ulnar artery.
- Biceps tendon.
- Beginning of posterior interosseous nerve.
- Supratrochlear lymph nodes.

Brachial Artery

It is a **continuation of the axillary artery and extends from the lower border of the teres major to the cubital fossa** and gives the following branches:

- Profunda brachii artery which accompanies radial nerve in the spiral groove and is injured in # of the mid shaft of the humerus.
- Superior ulnar collateral artery
- Inferior ulnar collateral artery which divides into anterior and posterior branches
- Radial artery
- Ulnar artery gives anterior and posterior ulnar recurrent

DERMATOMES

The area of skin supplied by one spinal nerve is called a dermatome.

There is varying degree of overlap of the adjoining dermatomes, so that the area of sensory loss following damage to the spinal cord or nerve roots is always less than the actual area of dermatome.

The dermatomes are complicated in the limbs because of embryological rotation.

On the trunk they extend round the body from posterior to anterior.

The tactile loss (light and crude touch) loss is greater than (hot, cold, pain) due to variability in the degree of overlapping. It is more for pain and thermal sensations.

The lines of cleavage or Langer's lines represent the direction of rows of collagen. They run longitudinally in the limbs and circumferentially in the trunk and neck.

The skin creases: The skin over joint folds is thin and firmly adherent to the underlying structures by fibrous tissue.

Upper Limb

- C4   Tip of shoulder
- C5   Lateral aspect of upper arm and upper part of forearm
- C6   Lateral aspect of lower part of forearm and lateral aspect of hand
- C7   Middle of hand (front and back)
- C8   Medial side of hand and lower part of forearm
- T1   Medial side of upper part of forearm and lower part of arm
- T2   Medial side of upper part of arm and floor of axilla

HAND

Muscles of Hand

The total number of muscles are twenty.
- **Group 1** Muscles of thenar eminence and adductor pollicis
- **Group 2** Muscles of hypothenar eminence and palmaris brevis
- **Group 3** Lumbricals
- **Group 4** Dorsal interossei
- **Group 5** Palmar interossei

Group 1

The muscles are **abductor pollicis brevis, flexor pollicis brevis and opponens pollicis.** They arise from the flexor retinaculum, scaphoid and trapezium and are inserted into the base of the proximal phalanx of thumb, but the opponens is inserted into the shaft of first metacarpal bone. **These are innervated by median nerve.**

The adductor pollicis arises by two heads the oblique and transverse heads. The oblique head arises from the bases of the second and third metacarpals. The transverse head arises from palmar surface of third metacarpal bone. Both the heads meet and are inserted into the base of the proximal phalanx of thumb after the intervention of the sesamoid bone. This muscle is innervated by the deep branch of ulnar nerve.

Group 2

The muscles are **abductor digiti minimi, flexor digiti minimi and opponens digiti minimi.** They arise from flexor retinaculum, pisiform and hamate. The abductor and flexor muscles are inserted into base of the proximal phalanx of little finger, but the opponens is inserted into the shaft of fifth metacarpal bone. All these muscles are **innervated by the ulnar nerve.**

1

Upper Limb

The palmaris brevis is a subcutaneous muscle and arises from the flexor retinaculum and palmar aponeurosis and is inserted into the skin of the medial border of hand. It deepens the cup of the hand and enables to have a firm grip. It is innervated by superficial branch of ulnar nerve.

Group 3

Includes lumbricals and look like the shape of earth worm. They are four in number and numbered from lateral to medial.

The first and second arise from the lateral side of tendon of flexor digitorum profundus tendon for index and middle fingers and are unipennate.

The third and fourth arise from the adjacent sides of the tendons of flexor digitorum profundus tendon for middle and ring fingers; ring and little fingers and are bipennate muscles.

They are all inserted into the dorsal digital expansions and bases of middle and distal phalanges of medial four fingers.

The 1st and 2nd are innervated by the median nerve and the 3rd and 4th by ulnar nerve.

These are flexors of metacarpophalangeal joints and extensors of interphalangeal joints and they are concerned with finer and skilful movements of hand.

Group 4

Includes dorsal interossei muscles are four and are bipennate. They arise from the palmar surfaces of shafts of adjacent metacarpal bones. The first from 1st and 2nd, the second from 2nd and 3rd, the third from 3rd and 4th, the fourth from 4th and 5th metacarpal bones.

The insertions are first into lateral side of base of proximal phalanx of index finger.

Second into lateral side of base of proximal phalanx of middle phalanx.

Third into the medial side of the base of proximal phalanx of middle finger.

Fourth into the medial side of the base of proximal phalanx of ring finger.

They are all innervated by deep branch of ulnar nerve.

Dorsal interossei are abductors of fingers, flexors of metacarpophalangeal and extensors of interphalangeal joints.

Group 5

Includes **palmar interossei, four in number. They are unipennate.**
They arise as follows:
- First from the medial side of the base of first metacarpal.
- Second from medial side of shaft of second metacarpal bone.
- Third from lateral side of shaft of fourth metacarpal bone.
- Fourth from lateral side of shaft of fifth metacarpal bone.

They are inserted as follows:

• First and second to medial side of bases of proximal phalanx of 1st and 2nd digits respectively.

• Third and fourth to lateral sides of bases of proximal phalanx of 3rd and 4th digits respectively.

They are all supplied by **deep branch of ulnar nerve**.

They are adductors of fingers and are flexors of metacarpophalangeal joints and extensors of interphalangeal joints.

Palmar Aponeurosis

It is the deep fascia of palm and is the continuation of palmaris longus.

It has three parts the lateral, medial and the central parts. The base of the central part divides into medial four slips and each slip divides into superficial and deep parts.

The superficial part fuses with the superficial transverse ligaments of the palm.

The deep part divides into two parts and they are attached into:

• Deep transverse ligament of palm
• Proximal and middle phalanx

Continuous with fibrous flexor sheaths

Dupuytren's Contracture

It is the inflammatory contracture of the palmar aponeurosis, characterized by fixing of the proximal and middle phalanx but the terminal phalanges are not involved. The ring finger is commonly affected.

Fibrous Flexor Sheaths

These are derived from the deep fascia of the fingers and present in all the five fingers. They are attached to the distal part of palmar aponeurosis and distally to sides of the phalanges and base of distal phalanx and so extends from head of metacarpal to base of distal phalanx. In the thumb it encloses the tendon of flexor pollicis longus and in the remaining four fingers the tendons of flexor digitorum superficialis and profundus tendons.

Retinacula

These are strong and thick bands of deep fascia and keep the tendons in proper position. There are two retinacula flexor and extensor retinacula on the flexor and extensor aspects respectively.

Flexor Retinaculum

Is attached medially to pisiform bone and hook of hamate and laterally to tubercle of scaphoid and crest of trapezium.

The structures crossing over it are:

- Palmaris longus tendon
- Palmar cutaneous branches of median and ulnar nerves
- Superficial palmar branch of radial artery
- Ulnar nerve and ulnar vessels

The structures deep to it are:

- Median nerve
- Tendon of flexor digitorum superficialis and profundus
- Flexor pollicis longus
- Flexor carpi radialis
- Radial and ulnar bursa

Carpal Tunnel

Is the passage formed by concavity of carpal bones bridged by flexor retinaculum. The structures passing deep to it are:

- Median nerve
- Ulnar bursa containing flexor digitorum superficialis and profundus.
- Radial bursa containing flexor pollicis longus
- Flexor carpi radialis

Carpal Tunnel Syndrome

Leads to sensory and motor symptoms due to the compression of the median nerve. It is caused by narrow of the size and shape of the tunnel, edema during pregnancy and bony swelling in osteoarthritis, myxoedema and dislocation of lunate. The effects of compression are painful paraesthesia, numbness of the digits on three and a half fingers, accumulation of fluid at night due to absence of pumping action of forearm muscles and loss of fine movements.

The anatomical changes include wasting of thenar muscles, hyperaesthesia of the palmar aspect of three and half digits but the skin of thenar eminence escapes as it is supplied by palmar cutaneous branch of median nerve which arises proximal to tunnel.

Extensor Retinaculum

Present on the dorsal aspect of the wrist. It is attached laterally to lower part of anterior border of radius. Medially attached to pisiform, triquetral.

Structures passing deep to the retinaculum are classified into **six osseo-fascial compartments and the structures passing from lateral to medial are:**

- APL, EPB
- ECRL, ECRB
- EPL
- ED, EI, posterior interosseous nerve, anterior interosseous artery
- EDM
- ECU

1

Upper Limb

Spaces of Hand

These are potential spaces lined by fascia due to the arrangement of fascia and fascial septa in hand and they are clinically important because they may be infected and pus may be collected.

The spaces are mainly three:
• Mid palmar space
• Thenar space
• Pulp space

Besides there are:
• Digital synovial sheaths
• Ulnar and radial bursae
• Space of parona in the forearm
• Dorsal subcutaneous
• Dorsal subaponeurotic spaces.

Mid palmar space: It is triangular, communicates proximally with space of Parona and distally with fascial sheath and the webs of the digits.

Medially lies the medial palmar septum and laterally the intermediate palmar septum.

Behind lies 2–5 metacarpal bones

In front lies the palmar aponeurosis

Thenar space: Communicates with fascial sheath of first lumbrical muscle.

Bounded in front by palmar aponeurosis

Behind fascia covering first dorsal interosseous and transverse head of adductor pollicis.

Laterally lateral palmar septum

Medially intermediate palmar septum

Pulp spaces: These are closed spaces in front of the distal phalanges of all the digits of hand and distal to fibrous sheaths of flexor tendons. It is divided into a number of tight compartments by fibrous septa from skin to periosteum of bone. The compartments contain subcutaneous fat and blood vessels. The proximal 1/5th of the distal phalanx is outside the space and gets its blood supply from a digital branch which does not pass through septa. The infection of pulp space is called **Whitlow** and causes severe pain due to increased tension and can cause necrosis of distal 3/4th. The pus can be drained by giving a lateral incision.

Dorsal subcutaneous space: It is the space between skin and superficial fascia of dorsum of hand. It contains dorsal venous arch.

Dorsal subaponeurotic space: It is the space between deep fascia and dorsal surface of metacarpal bones and interossei muscles.

Paronas space: It is a potential space situated deep to the long flexor tendons of the forearm. Posteriorly lies the interosseous membrane and pronator quadratus. Inferiorly the flexor retinaculum.

Ulnar bursa: Encloses **flexor digitorum superficialis and profundus** and extends from about 2.5 cm above flexor retinaculum to about half way of the metacarpal bones.

Radial bursa: Encloses **flexor pollicis longus** and extends from 2.5 cm above flexor retinaculum to the base of the distal phalanx of thumb.

Anatomical Snuff Box

A **depressed triangular area** on the lateral side of the wrist and is seen clearly when thumb is extended. It is bounded **laterally by abductor pollicis longus and extensor pollicis brevis, medially by tendon of extensor pollicis longus**.

The floor is formed by scaphoid, trapezium and base of 1st metacarpal bone.

The contents are:
- **Cephalic vein**
- **Radial artery**
- **Superficial branch of radial nerve**

Cranio-cleido Dysostosis

It is a rare abnormality. There is congenital absence of one or both clavicles. The patient can bring both the shoulders close to each other in front of the chest. There is faulty ossification of membranous bones. Thus, the patient may show additional abnormalities involving skull bones.

Winging of Scapula

Serratus anterior muscle keeps the medial border of scapula closely applied to the chest wall. Injury to long thoracic nerve of bell causes paralysis of serratus anterior muscle. The patient experiences difficulty in raising the arm above the head as serratus anterior is used in overhead abduction and pushing and punching movements. When the patient is asked to place his hands on the wall in front and asked to push, the medial border of the scapula on the affected side stands out-winged scapula.

Pulsating Scapula

The arterial anastomosis around the scapula supplies the muscles around the scapula. When the circulation in the axillary/brachial artery is affected (coarctation of aorta or blockade in the main vessels) it necessitates opening up the collaterals. It leads to dilatation and tortuosity of the collaterals that makes the scapula pulsatile.

Klippel-Feil Syndrome

There is bilateral failure of descent of scapula. Other associated anomalies are failure of fusion of occipital bone and defect in cervical spine. This results in webbing of neck and gross limitation of movements of neck.

Triangle of Auscultation

This triangle is bounded by the trapezius, latissimus dorsi and medial border of scapula with rhomboid major forming the floor. This triangle may be used for auscultating breath sounds as this area is least covered with muscles.

Rotator Cuff Tears

The rotator cuff is composed of the tendons of the **supraspinatus, infraspinatus, subscapularis and teres minor**. These are attached to the anterior, superior and posterior aspect of upper end of humerus.

Functions

- Infraspinatus and teres minor are lateral rotators of the shoulder joint.
- Resists shearing forces of the deltoid muscle during abduction and forward flexion.
- Stabilizes humeral head during the movement of the shoulder joint
- Subscapularis is a medial rotator
- Supraspinatus initiates abduction.

Subacromial Bursitis

Supraspinatus tendon may cause inflammation of subacromial bursa. This is due to inflamed and calcified tendon of supraspinatus. Thus in first fifteen degree abduction there is pain at the shoulder joint as the supraspinatus tendon and the bursa beneath it is affected. The abduction beyond fifteen degree does not cause pain as the inflamed bursa is away from supraspinatus tendon.

Painful Arc Syndrome (Supraspinatus Syndrome)

It is characterized by

1. Pain in 60–120 degree abduction
2. Chronic thickening of supraspinatus tendon causing impingement of tendon against coracoacromial arch.

Causes of the syndrome

- Violent dislocation of shoulder
- Tear of supraspinatus tendon
- Calcified deposit in supraspinatus tendon
- Subacromial bursitis
- Injury of greater tubercle

Frozen Shoulder (Adhesive Capsulitis or Periarthritis)

It is due to tendinitis involving rotator cuff. All shoulder movements are restricted due to adhesions, its cause is unknown.

Spontaneous recovery is seen in six to twelve months.

Volkmann's Ischaemic Contracture

Flexion deformity of wrist and fingers resulting from fixed contracture (shortening) of flexor muscles of forearm.

Causes

The ischaemia of flexor muscles because of

1. Injury to brachial artery/spasm/obstruction of artery near elbow
2. Supracondylar fracture with displacement
3. Tight plaster cast/bandage
4. Improper use of tourniquet
5. Tense oedema of soft tissue of forearm within unyielding fascial compartment.

Injury to the artery leads to interruption of blood flow which causes ischaemia. This results in paralysis of deep flexor muscles (FDP and FPL). This is irreversible after six hours.

Necrosis of muscles is replaced by fibrosis. The muscles are permanently shortened, resulting in flexion deformity.

Pronator Syndrome

This is the uncommon entrapment neuropathy of medium nerve.

Can occur as nerve passes

1. Deep to biceps aponeurosis
2. Between two heads of pronator teres
3. Through a fibrous arch of flexor digitorum superficialis.

Clinical Features

1. Pain and tenderness in proximal aspect of anterior forearm.
2. Symptoms often follow activities that involve repeated elbow movements.
3. Weakness of all muscles innervated by median nerve including abductor pollicis brevis and long finger flexors.
4. Sensory impairment on palm.

Cubital Tunnel Syndrome

Entrapment neuropathy of ulnar nerve

It is seen in the tunnel formed by tendinous arch connecting two heads of flexor carpi ulnaris at their humeral and ulnar attachments.

Students Elbow

There is inflammation of subcutaneous olecranon bursa which causes a round, fluctuating, and painful swelling of about 1 inch over olecranon.

1

Upper Limb

It is due to
- Repeated friction
- Trauma during fall on elbow
- Infection from abrasions of skin covering olecranon process

Cubitus Valgus

This results in increase in carrying angle at elbow. It is one of the clinical manifestations of Turner's syndrome (45, XO constitution).

Tennis Elbow

This is due to inflammation of tissues surrounding lateral epicondyle of humerus. It is the most common cause if elbow pain in orthopaedic OPD.

Causes Include

1. Spasm of radial collateral ligament
2. Tearing of fibres of ECRB
3. Inflammation of bursa underneath ECRB
4. Stain/tear of common extensor origin

Mechanism

Repeated violent extension of wrist with forearm pronated (backhand stroke in lawn tennis)

Clinical Features

1. Pain and tenderness over lateral epicondyle
2. Pain generally occurs on extension of elbow when forearm is pronated.

Golfer's Elbow

There is inflammation in region of medial epicondyle.
Causes include
- **Spasm of ulnar collateral ligament**
- **Partial tear of ulnar collateral ligament**
- **Partial tear of common flexor origin**

Clinical Features

Pain and tenderness over anterior aspect of medial epicondyle.

Pain is aggravated by putting flexor tendons on stretch by forcible extension of wrist while patient flexes it.

Subluxation of Radial Head/Pulled Elbow

This is common in young children. *The Annular ligament is funnel shaped in adults while it is tubular/vertical in children.*

When child is suddenly lifted or pulled up by forearm (when forearm is pronated) in following circumstances

- To remove child from danger
- To pull child upstairs
- When child indulges in temper tantrum

The radial head slips out of annular ligament termed incomplete dislocation (subluxation)

Clinical Features

- Inability to use the limb from a fall or jerk is highly suggestive
- Child complains of pain and limitation of supination
- Child keeps elbow fixed/supported in slight flexion and pronation.

Carpal Tunnel Syndrome

Most common entrapment mononeuropathy

Compression of median nerve as it passes through fibro-osseous tunnel beneath flexor retinaculum.

Tunnel may be narrowed by:

- **Arthritic changes in wrist joint (rheumatoid arthritis)**
- **Anterior dislocation of lunate/complication of Colles fracture**
- **Soft tissue thickening in myxoedema and acromegaly.**
- **Oedema and obesity including pregnancy.**
  - **Clinical features:** These start with impairment of finer movements (sewing, knitting, picking a pin) and attacks of pain, tingling and numbness of affected hand
  - **Wasting of thenar eminence:** Partial atrophy confined to radial half of thenar eminence: abductor pollicis brevis and opponens pollicis are affected.
  - **Hyperaesthesia:** Along the distribution of median nerve
  - **Tinels sign:** Percussion of median nerve gently at wrist causes tingling sensation radiating into hand.
  - **Wrist flexion test (Phalens sign):** Exacerbation of symptoms when patient is asked to flex wrist. Symptoms disappear as wrist is straightened.
  - No sensory impairment noticed over palm as the palmar cutaneous branch which is given superficial to retinaculum is spared.
  - **Surgical treatment:** Carpal tunnel release: Partial or complete division of flexor retinaculum.

Dupuytren's Contracture

It is a **progressive thickening and shortening of the palmar aponeurosis which results in flexion deformities of the fingers and distal palm.**

Dupuytren's contracture mainly affects middle-aged men.

It most commonly affects the ring and little fingers, followed by middle finger.

Dupuytren's contracture may be seen in association with

- **Epilepsy**
- **Diabetes mellitus**
- **Alcoholism**

The first sign of the condition is a **slowly enlarging, nodule that appears under the skin near the distal palmar crease opposite the ring finger. Flexion contractures gradually develop in the metacarpophalangeal joint and later in the proximal interphalangeal joint of the involved finger.**

As the flexion deformity progresses, secondary contractures affect skin, nerves, blood vessels, joint capsules

Made Lung Deformity

There is **subluxation of lower end of ulna.** Usually it is consequent to repeated trauma of the lower end of the radius in young adults. Thus the radius growth is delayed where as ulna continues to grow. This unequal growth forces the lower end of ulna to subluxate.

Tenosynovitis

It is an **inflammation of a tendon and its surrounding synovial sheath. Purulent tenosynovitis is a serious infection because it produces adhesions within the tenosynovial canal.** When treatment is delayed, the infection passes to a sub-acute state that produces progressive destruction. The infection is usually secondary to a puncture wound. The onset is insidious.

Signs of Tendon Sheath Infection

- **Uniform swelling**
- **Fixed flexion where the finger is held in slight flexion**
- **Pain on attempted passive extension of the partly flexed finger.**
- **Tenderness along the course of the tendon sheath into the distal palm.**
    - The tendons of the 2nd, 3rd and 4th digits have separate digital synovial tendon sheaths thus the infection is usually confined to that digit.
    - In untreated infections the proximal ends of these sheaths may rupture. The infection spreads into the thenar or midpalmar spaces.
    - The tendinous sheath of the flexor pollicis longus continues into the palm and through the carpal tunnel as the radial bursa

- The tendinous sheath of little finger is continuous with the common flexor sheath or ulnar bursa.
- An infection of either can spread well into the distal forearm and into the subtendinous space of parona (a potential space between the flexor tendon sheaths and the pronator quadrates muscle in the distal forearm).
- A frequent communication between the two bursae may lead to the formation of a horseshoe abscess that affects both the thumb and little finger.

"Trigger" Finger

It is due to localized inflammation of a Tendon and its enveloping synovial sheath (Tenosynovitis) of the superficial and deep flexor tendons over the metacarpal head.

There is thickening and narrowing of the sheath, and a nodular enlargement develops in the tendons distal to the pulley. These changes interfere with the smooth gliding of the tendons through the fibrous sheath.

It occurs most often in the middle or ring fingers. It is generally seen in middle-aged women. Its exact cause is not known.

Trigger finger may be associated with rheumatoid arthritis involving several fingers.

"Scaphoid" Fracture

Most fractures of the scaphoid waist result from a **fall on the outstretched hand,** which produces a break through the waist of the scaphoid.

Signs and Symptoms

- **Tenderness and pain over the anatomical snuffbox**
- **Swelling and loss of the normal concavity of the dorsoradial region of the wrist**
- **Discomfort during thumb movements**

The blood supply to the bone plays an important role in the healing of fractures. **Avascular necrosis** is a complication of scaphoid fractures.

- The major blood supply to the scaphoid (nutrient branches of radial artery) enters the distal pole on the dorsal aspect of the bone. Thus the proximal pole has a relatively poor blood supply.
- Fractures through the waist of the scaphoid may disrupt most of the blood supply to the proximal pole leading to avascular necrosis.

"Mallet" Finger

This is caused by "Hyper-flexion that disrupts the extensor mechanism of the distal phalanx. It is common in baseball players."

It can be a result of:

- Stretching of the **extensor tendon**
- Complete disruption of the **extensor tendon**
- Avulsion fracture of the base of the **distal phalanx**

Signs Include

- Tenderness over the dorsum of distal IP joint.
- Inability to actively extend the distal phalanx.
- Treatment consists of splinting the distal interphalangeal joint in extension.
- Mallet finger with avulsion of a large bone fragment may be associated with palmar subluxation of the distal interphalangeal joint.

"Claw Hand": It is characterized by:

- *Extension at wrist joint-unopposed action of extensors at the wrist*
- *Hyperextension at MP joint*
- *Flexion at IP joint*

The lumbricals cause flexion at MP joint and extension at IP joint due to insertion in the dorsal digital expansion. The paralysis of lumbricals would result in unopposed action of ling extensors and flexors leading to hyperextension at MP joint and flexion of IP joints respectively. The flexion at IP joint is possible by the unaffected long flexors because long flexors are innervated proximal to the wrist.

"Ape Thumb" Deformity

When the **median nerve is injured proximal to the wrist, the thenar muscles are paralyzed. It leads to flattening of the thenar eminence.** The thumb assumes the position in line with other metacarpals. This is called ape thumb deformity.

"Ganglion" Cyst

It is a cystic lesion found in close association with a joint capsule or tendon sheath. The most common site is the **dorsum of the wrist** just lateral to the common extensor tendons of the fingers.

It is considered that a ganglion results **from cystic degeneration of connective tissue near joints or tendon sheaths. On examination the features are:**

- Cyst is firm, smooth, round, slightly fluctuant which may be tender.
- Usually fixed but may be slightly movable if it involves a tendon sheath.

Treatment is complete **surgical excision of the Ganglion.**

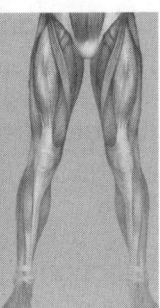

2

Lower Limb

THIGH

Midinguinal Point and its Importance

Midinguinal point is a **point midway between anterior superior iliac spine and the pubic symphysis.** It is an important landmark. **The Femoral artery and head of femur lie beneath the midinguinal point.**

"Holdens Line" and its Importance

The deep layer of superficial fascia is firmly attached to the deep fascia of thigh along a horizontal line a little lateral to pubic tubercle and extends for about 8 cm. laterally; **"This line of Firm Attachment" is called Holdens Line.**

Clinical importance: "The Extravasation of urine between these two layers cannot extend into the Thigh" because of the firm attachment.

Patellar Plexus

It is a **plexus of nerves in front of patella** and upper end of tibia. It is formed by:
- **Anterior division of lateral and medial cutaneous nerve**
- **Intermediate cutaneous nerve**
- **Infrapatellar branch of saphenous nerve**

Housemaids Knee

Chronic enlargement of "Prepatellar bursa" is known as Housemaids knee because it commonly occurs in housemaids who have to kneel regularly for sweeping the floor.

Miner's Beat Knee

It is **Acute suppurative prepatellar bursitis in miners.**

Clergyman's Knee

It is enlargement of **subcutaneous infrapatellar bursa in clergyman.**

Iliotibial Tract

The **thickening of fascia lata on the lateral side of the thigh is called the illiotibial tract.**

Functions

- Iliotibial tract **stabilizes knee both in extension and partial flexion**, i.e during walking and running.
- In leaning forwards with slightly flexed knees, it is the only antigravity force to support the knee.

The modifications of deep fascia of thigh

- **Saphenous opening:** Oval gap 4 cm below and lateral to pubic tubercle. Upper lateral and lower margins form a crescentic sharp edge and medially deep part of fascia passes behind the femoral sheath.
- **Cribriform fascia:** Covers the saphenous opening and is pierced by great saphenous vein, two superficial arteries and lymphatics.
- **Iliotibial tract:** Receives insertion of ¾ of gluteus maximus and tensor fascial lata.

Superficial fascia with 2 layers
- Superficial fatty: **Campers fascia**
- Deep membranous layer: **Scarpas fascia**

The deep layer of superficial fascia is firmly attached to deep fascia of thigh along a horizontal line a little lateral to pubic tubercle and extends about 8 cm laterally. This line of firm attachment is called as **Holden's line**. The extravasation of urine cannot extend into the thigh because of firm attachment between two layers along this line.

Fascia lata: With iliotibial tract which is a thickened part laterally. Two muscles are attached to it namely gluteus maximus and tensor fascia lata. It stabilizes the knee both in extension and in partial flexion.

Saphenous Opening

Oval opening in the fascia lata. The center lies 4 cm below and lateral to pubic tubercle. The lateral margin of the opening is sharp. The opening is closed by the cribriform fascia.

Intermuscular Septa

Three intermuscular septa namely lateral, medial and posterior intermuscular septa divide the thigh into compartments.
Front of thigh
Medial side of thigh
Back of thigh

Muscles of the Front of Thigh

The articularis genu pulls the synovial membrane upwards during extension of knee.

The iliacus and psoas are the muscles of the iliac region and also the part of posterior abdominal wall. They are the chief and powerful flexors of the hip. They are supplied by spinal segments from L2, 3.

Muscle	Action	Nerve supply
Sartorius	Adductor and lateral rotator of thigh and flexor of leg	Femoral nerve (L 2, 3, 4)
Quadriceps femoris	Extensor of the leg	Femoral nerve
Rectus femoris	Flexes the hip	
Vastus lateralis		
Vastus medialis	Prevents lateral displacement of the patella	
Vastus intermedius		

Gluteal Region

Muscle	Action	Nerve supply
Gluteus maximus	Chief extensor of the thigh at the hip	Inferior gluteal
Gluteus medius	Abductor of thigh	Superior gluteal
Gluteus minimus	Abductor of thigh	Superior gluteal
Piriformis	Lateral rotator of thigh	Ventral ramus of S1, 2.
Gamellus superior	Lateral rotator of thigh	Nerve to obturator internus
Gamellus inferior	Lateral rotator of thigh	Nerve to quadratus femoris
Obturator internus	Lateral rotator of thigh	Nerve to obturator internus
Quadratus femoris	Lateral rotator of thigh	Nerve to quadratus femoris
Obturator externus	Lateral rotator of thigh	Posterior division of obturator nerve
Tensor fascia lata	Abductor and medial rotator of thigh	Superior gluteal

Muscles of Back of Thigh

Muscle	Action	Nerve supply
Semitendinosus	Chief flexors of knee	Tibial part of sciatic nerve
Semimembranosus	Chief flexors of knee	Tibial part of sciatic nerve
Biceps femoris	Chief flexors of knee	Long head from tibial part of sciatic nerve and short head from common peroneal part of sciatic nerve

Adductor Compartment of Thigh

Muscle	Action	Nerve supply
Adductor longus	Adductors of thigh flexion and lateral rotation of thigh	Obturator nerve
Adductor brevis	Adductors of thigh flexion and lateral rotation of thigh	Obturator nerve
Adductor magnus	Extends the thigh	Obturator nerve and tibial part of sciatic nerve
Gracilis	Flexor and medial rotator of thigh	Obturator nerve
Pectineus		Femoral nerve and obturator nerve

Femoral Triangle

It is known as scarpa's triangle

The boundaries of femoral triangle are:

Laterally: Medial border of sartorius.

Medially: Medial border of adductor longus

Base: Inguinal ligament

Apex: Directed downwards and is formed by meeting of medial and lateral boundaries.

Roof

- Skin
- Superficial fascia
- Deep fascia

Floor

- Laterally by iliacus and psoas major
- Medially by adductor longus and pectineus.

The contents of femoral triangle are:

1. Femoral artery
2. Branches of femoral artery:
   (a) **Deep branches:** Profunda femoris, deep external pudendal and muscular
   (b) **Superficial branches:** Superficial external pudendal, superficial epigastric and superficial circumflex iliac.
3. Femoral vein (medial to artery) and its tributaries.
4. Femoral sheath
5. Femoral nerve
6. Nerve to pectineus

7. Femoral branch of genitofemoral nerve
8. Lateral cutaneous nerve of thigh
9. Deep inguinal lymph nodes.

Femoral Sheath

- It is a **funnel shaped fascial sleeve** enclosing the upper 1½ inches of the femoral vessels.
- It is formed by the downward extension of the abdominal fasciae.
- The anterior wall is formed by fascia transversalis and posterior wall by fascia iliaca.

The Relations of Femoral Sheath

Anterior
- Skin
- Superficial fascia, and
- Deep fascia with saphenous opening and great saphenous vein

Posterior
- Iliopectineal fascia
- Pectineus and
- Iliopsoas

Lateral
- Femoral nerve and
- Iliacus

Medial
- Lacunar ligament
- Pectineus and
- Pubic bones

Femoral Canal

It is the **medial compartment of the femoral sheath**. It is conical and ½ inch wide at base and ½ inch long.

Femoral Ring

The "**Base or upper end of the femoral canal is called the femoral ring**". The femoral ring is filled by condensed extra peritoneal tissue, the femoral septum, containing a lymph node and covered by parietal peritoneum.

The boundaries of the femoral ring are
- **Anterior:** Inguinal ligament
- **Posterior:** Pectineus and its fascia

2

- **Lateral:** Septum separating it from the femoral vein.
- **Medial:** Concave margin of lacunar ligament.

The contents of femoral canal: L3
- Lymph node (of Cloquet or of Rosenmüller)
- Lymphatics
- Loose areolar tissue

The functions of femoral canal
- It serves as a dead space for expansion of the femoral vein.
- It allows a lymphatic pathway from the lower limb to the external iliac lymph nodes.

The clinical importance of the femoral canal
The femoral canal is a potential point of weakness in the lower abdominal wall through which a viscus (intestines or urinary bladder) may protrude and give rise to a femoral hernia.

Why femoral hernia is more commoner in females
Because the femoral canal is larger in the females due to the greater width of the pelvis and smaller size of the femoral vessels. In the females, there is a rise in intra-abdominal pressure due to pregnancy predisposing to femoral hernia.

Strangulation is more common in femoral hernia: Because the neck of the femoral canal is narrow.

The risk of enlarging the opening of the femoral canal in releasing the strangulation of a femoral hernia.

In order to enlarge the opening of the femoral canal the sharp lateral edge of the **Lacunar (Gimbernat's) ligament** may require incision. **An abnormal obturator artery may occasionally be present, which passes behind the lacunar ligament and is then in danger of being cut.**

The coverings of femoral hernia are:
From within outwards:
- *Peritoneum*
- *Femoral septum*
- *Femoral sheath*
- *Cribriform fascia*
- *Superficial fascia*
- *Skin*

Adductor Canal

The boundaries of the adductor canal
Posteriorly:
  (a) Adductor longus above
  (b) Adductor magnus below
Anteriorly: Vastus medialis

Medially: Sartorius which lies on a fascial sheet extending across the anterior and posterior walls.

The extent of the adductor canal: It extends from the apex of the femoral triangle to the tendinous opening in the adductor magnus.

The contents of the adductor canal are:
- **Femoral artery**
- **Femoral vein**
- **Descending genicular branch of the femoral artery**
- **Saphenous nerve**
- **Nerve to vastus medialis**
- **Obturator nerve**

Popliteal Fossa

The boundaries of the popliteal fossa
- **Superolaterally:** Biceps femoris tendon
- **Superomedially:** Semimembranosus and semitendinosus
- **Inferomedially:** Medial head of gastrocnemius
- **Inferolaterally:** Lateral head of gastrocnemius and plantaris.

Structures form the floor of the popliteal fossa: From above downwards:
- The popliteal surface of the femur
- The capsule of the knee joint
- Popliteal fascia

The relationship between the tibial nerve and popliteal vessels in the popliteal fossa: From superficial to deep lie, the tibial nerve, popliteal vein and popliteal artery. The popliteal artery is crossed by the popliteal vein and tibial nerve posteriorly from the lateral to medial side.

The contents of popliteal fossa are:
- Popliteal artery and its branches
- Popliteal vein and its tributaries
- Tibial nerve and its branches
- Common peroneal nerve and its branches
- Genicular branch of obturator nerve
- Posterior cutaneous nerve of thigh
- Popliteal lymph nodes
- Fat

Gluteal Region

The structures passing through greater sciatic foramen are:
Structures passing above piriformis
- Superior gluteal nerve
- Superior gluteal vessels

Structures passing below piriformis
- Inferior gluteal vessels
- Internal pudendal vessels
- Inferior gluteal nerve
- Sciatic nerve
- Posterior cutaneous nerve of thigh
- Nerve to quadratus femoris
- Pudendal nerve
- Nerve to obturator internus.

The structures passing through lesser sciatic foramen
- Tendon of obturator internus
- Internal pudendal vessels
- Pudendal nerve
- Nerve to obturator internus

The structures lying under cover of gluteus minimus
- Reflected head of rectus femoris
- Capsule of hip joint

The structures lying under cover of gluteus medius
- Superior gluteal nerve
- Deep branch of superior gluteal artery
- Gluteus minimus
- Trochanteric bursa of gluteus medius.

The structures lying under the cover of gluteus maximus
Ligaments
- Sacrotuberous
- Sacrospinous
- Ischiofemoral

Bones and joints
- Ilium
- Ischium with ischial tuberosity
- Upper end of femur with greater trochanter
- Sacrum
- Coccyx
- Hip joint
- Sacroiliac joint

Bursae
- Trochanteric bursa of gluteus maximus
- Bursa over ischial tuberosity
- Bursa between gluteus maximus and vastus lateralis

Muscles
- Gluteus medius
- Gluteus minimus
- Reflected head of rectus femoris
- Insertion of adductor magnus.
- Obturator externus
- Obturator internus
- Origin of hamstrings
- Piriformis
- Quadratus femoris
- Superior and inferior gemelli

Vessels
- Superior gluteal vessels
- Inferior gluteal vessels
- Ascending branch of medial circumflex femoral artery
- Cruciate anastomosis
- First perforating artery
- Internal pudendal vessels
- Trochanteric anastomosis

Nerves
1. Superior gluteal (L4, 5, S1)
2. Inferior gluteal (L5, S1, 2)
3. Sciatic (L4, 5, S1, 2, 3)
4. Nerve to obturator internus (L5, S1, 2)
5. Nerve to quadratus femoris (L4, 5, S1)
6. Perforating cutaneous nerve (S2, 3).
7. Posterior cutaneous nerve of thigh (S1, 2, 3)
8. Pudendal nerve (S2, 3, 4)

Waddling Gait

Results from **Bilateral paralysis of gluteus medius and minimus** so that the patient walks with swaying to clear the feet off the ground when unilateral then it is known as lurching gait.

LEG AND FOOT

The Parts of Deep Fascia of Leg

Intermuscular septa:
- Anterior and posterior intermuscular septa: Divide leg into three compartments anterior, lateral and posterior

- Superficial transverse fascial septum: Separates superficial and deep muscles of back of leg. Also forms flexor retinacula
- Deep transverse facial septum: Separates tibialis posterior from long flexors of toes.

Retinacula

- Extensor retinacula: Superior and inferior
- Peroneal retinacula: Superior and inferior

The attachments of inferior extensor retinacula

- It is Y-shaped retinacula
- **Stem:** Attached to anterior nonarticular part of superior surface of calcaneum
- **Upper band:** Attached to anterior border of medial malleolus
- **Lower band:** Attached to plantar aponeurosis

The structures passing deep to inferior extensor retinacula

- Tibialis anterior
- Extensor hallucis longus
- Deep peroneal nerve
- Anterior tibial vessels

The Muscles of Posterior Compartment of Leg

Superficial muscles:

- Gastrocnemius
- Soleus
- Plantaris

Deep muscles:

- Popliteus
- Flexor digitorum longus
- Flexor hallucis longus
- Tibialis posterior

Tendocalcaneous: It is a long tendon, receiving the insertion of fibres of soleus

The muscles found in different layers of sole of foot

From Without Inwards

First layer

- Flexor digitorum brevis
- Abductor hallucis
- Abductor digiti minimi

Second layer

- Flexor digitorum accessories
- Lumbricals: Four in number

Third layer
- Flexor hallucis brevis
- Flexor digiti minimi brevis
- Adductor hallucis

Fourth layer
Three plantar and four dorsal interossei.

Plantar Aponeurosis and its Functions
It is the thickened central part of the deep fascia of sole.

Functions
- Gives origin to muscles of first layer of sole
- Helps in maintaining the longitudinal arch of the foot
- Protects the digital vessels and nerves and deeper muscles
- Provides attachment to skin of sole

The functions of interossei of sole
- **Dorsal** interossei: Abductors of the toes
- **Plantar** interossei: Adductors of the toes

ARTERIAL SUPPLY OF LOWER LIMB

The branches of profunda femoris are:
- Lateral circumflex femoral artery
- Medial circumflex femoral artery
- Perforating arteries
- Muscular branches
- Descending genicular artery.

The branches of popliteal artery are:
- Cutaneous branches
- Superior muscular branches
- Sural arteries
- Superior genicular arteries: Medial and lateral
- Middle genicular artery
- Inferior genicular arteries: Medial and lateral
- Terminal branches: Anterior and posterior tibial.

The branches of anterior tibial artery are:
- Muscular branches
- Recurrent branches: Anterior and posterior tibial.
- Malleolar branches: Anterior medial and anterior lateral

2

Lower Limb

Dorsalis pedis artery: It is the continuation of anterior tibial artery in front of ankle between the two malleoli.

The branches of dorsalis pedis artery are:

- Lateral tarsal artery
- Medial tarsal branches: 2–3
- Arcuate artery
- First dorsal metatarsal artery.

The pulsations of dorsalis pedis artery are felt between the tendon of extensor hallucis longus and first tendon of extensor digitorum longus on dorsum of foot about 5 cm distal to medial and lateral malleoli, over intermediate cuneiform bone.

The branches of posterior tibial artery are:

- Peroneal
- Muscular
- Nutrient artery to tibia
- *Anastomotic branches:*
  - Circumflex fibular
  - Communicating branch to peroneal
  - Medial malleolar
  - Calcanean
- *Terminal branches:* Medial and lateral plantar.

VENOUS DRAINAGE OF LOWER LIMB

The different factors which facilitate the return of venous blood to heart
Local factors:

- Veins of lower limb are larger than veins of other parts of body. They also have greater number of valves, which prevent the back flow of blood.
- Muscular contraction compresses the deep veins and drives the blood upwards
- Muscular compression of veins is made more effective by tight deep fascia

General factors:

- The valves which maintain a unidirectional flow.
- Negative intrathoracic pressure, which pulls the column of blood up and it is made more negative during inspiration.
- Vis-a-tergo (compulsion from behind) produced by arterial pressure and overflow from capillary bed.

The perforators in lower limb

There are the veins connecting the superficial veins with the deep veins and they permit only unidirectional flow of blood, from superficial to the deep veins by means of valves.

Calf pump or peripheral heart

In upright position, venous return from lower limb depends largely on the contraction of calf muscles, these are known as calf pump. The soleus is called peripheral heart for same reason.

Varicose veins

If the valves in veins become incompetent, the pressure during muscular contraction is transmitted from deep veins to the superficial veins (leakage of blood). This causes dilatation of the superficial veins, known as varicose veins. Later on gradual degeneration occurs, leading to varicose ulcers.

NERVES OF LOWER LIMB

Lumbar Plexus

By the ventral rami L1–3 and greater part of ventral ramus of L4. The first lumbar nerve also receives a branch from T12 nerve.

The branches of lumbar plexus are:

1. *Muscular:*

   To quadratus lumborum (T12, L1–3)

   Psoas minor (L1)

   Psoas major (L2, 3)

   Iliacs (L2, 3)

2. Iliohypogastric nerve (L1)

3. Ilioinguinal nerve (L1)

4. Genitofemoral nerve (L1, 2)

5. Lateral cutaneous nerve of thigh (dorsal division of ventral primary rami of L2, 3)

6. Femoral nerve (dorsal division of ventral primary rami of L2–4)

7. Obturator (ventral division of ventral primary rami of L2–4)

8. Accessory obturator (ventral division of ventral primary rami of L3, 4)

The Branches of Obturator Nerve

(a) Anterior branch supplies

1. Muscular branches: To adductor longus, gracilis, adductor brevis, pectineus.

2. Articular: To hip joint

3. Cutaneous: To subsartorial plexus

4. Communicating branch.

(b) Posterior branch supplies:

1. Muscular branches: To obturator externus, adductor magnus

2. Articular: To knee joint

The Branches of Femoral Nerve

A. **Anterior division** supplies:

1. Nerve to pectineus
2. Intermediate cutaneous nerve of thigh
3. Medial cutaneous nerve of thigh
4. Nerve to sartorius

B. **Posterior division** supplies:

1. Saphenous nerve
2. Muscular branches to quadriceps femoris
3. Vascular branches to femoral artery.

Meralgia Paresthetica

It is a clinical condition characterized by pain, tingling, numbness or anaesthesia in the area of distribution of the lateral cutaneous nerve of the thigh. This nerve (a branch of the lumbar plexus) usually enters the thigh by passing deep to the inguinal ligament. Occasionally, the nerve pierces the ligament and may then be compressed by it with resultant irritation of the nerve.

The Adductor Spasm

It is **spasm of the adductor muscles of the thigh and occurs in spastic paraplegia.**

Referred pain: A patient sometimes complain of pain in the knee when the disease is actually in the hip joint.

This is a referred pain because both the hip and knee joints are supplied by the same nerves, i.e. the femoral and obturator nerves.

Sciatic Nerve

The sciatic nerve is the **continuation of the sacral plexus and derives its fibres from the L4, 5, S1, 2, 3. It is the largest nerve in the body. The main trunk of the sciatic nerve is the nerve of the flexor compartment of the thigh.**

Branches

1. Articular: To hip joint
2. Muscular: To biceps femoris, semitendinosus, semimembranosus and ischial head of adductor magnus.
3. Terminal:
    1. The tibial nerve is the nerve of the flexor compartments of the thigh (through the parent trunk) leg and sole of the foot. It receives fibres from the anterior divisions of L4, 5, S1, 2,3.
    2. The common peroneal nerve is the nerve of the extensor and peroneal compartments of the leg and dorsum of the foot. It is derived from the posterior divisions of L4, 5, S1, 2.

The effect of a complete lesion of the sciatic nerve in the gluteal region

Motor loss:

- Loss of flexion of the knee due to paralysis of the hamstring muscles, but some weak movement is possible due to the action of the sartorius (femoral nerve) and gracilis (obturator nerve).
- Loss of all movements below the knee due to paralysis of all the muscles of the leg and foot. There will be a foot drop deformity.
- Loss of Achilles jerk and plantar reflex.

Sensory loss: on the outer side of the leg and almost the entire foot.

Sciatica

Sciatica is the term applied when pain is felt along the course and distribution of the sciatic nerve, i.e in the buttock, posterior aspect of the thigh and leg, and lateral aspect of the leg and foot. This is due to irritation of one or more of the roots of the sciatic nerve, and commonly occurs due to a prolapsed intervertebral disc in the lumbar region.

Foot drop: The common peroneal (lateral popliteal) nerve commonly injured and the common causes of the injury.

The nerve is commonly injured where it winds round the neck of the fibula. It may be damaged at this site by the pressure of a tight bandage of plaster cast, in severe adduction injury to the knee or from direct trauma.

The effects of a complete section of the common peroneal (lateral popliteal) nerve at the level of the neck of the fibula.

Motor loss:

1. Inability to extend the foot or toes due to paralysis of the ankle and foot extensors (tibialis anterior, extensor hallucis longus, extensor digitorum longus, peroneus tertius and extensor digitorum brevis). This results in foot drop which is characteristic of the common peroneal nerve injury.
2. Inability to evert the foot due to paralysis of the peroneal muscles.

Paralysis of the extensor and evertor muscles of the foot causes the foot to assume a position of equinovarus (equinus = plantar flexion; varus = inversion), results in a slapping or high steppage gait (the patient raises the knee high, and the foot hangs flexed and inverted.

Sensory loss: Over the anterior and lateral aspects of the leg and foot. The lateral border of the foot and the lateral side of the little toe are unaffected since they are supplied by the sural branch of the tibial nerve.

The structures supplied by deep peroneal nerve are:

Muscular branches:

- Tibialis anterior
- Extensor hallucis longus
- Extensor digitorum longus
- Peroneus tertius

- Extensor digitorum brevis and
- First and second dorsal interossei

Cutaneous branches: To adjacent sides of first and second toes.

Articular branches: To ankle joint, tarsal joint.

The effect of lesion of deep peroneal nerve

- Sensory loss: adjacent sides of I and II toe.
- Motor loss: Paralysis of muscles supplied by it. So over activity of peroneal and flexor muscles leads to talipes equinovalgus.

The Branches of superficial peroneal nerve are:

- **Muscular branches: To peroneus longus and peroneous brevis.**
- **Cutaneous branches:** To lower 1/3 of lateral side of leg.

Dorsum of foot: Medial side of I toe, lateral side of II toe and III, IV, V, toe.

Communicating branches: To sural, deep peroneal and saphenous nerve.

If nerve supply to peroneal muscles is cut off: Talipes varus

The tibial (medial popliteal) nerve commonly injured the common causes of the injury: The tibial nerve may be damage in or below the popliteal fossa by automobile accident, fractures of leg or by gunshot or stab wounds. The frequency of injuries to the tibial nerve is far less than the common peroneal nerve because of its deeper position and more protected course.

The effects of a complete section of the tibial (medial popliteal) nerve in the popliteal fossa.

Motor Loss

- Inability to fully flex the ankle joint due to paralysis of the gastocnemius and soleus. A small degree of flexion is possible by the peroneus longus (which is supplied by the superficial peroneal nerve).
- Inability to invert the foot against resistance due to paralysis of the tibialis posterior. The foot assumes the position of a calcaneovalgus (calcaneus = dorsiflexion; valgus = eversion) by the unopposed action of the extensors and evertors. The patient cannot stand on tip-toe. Walking is difficult due to difficulty in taking off.
- Inability to flex the toes due to paralysis of both the long and short flexors of the toes.
- Ankle jerk is absent.

Sensory loss over the sole (except the inner border)

Vasomotor and trophic changes are common. The foot becomes oedematous, discolored and cold. Trophic ulcers are almost inevitable.

The Cutaneous Nerve Supply of Back of Leg

- **Saphenous nerve (L3, 4):** Branch of posterior division of femoral nerve
  Supplies skin of medial area of leg and medial border of foot up to ball of I toe.

- **Posterior division of medial cutaneous nerve of thigh (L2, 3):** Supplies upper most part of medial area of calf.
- **Posterior cutaneous nerve of thigh (S1, 2, 3):** Supplies upper ½ of central area of calf.
- **Sural nerve (L5, S1, 2):** Branch of tibial nerve. Supplies lower ½ of central area and lower 1/3 of lateral area of calf and lateral border of foot.
- **Lateral cutaneous nerve of calf (L4, 5 S1):** Branch of common peroneal nerve. Supplies skin of upper 2/3 of lateral area of leg.
- **Peroneal (sural) communicating nerve (L5 S1, 2):** Branch of common peroneal nerve. Supplies skin of lateral area of calf
- **Medial calcaneon branches (S1, 2):** Supplies skin of heel and medial side of sole of foot.

2

Lower Limb

JOINTS OF LOWER LIMB

Hip Joint

Hip joint is a ball and socket type of synovial joint.

The factors which increase the stability of the hip joint

The stability of hip joint is increased by the following factors:
- Depth of acetabulum with a narrow mouth is made by acetabular labrum
- Tension and strength of ligaments
- Strength of the surrounding muscles
- Length and obliquity of neck of femur

The wide range of mobility depends upon the neck of femur which is narrower than the equatorial diameter of the head.

The relations of the hip joint are:
- **Anteriorly:** Lateral fibres are pectineus, iliopsoas, straight head of rectus femoris.
- **Posteriorly:** Quadratus femoris covering obturator externus and ascending branch of medial circumflex femoral artery, the piriformis, obturator internus with two gemelli separate the sciatic nerve from the nerve to quadratus femoris.
- **Superior:** Reflected head of rectus femoris covered by gluteus minimus.
- **Inferior:** Lateral fibres of pectineus and obturator externus.

The axis of different movements of hip joint
- For rotation, vertical axis passing through the centre of head of femur and its lateral condyle.
- Extension and flexion occur around a transverse axis.
- Adduction and abduction occur around an anteroposterior axis.

The range of movements at the hip joint
- Flexion is limited by contact of thigh with anterior abdominal wall.

- Adduction is limited by contact with opposite limb. Range of other movements: lateral rotation 60° and medial rotation 25°
- Abduction 50° and extension 15°.

The nerves supplying the hip joint

The hip joint is supplied by:

- **Femoral nerve, through nerve to rectus femoris**
- **Anterior division of obturator nerve**
- **Accessory obturator nerve**
- **Nerve to quadratus femoris**
- **Superior gluteal nerve.**

   The different muscles producing extension of the hip joint: Gluteus maximus and hamstrings.

Muscles produce abduction of the hip joint

- Chief muscles: Gluteus medius and minimus.
- Accessory muscles: Tensor fasciae lata and sartorius

Trendelenburg Test

This test is employed for testing the stability of the hip joint. A positive test indicates a defect in osseomuscular stability especially abductors of hip joint and the patient has a lurching gait. If the patient is asked to stand on one leg. If the abductors of thigh are paralysed on that side, they will be unable to sustain the pelvis against the body weight and pelvis tilts downwards on unsupported side.

   Injury of the hip joint in which sciatic nerve likely to be damaged

   It is likely to be injured in the posterior dislocation of the hip joint associated with fracture of the posterior lip of the acetabulum, to which the nerve is closely related.

Knee Joint

Compound synovial joint, having

- Condylar synovial joint: Between the condyles of femur and tibia
- Saddle syonovial joint: Between femur and patella

The articular surfaces in knee joint are:

- Condyles of femur
- Condyles of tibia
- Patella

The ligaments of knee joint are:

- **Fibrous capsule**
- **Ligamentum patellae**
- **Collateral ligaments: Tibial and fibular**
- **Popliteal ligaments: Oblique and arcuate**
- **Cruciate ligaments: Anterior and posterior**

- **Meniscus: Medial and lateral**
- **Transverse ligament**
- **Coronary ligament: It is the part of fibrous capsule lying between the menisci and tibia**

The openings in the fibrous capsule of knee joint

- For suprapatellar bursa
- For the exit of tendon of popliteus with its synovial bursa

The attachments of oblique popliteal ligament

It arises as an expansion from the tendon of semimembranous. It blends with the posterior surface of fibrous capsule and is attached to the intercondylar line and lateral condyle of femur.

The structures piercing oblique popliteal ligament

- *Posterior division of obturator nerve*
- *Middle genicular nerve and vessels.*

Menisci and their functions

These are two fibrocartilaginous structures, semilunar in shape, which make the tibial articular surface deeper and divide the joint cavity partially into upper and lower compartment.

Functions:

- They act as shock absorbers
- They make the articular surfaces more congruent.

They can adapt to varying curvatures of different parts of femoral condyles.

The arterial supply of knee joint:

- Genicular branches of popliteal artery
- Descending genicular branch of femoral artery
- Descending branch of lateral circumflex femoral artery
- Recurrent branches of anterior tibial artery and
- Circumflex fibular branch of posterior tibial artery.

The arteries forming the anastomosis around the knee joint

Medially:

- Descending genicular
- Superior medial genicular
- Inferior medial genicular

Laterally:

- Descending branch of lateral circumflex femoral
- Superior lateral genicular
- Inferior lateral genicular
- Anterior lateral recurrent
- Posterior lateral recurrent
- Circumflex fibular

2

Lower Limb

The nerve supply of knee joint
- Femoral nerve
- Genicular branches of tibial and common peroneal nerves and
- Posterior division of obturator nerve

The movements possible at knee joint
- Flexion
- Extension
- Medial and lateral rotation

Conjunct and Adjunct Rotation

- Conjunct rotation: Rotation of knee joint combined with flexion and extension
- Adjunct rotation: Rotation of knee joint occurring independently in a partially flexed knee.

The changes in the axis of movement of the knee joint with flexion and extension: The flexion and extension of the knee joint takes place on a transverse axis which shifts along with the movements. Because of the spiral profiles of the femoral condyles, the axis shifts upwards and forwards during extension and backwards and downwards during flexion.

The Mechanism of Locking and Unlocking Movements of the Knee Joint

In full extension from the position of flexion the last 30° of extension is accompanied by medial rotation of the femur on the tibia or lateral rotation of the tibia on the femur depending on whether the tibia or the femur is fixed. This is conjunct rotation and occurs passively as a part of the extension movement, is described as locking of the knee joint.

From the position of full extension, the beginning of flexion is accompanied by lateral rotation of the femur or medial rotation of the tibia depending on whether the tibia or the femur is fixed. This rotation is called unlocking of the knee joint. The contraction of popliteus is responsible for this unlocking movement.

The intra-articular structures of the knee joint
- **Cruciate ligaments: Anterior and posterior**
- **Menisci: Medial and lateral**
- **Infrapatellar pad of fat**
- **Synovial membrane**
- **Origin of popliteus**

The bursa around knee joint
Anteriorly:
- Subcutaneous prepatellar bursa
- Subcutaneous infrapatellar bursa
- Deep infrapatellar bursa
- Suprapatellar bursa

Medially:
- Bursa deep to medial head of gastrocnemius
- Bursa deep to tibial collateral ligament
- Semimembranosus bursa
- Anserine bursa
- Occasionally, bursa between tendons of semitendinosus and semimembranosus.

Laterally:
- Bursa deep to lateral head of gastrocnemius
- Bursa between fibular collateral ligament and tendon of popliteus.
- Bursa between fibular collateral ligament and biceps femoris
- Bursa between tendon of popliteus and lateral condyle of tibia

The bursa communicating with the knee joint
- Suprapatellar bursa
- Popliteal bursa
- Bursa deep to medial head of gastrocnemius

Anserine Bursa

It is a bursa with several diverticula which separate the tendons of sartorius, gracilis and semitendinosus from bony surface of tibia.

The different muscles producing movements of knee joint

Extension • Quadriceps femoris • Tensor fasciae lata
Flexion • Semitendinosus • Sartorius • Biceps femoris • Gracilis • Semimembranosus • Popliteus • Gastrocnemius
Medial rotation • Semitendinosus • Sartorius • Biceps femoris • Gracilis • Semimembranosus
Lateral rotation • Biceps femoris

2

Lower Limb

Ligaments which become taut in full extension and flexion of the knee joint

In full extension:

- Anterior cruciate ligament
- Tibial and fibular collateral ligament
- Oblique popliteal ligament

In full flexion:

- Posterior cruciate ligament.

Causes of a tear of the menisci (semilunar cartilages) of the knee joint

The menisci are usually torn by a twisting force with the knee flexed. When the flexed knee is forcibly abducted and externally rotated, the medial meniscus is trapped between the medial condyles of the femur and tibia and is torn.

A severe adduction and internal rotation of the flexed knee may result in a tear of the lateral meniscus. But this injury is less common.

The tears of medial meniscus are more frequent than that of lateral meniscus

Because the medial meniscus is more firmly attached to the upper surface of the tibia, capsule and the tibial collateral ligament and therefore, is less able to adapt itself to sudden changes of position. The lateral meniscus on the other hand, is drawn backwards and downwards on the groove on the posterior aspect of the lateral tibial condyle by the medial fibres of popliteus. This prevents the lateral meniscus from being impacted between the articular surfaces of the femur and the tibia during movements of the knee joint.

Tear of medial meniscus there is locking of the knee before it is fully extended

Because the torn segment of the cartilage is displaced and lodges between the femoral and tibial condyles and prevents full extension of the knee.

The pain of hip joint is referred to the knee: Because of the common nerve supply of the two joints.

Meniscal Tear

- **Medial meniscus is 20 times more prone to injury than lateral meniscus.** The medial meniscus is firmly adherent to the deep part of tibial collateral ligament. In forceful strains (adduction and lateral rotation of the femur over the tibia with the foot firmly placed on the ground) the medial meniscus gets torn. It is because:
- The medial collateral ligament does not allow the meniscus to move away from under the femoral condyle.
- It gets compressed crushed between femoral and tibial condyles that are moving with great force.
- Part of the torn cartilage may get displaced. This small piece floats in the joint cavity. It may get lodged between femoral and tibial condyles causing locking of knee joint in flexed position.
- The tear in the medial meniscus may be in the longitudinal direction (bucket handle tear) or transverse.

- Injury to the lateral meniscus is less common because the meniscus is relatively mobile due to pull of: Tendon of popliteus
- In severe adduction and internal rotation of the knee there could be tearing in the lateral semilunar cartilage.

Management

These are treated arthroscopically

Meniscal tears are usually treated by partial meniscectomy

Preservation of the meniscus is important to the function of the joint

Peripheral meniscus tears have potential for healing. These should be re-attached.

A small undisplaced tear may heal with protection alone immobilisation.

Ankle Joint

Hinge variety of synovial joint.

The articular surfaces of ankle joint

From above:

- Lower end of tibia with medial malleolus
- Lateral malleolus
- Inferior transverse tibiofibular ligaments.

From below: Body of talus.

The ligament of ankle joint

Lateral ligament: Consists of—

- Anterior talofibular ligament
- Posterior talofibular ligament
- Calcaneofibular ligament.

Medial (deltoid) ligament: It has

Superficial part: Consists—

- Anterior fibres (tibionavicular)
- Middle fibres (tibiocalcanean) and
- Posterior fibres (posterior tibiotalar)

Deep part (anterior tibiotalar)

The tendons crossing the deltoid ligament

- Tibialis posterior
- Flexor digitorum longus

The structures related to ankle joint

Anteriorly: From medial to lateral side:

- **Tibialis anterior**

2

- Extensor hallucis longus
- Anterior tibial vessels
- Deep peroneal nerve
- Extensor digitorum longus
- Peroneus tertius

Posteriorly: From medial to lateral side
- Tibialis posterior
- Flexor digitorum longus
- Posterior tibial vessels
- Tibial nerve
- Flexor hallucis longus
- Peroneus brevis
- Peroneus longus.

The movements produced at ankle joint
- Dorsiflexion
- Plantar flexion
- Accessory movements: With plantar flexion slight amount of side to side gliding, abduction and adduction are permitted.

The muscles producing movements at ankle joint

Dorsiflexion

Main muscle: Tibialis anterior
Accessory muscles:
- Extensor digitorum longus
- Extensor hallucis longus
- Peroneus tertius

Plantar Flexion

Main muscles:
- Gastrocnemius
- Soleus

Accessory muscles:
- Flexor digitorum longus
- Flexor hallucis longus
- Tibialis posterior
- Plantaris

   Most frequent fracture at the ankle joint: Pott's fracture, usually produced by an abduction external rotation injury.

Tibiofibular Joints

Type of joints
- Superior tibiofibular joint: Plane synovial joint
- Lower tibiofibular joint: Syndesmosis type of fibrous joint

The structures passing through interosseous membrane of tibiofibular joint
- Anterior tibial vessels
- Perforating branch of peroneal artery

Joints of Foot

Inversion and eversion of foot
- **Inversion:** Movement in which medial border of foot is elevated and sole faces medially and inwards
- **Eversion:** Movement in which lateral border of foot is elevated and sole faces laterally and outwards.

The joints at which inversion and eversion takes place
- Subtalar (talocalcanean) joint
- Talocalcaneonavicular joint.

    The axis of inversion and eversion: Oblique axis which runs forwards, upwards and medially. It passes between back of calcaneum, sinus tarsi and superomedial aspect of neck of talus.

The Evertors of Foot

Mainly by, peroneus brevis and longus. Also, by peroneus tertius.

The Invertors of Foot

Principal muscles
- Tibialis anterior
- Tibialis posterior

Accessory muscles
- Flexor hallucis longus
- Flexor digitorum longus

Arches of Foot

Longitudinal arches: There are two longitudinal arches
- Medial
- Lateral

Transverse arch

The arches of foot are maintained by:
- The configuration of **articulating bones** forming the arch

2

Lower Limb

- The **ligaments and muscles** binding the adjacent bones and ends of an arch.
- **Tendons of muscle** which act as sling and thus help to suspend the arch from above.

The functions of arches of foot are:

✓ Provide a **rigid support** for the sustaining the weight of body in standing position

✓ As **mobile spring board** during walking and running

✓ As **shock absorber** in jumping

✓ **Protects the soft tissues** of sole foot.

The **"medial" longitudinal arch is formed** by: Calcaneum, talus, navicular, three cuneiforms and three medial metatarsals.

The "lateral" longitudinal arch is formed by: Calcaneum, cuboid and lateral two metatarsals.

The "transverse" arch is formed by the bases of the five metatarsals and the adjacent cuboid and cuneiforms of both feet.

Structures that maintain the medial longitudinal arch:

The bony configurations do not contribute to the maintenance of this arch.

Ligaments:

- The medial part of the **plantar aponeurosis** acts as a tie-beam.
- The **plantar calcaneonavicular (spring) ligament** supports head of talus and forms intersegmental ties (connect adjacent bones).

Muscles:

- **Medial half of the flexor digitorum brevis and abductor hallucis** act as tie-beams (connect ends of arch)
- **Tibialis anterior, tibialis posterior and flexor hallucis longus** act by forming sling and suspend the arch.

The lateral longitudinal arch of the foot is maintained by:

Ligaments:

- The short plantar ligament, long plantar ligament and dorsal ligaments form intersegmental lies.
- Lateral part of the plantar aponeurosis acts as a tie-beam.

Muscles:

- The peroneus longus and peroneus brevis muscles form the slings
- Lateral half of the flexor digitorum brevis and abductor digiti minimi act as tie-beam.

The transverse arch of the foot is maintained by:

Tarsal and metatarsal bones contribute in maintaining the concavity of arch.

Ligaments:

1. Ligaments that bind together the cuneiforms and the bases of the metatarsals form intersegmental ties.
2. Superficial and deep transverse metatarsal ligaments act as tie-beams.

Muscles:
- The peroneus longus and tibialis posterior form slings
- Abductor hallucis acts as tie beam.

The deformities of the foot resulting from defects of the longitudinal arches of the foot

Pes "planus" (flat foot): Due to flattening of the longitudinal arch, in particular the medial arch

Pes "cavus" (high arched foot): The congenital form is probably due to shortness of the plantar fascia (aponeurosis). The acquired form can be due to paralysis of the intrinsic muscles of the foot due to a lesion of the tibial nerve.

The Talipes Deformity of the Foot

In talipes the foot does not lie in plantigrade position. **The person walks either on the heels or on the toes.**

When he walks on the heel the condition is known as **talipes calcaneus** while walking on the toes is known as **talipes equines**. In both these conditions the foot may be **inverted (varus) or everted (valgus).**

Hallus Valgus

In hallux valgus, there is **Lateral deviation of the great toe at the metatarsophalangeal joint.**

Ganglion

It is a **cystic lesion found in close association with a joint capsule or tendon sheath.**

The most common site is the dorsum of the wrist just lateral to the common extensor tendons of the fingers.

It is considered that a ganglion results from cystic degeneration of connective tissue near joints or tendon sheaths.

The only finding may be a slowly growing localized swelling. Most patients report intermittent aching and mild weakness.

On Examination
- Cyst is firm, smooth, round, slightly fluctuant which may be tender.
- Usually fixed but may be slightly movable if it involves a tendon sheath.

Treatment
Complete surgical excision of the ganglion and the ligament us tissue at its base.

Psoas Abscess

Tuberculous disease of body of any of the thoracic or lumbar vertebrae gives rise to a cold abscess (no signs of inflammation). This abscess trickles under the psoas sheath up to the insertion of psoas major. This painless swelling may be mistaken for a femoral hernia and flexion deformity of hip it due to spasm of psoas.

Trendelenburgs Sign

This test is used to **detect incompetent valves in a suspected case of varicose veins**. The person lies down and the affected leg is elevated to empty the vein. Then the person is asked to stand up and the filling of the veins is observed.

If the valves are incompetent, the vein fills from above.

If the valves are normal, they do not allow backflow of blood, and the vein fills from below.

Meralgia Paresthetica

It is a common sensory neuropathy caused by compression of the lateral femoral cutaneous nerve of thigh as it passes through or deep to the lateral end of the inguinal ligament.

It may develop spontaneously. It is commonly seen in obese patients wearing tight-fitting garments. Usually it occurs unilaterally.

Patients complain of paresthesia on the lateral aspect of the thigh which is associated with long periods of standing. The symptoms usually resolve spontaneously.

Iliotibial Tract Friction Syndrome

It is caused by the **tense iliotibial tract rubbing the lateral femoral condyle during running.** It induces an inflammatory response. The resulting lateral knee pain is felt above the joint. Iliotibial tract friction syndrome usually occurs in:

• Bowlegged runners (joggers) with pronated feet

• Wearing shoes with worn lateral soles

Pain and tenderness at the insertion of the iliotibial tract into the lateral tibial condyle may result from stress chronic bursitis.

Surgery

Excision of an bursa (deep to the tract)

Tenotomy of the iliotibial tract

Trendelenburg Gait

This is also called **uncompensated gluteal gait**. This is an abnormal gait associated with a weakness of the gluteus medius.

This is characterized by the **dropping of the pelvis on the unaffected side of the body at the moment of heel-strike on the affected side.** In this deviation, the pelvis drops during the walking cycle and it lasts until heel-strike on the unaffected side. It is accompanied by an apparent lateral protrusion of the affected hip. **The person with a trendelenburg gait displays a lateral deviation of the entire trunk and the affected side during the stance phase of the affected lower limb.**

Weavers Bottom

A **bursa between gluteus maximus and ischial tuberosity gets inflamed in individuals who work in a sitting position with constant movements of lower limbs**. The local friction accounts for bursitis. This is commonly seen in weavers.

Calcar Femorale

The internal structure of upper end of femur is characterized by presence of **trabeculae—thin sheets of compact bone. Inferior cortex of base of neck of femur. The trabeculae join to form plates termed lamellae.** The arrangement and nature of these bony plates is to strengthen the bone and offer resistance to the tensile or shearing force. **Thus extending from the linea aspera into the neck is a well defined vertical plate of bone called calcar femorale.** It merges medially with the posterior wall of the neck and laterally with greater trochanter.

Perthes Disease

It is also known **coxa plana of Legg-Calve-Certhes disease.**

Here there is **osteochondrosis of the head of the femur in children** which is characterized by initial epiphyseal necrosis or degeneration followed by regeneration or recalcification. Flattening of head thickening of neck of femur.

Coxa Vera

In adult males the **neck shaft angle of femur is about 135°**. In females, it is less. With age the angle gradually diminishes in both sexes. In trauma or local or general disease of the bone, there is reduction of this angle. **This reduction of neck shaft angle is termed as coxa vera.**

Coxa Valga

It is a rare deformity. **It is the reverse deformity causing increase in neck shaft angle of femur.** Here the **limb is abducted and externally rotated.** It occurs in old cases of infantile paralysis. Even in below knee amputee, the weight of the dragging limb causes this deformity.

Popliteal Artery Aneurysm

A **localized dilatation of the popliteal artery is termed as aneurysm**. Due to decline in the definitive causative reasons (syphilis) now aneurysm of popliteal artery are far less common. For surgical correction of this condition, femoral artery is ligated in the adductor canal.

Bone Graft

To facilitate repair and to compensate for the bone loss, fragments of bone are put at the fractured/affected site (bone graft). **The Fibula is commonly chosen for bone grafting as partial removal of fibula does not affect locomotion.** The repair at the fracture site is facilitated due to the restoration of blood supply to the bone as the piece of fibula is alive with its periosteal and nutrient arteries.

Footballers Ankle

Football goalkeeper kicks the ball mostly from close to **proximal part of dorsum of foot in a plantar-flexed position.** Over a period of time, the repeated impact initiates formation of bony spicule on the front of neck of talus. **This makes the ankle painful termed as Footballers ankle.**

Tarsal Tunnel Syndrome

Paraesthesia and pain in the sole of the foot due to compression of tibial nerve under the flexor retinaculum of the ankle is termed as tarsal tunnel syndrome. The posterior tibial nerve passes through a tunnel analogous to the carpal tunnel in the wrist. Compression within the tunnel leads to **pain, numbness and paraesthesiae in the sole of the foot.**

Calcaneal Spur

Increased body weight due to obesity/pregnancy may cause tear in the plantar fascia at its attachment on the medial tubercle of calcaneus. Haemorrhage into the periosteum and repeated tears result in calcification. Later, a spike of bone-calcaneal spur is formed. Pain in the heel is not due to the spur but the reactive fibrosis involving the periosteum. Right heal is affected twice because of normal tendency of weight bearing. **The letter "F" illustrates the preferential reasons for occurrence of calcaneal spur (fat, fertile, females of forty with flat feet).**

Other sites of calcaneal spur:

On the undersurface of the bone at the attachment of short plantar ligament.

On the posterior surface of the bone at the attachment tendocalcaneus

• Degenerative

• Using hard sole shoes

In individuals who are required to stand for a long period there is tendency of medial longitudinal arch to flatten. **This causes stretching of plantar aponeurosis. The stretched aponeurosis may get inflammed (fascitis) or get torn at its attachment to the medial tubercle of calcaneus.** This causes pain in the affected heel while standing for long duration—**policemen heel.**

3

Thorax

Thoracic Cage
- Anteriorly: Sternum
- Posteriorly: Twelve thoracic vertebrae and intervertebral discs
- One each side: Twelve ribs with their cartilages

Thoracic cage with age changes
- In adults, in transverse section thorax is reniform, with a greater transverse diameter than anteroposterior. In infants, circular in transverse section
- In adults, ribs are oblique. In infants, ribs are horizontal.

The boundaries of thoracic inlet
- Anteriorly: Upper border of manubrium sterni
- Posteriorly: Upper border of body of T1 vertebra
- One each side: First rib with its cartilage.

The direction of plane of inlet of thorax
Downwards and forwards with a obliquity of about 45 degrees. The upper border of manubrium sterni lies at level of upper border of T3 vertebra.

Sibson's Fascia and its Attachments
It is a triangular membrane at thoracic inlet (diaphragm of inlet of thorax).

Attachments
- **Apex: Tip of transverse process of C7 vertebra.**
- **Base: Inner border of first rib and its cartilage**
- **Inferior surface: Fused with cervical pleura**

THORACIC INLET

The Structures Passing through Thoracic Inlet
Muscles
- Sternohyoid

57

- Sternothyroid
- Longus colli

Arteries

- Right and left internal thoracic arteries
- Brachiocephalic artery
- Left common carotid
- Left subclavian
- Right and left superior intercostal arteries

Nerves

- Left recurrent laryngeal nerves
- Right and left phrenic nerves
- Right and left vagus nerves
- Right and left first thoracic nerves
- Right and left sympathetic chain

Veins

- Right and left brachiocephalic veins
- Right and left first posterior intercostal veins
- Inferior thyroid veins

Others

- Thymus
- Trachea
- Esophagus
- Anterior longitudinal ligament
- Right and left pleurae
- Apex of right and left lungs.

The Boundaries of Outlet of Thorax

- Anteriorly: Infrasternal (subcostal) angle between two costal margins
- Posteriorly: Inferior surface of body of 12th thoracic vertebra
- On each side: Costal margin formed by 7th, 8th, 9th and 10th costal cartilage and 11th and 12th ribs.

Rib Fractures

Fracture of the ribs is the most common thoracic injury with simple fractures; pain on inspiration is the principal symptom. Localized pain, tenderness, and occasionally crepitus confirm the diagnosis. A chest X-ray should be obtained to exclude other intrathoracic injuries and not necessarily to identify a rib fracture.

Stove in Chest

This is produced in severe crush injuries in which multiple rib fractures are produced along with permanent indentation of chest wall.

Flail Chest

This results from more severe injury to chest. Multiple rib fractures result in unstable chest wall in which flail area sucked inwards during inspiration and pushed out in expiration.

Cervical Rib

It is attached to the transverse process of 7th cervical vertebra and its distal extremity is free or articulates with first thoracic rib. It may press on the lower trunk of brachial plexus producing paraesthesiae along ulnar border of forearm and wasting of small muscles of hand. Less commonly, vascular changes are produced due to pressure on subclavian artery.

Pneumothorax

Pneumothorax results from lacerations of the chest wall or lung, or rupture of alveoli (paper bag effect) and can be caused by either penetrating or blunt trauma. Tension pneumothorax develops when a flap valve leak allows air to enter the pleural space but prevents its escape. Intrapleural pressure rises, causing total lung collapse and a shift of the mediastinum to the opposite side.

Hemothorax

Hemorrhage into the pleural space occurs in some quantity in almost every patient with a diagnosable chest injury. Blood loss may vary from slight to extensive. Although an upright chest X-ray examination can diagnose an intrathoracic accumulation of more than 200 ml of blood. Bleeding may be from any intrathoracic structure, although massive hemothorax generally signals a systemic arterial or major pulmonary vascular injury.

Cardiac Tamponade

It is most frequently caused by penetrating thoracic injuries, but occasionally it is observed in blunt thoracic trauma from myocardial rupture, coronary artery laceration, or ascending dissection of an aortic tear. Accumulation of as little as 150 ml of blood in the pericardial sack may impair diastolic filling enough to produce distended neck veins, shock, and cyanosis. Beck's classic diagnostic triad of distended neck veins, muffled heart sounds, and hypotension is present in only one third of patients with tamponade.

Rupture of the Thoracic Aorta

It is the most lethal injury following blunt chest trauma. Here the aortic arch at the descending aorta is believed to undergo flexion or torsion, disrupting the aortic wall at the ligamentum arteriosum immediately distal to the left subclavian artery. Occasionally, the ascending aorta at the root of the heart may be injured.

Blunt Injury of the Esophagus

It is rare, and penetrating injuries are rarely isolated. The most common symptom of esophageal perforation is extreme pain with the slow evolution of fever several hours later. Regurgitation of blood, hoarseness, dysphagia, or respiratory distress may also be present because of injuries to the trachea. Suspicious radiographic findings are mediastinal air and widening or presence of a foreign body.

Blunt Tracheal or Bronchial Injuries

Are often due to compression of the airway between the sternum and the vertebral column in decelerating steering wheel motor vehicle accidents with resultant shearing of the right main stem bronchus from the carina or transverse lacerations of the trachea. Alternatively, a blow-out injury to the membranous trachea may occur during chest wall compression with a closed glottis. Patients with tracheal injuries may present with mediastinal and deep cervical emphysema or pneumothorax with a massive air leak.

Jugular notch: Also called suprasternal notch, present in middle of superior border of manubrium.

The level of jugular notch: It lies at level of intervertebral disc between T2 and T3 vertebrae

Sternal Angle (Angle of Louis)

It is the angle formed at the junction of manubrium and body of sternum. It is convex forwards.

The level of sternal angle: Intervertebral disc between T4 and T5 vertebrae

The clinical significance of sternal angle

It is an important land mark for counting ribs as 2nd costal cartilages articulates with sternum of this level.

The structures lying at level of sternal angle

- Arch of aorta begins and also ends
- Ascending aorta ends
- Azygous vein opens into superior vena cava
- Descending aorta begins
- Marks the upper limit of base of heart
- Pulmonary trunk divides into two pulmonary arteries
- Trachea divides into two principal bronchi.

Funnel chest: *Deformity of chest in which the body of sternum and xiphoid process is depressed. This predisposes to respiratory and cardiovascular disturbances.*

Pigeon chest: *It is condition in which deformity of chest occurs due to forward projection of sternum and flattening of chest on either side.*

INTERCOSTAL SPACES

Gaps between ribs and their costal cartilages are called intercostal spaces.

Typical Intercostal Spaces

The 3rd to 8th spaces are typical intercostal spaces. The blood and nerve supply of 3rd to 6th intercostal spaces is limited only to the thoracic while those of lower spaces extend into the abdomen.

The contents of a typical intercostal space

A. Muscles:
- External intercostal
- Internal intercostal
- Transversus thoracis (innermost intercostal)

A. Intercostal nerve

B. Intercostal vessels and lymphatics.

The Attachment and Extent of External Intercostal Muscle

Attachment

Origin: Lower border of the rib above.

Insertion: Outer lip of the upper border of the rib below.

Fibres run downward and medially in anterior part and downwards and laterally in posterior part.

Extent: From the tubercle of rib behind to its costochondral junction in front where it continues as external intercostals membrane.

The Attachment and Extent of Internal Intercostal Muscle

Attachment

- *Origin:* Floor of the costal groove of the rib above.
- *Insertion:* Inner lip of the upper border of the rib below.
- Fibres are at right angles to those of external intercostal

Extent: From the lateral margin of the sternum to the angle of the rib where it continues as the internal intercostal membrane.

The muscles which comprise the transversus thoracic group

- Subcostalis
- Intercostalis intimi
- Sternocostalis

The attachment of muscles comprising transversus thoracic group of muscles.

They form the innermost layer of the muscles of the thoracic wall.

- **Subcostalis:** Present in posterior parts of the lower spaces. They are attached to the inner surface of rib near angle and to the inner surface of the second or third rib below.

- **Intercostalis intimi:** Present in the middle 2/4 of the upper spaces, except in the 1st space. They arise from inner surface of the upper rib and are inserted into the inner surface of the rib below.
- **Sternocostalis:** Present in the anterior part of the upper spaces, except in the 1st space. They arise from the lower part of the posterior surface of the body of the sternum and the xiphoid process and the adjacent costal cartilages. They pass upwards and laterally and are inserted by slips to the costal cartilages of the 2nd to 6th ribs. The direction of fibres of these three parts is same as internal intercostals muscle.

The position of neurovascular plane of thorax: Between internal intercostal muscle and intercostalis intimi and posteriorly between pleura and internal intercostal membrane.

If intercostal muscles are paralysed: There will a retraction of intercostal spaces during inspiration and bulging during expiration.

Intercostal Nerves are formed and How they are Distributed

- These are the veneral primary rami of T1–T11 nerves.
- The ventral primary rain of T12 forms subcostal nerve.
- T1 and T2 supply the upper limb.
- T3 to T6 supply thoracic wall (typical intercostals nerves)
- T7 to T11 supply abdominal wall.

The branches of a typical intercostal nerve

1. *Communicating:*
   a. White ramus communicans connected to
   b. Grey ramus communicans sympathetic ganglion
2. *Muscular:*
   a. Muscular branches: Supplies intercostal muscles, serratus posterior superior
   b. Collateral branch: Supplies intercostal muscles, parietal pleura and periosteum of rib.
3. *Cutaneous:*
   a. Lateral cutaneous branch: Emerges at mid axillary line
   b. Anterior cutaneous branch: Emerges at lateral border of sternum.

The pain due to irritation of intercostal nerves is referred

To the front of chest or abdomen, i.e. at the peripheral termination of nerve

The course of pus from vertebral column around the thorax

The pus may track along the course of neurovascular bundle and may point at the exit of cutaneous branches of intercostals nerve, i.e. lateral to erector spinae, in mid axillary line and just lateral to the sternum.

The Arteries of Intercostal Space

1. One posterior intercostal artery
2. Two anterior intercostal arteries

The branches of posterior intercostal arteries

1. Dorsal branch
2. Muscular branches
3. Collateral intercostal branch
4. Lateral cutaneous branch
5. Mammary branches: of 2nd, 3rd, and 4th arteries.

The origins of intercostal arteries

a. Posterior intercostals arteries:

Ist and 2nd: From superior intercostals artery which is a branch of costocervical trunk.

3rd to 11th: From descending thoracic aorta.

b. Anterior intercostals arteries:

Of Ist to 6th space: From internal thoracic artery

Of 7th to 9th space: From musculophrenic artery

10th and 11th spaces do not have anterior intercostal arteries.

The Intercostal Veins

a. Anterior intercostals veins: Two in each of upper nine spaces.

In upper six spaces: Drain into internal thoracic vein.

In lower three spaces: Into musculophrenic vein.

b. Posterior intercostals vein: One in each of eleven spaces.

Mode of termination is:

On left side:

Ist: Into left brachiocephalic vein.

2nd to 4th: Form left superior intercostals vein which drains into left brachiocephalic vein.

5th to 8th: Into accessory hemiazygous vein.

9th to 11th and subcostal veins: Into hemiazygous vein.

On right side:

Ist: Into right brachiocephalic vein.

2nd to 4th: Form right superior intercostals vein which drains into right brachiocephalic.

5th to 11th and subcostal vein: Into azygous vein.

The Branches of Internal Thoracic Artery

- Pericardiophrenic
- Mediastinal
- Anterior intercostal of upper six spaces
- Perforating
- Superior epigastric
- Musculophrenic

3

Thorax

PLEURA

It is a serous membrane, lined by mesothelium. There are two pleural sacs, one on either side of mediastinum.

- Each lung is covered by a smooth glistening layer which is a serous covering also thin and delicate and also lines the walls of the thorax.
- It has two layers the parietal and visceral layers and at the root of the lung both the layers are continuous with each other. This arrangement arises because the embryonic lung grows laterally into the pleural cavity and carries the medial wall of that cavity with it as a covering the pulmonary pleura. The lung then expands outwards to fill the cavity which is reduced to a mere slit between the outer wall of the cavity (parietal pleura) and the surface of the lung (pulmonary pleura).
- At the root of the lung the parietal and visceral layers of the pleura which are continuous with each other and form a tube of pleura which encloses the bronchus and the pulmonary vessels is going downwards and forms a sleeve or a fold called the pulmonary ligament.
- Normally the parietal and the visceral layers are in contact with each other separated by a potential space called the pleural cavity.
- The parietal pleura is divided into costal, diaphragmatic, mediastinal and cervical pleura.
- The visceral pleura covers the lung, is often adherent to it and covers its lobes and enters its fissures.

The parts of pleura
- Outer layer: Parietal pleura
- Inner layer: Visceral pleura
- The two layers are continuous with each other at the hilum of lung.
- The two layers enclose between them a potential space known as pleural cavity.

The parts of parietal pleura
1. **Costal:** Lines the thoracic wall and is loosely attached to it by areolar tissue
2. **Diaphragmatic:** Lines upper surface of diaphragm.
3. **Mediastinal:** Lines mediastinum
4. **Cervical:** Extends into neck and covers apex of lung. Covered by Sibson's fascia.

The extent of cervical pleura in neck
It extends two inches above the first costal cartilage and one inch above medial ½ of clavicle.

The relations of cervical pleura
- Anteriorly: Subclavian artery and scalenus anterior muscle,
- Posteriorly: Neck of first rib with its relations.
- Medially: Large vessels of neck.
- Laterally: Scalenus medius.

Pulmonary Ligament—its Functions

It is parietal pleura surrounding the root of lung which hangs down as a fold called pulmonary ligament.

Functions

• *It provides dead space into which veins of lung can expand when venous return increases.*
• *Because of it, lung root can descend with the descent of diaphragm.*

The recesses of pleura

These are folds of parietal pleura, which act as reserve spaces, into which lungs can expand during deep inspiration.

Three in number:

• **Costo-mediastinal recess:** Present in cardiac notch of left lung anteriorly, between costal and mediastinal pleurae.
• **Costo-diaphragmatic recess:** On both sides inferiorly, between costal and diaphragmatic pleurae.

The parts of lungs not covered with visceral pleura: At hilum and along the attachment of pulm on ary ligament where it is continuous with parietal pleura.

The Nerve Supply of Pleura

Parietal pleura: Intercostal nerves: Costal and diaphragmatic pleurae at periphery.
Phenric nerves: Mediastinal and central part of diaphragmatic pleurae. Pain sensitive
Visceral pleura: Sympathetic nerves: T2–T5. Pain insensitive.

The Arterial Supply of Pleura

• Parietal pleura: Intercostal arteries
• Internal thoracic arteries
• Musculophrenic arteries
• Visceral pleura: Bronchial arteries

The Lymphatic Drainage of Pleura

• **Parietal pleura:** Lymphatics drain into intercostal, internal mammary, mediastinal and diaphragmatic lymph nodes.
• **Visceral pleura:** Drained by bronchopulmonary lymph nodes.

The Developmental Origin of Pleura

• **Parietal pleura:** Somatopleural layer of lateral plate mesoderm.
• **Visceral pleura:** Splanchnopleural layer of lateral plate mesoderm.

The Surface Marking of Pleura

Cervical pleura: Curved line forming a dome over the medial 1/3 of clavicle. The apex of curve lies 2.5 cm above the clavicle.

3

Thorax

Anterior margin:

1. On right side: From sternoclavicular joint downwards and medially to midpoint of sterna angle, where it continues vertically downwards to midpoint of xiphisternal joint.

2. On left side: Same course up to fourth costal cartilage, where it arches and descends along sternal margin of 6th costal cartilage.

Inferior margin: Laterally from lower limit of anterior margin, so that it crosses 8th rib in midclavicular line, 10th rib in mid axillary line and 12th rib at lateral border of sacrospinalis. Then horizontally to lower border of T12 vertebra.

Posterior margin: From a point 2 cm, lateral to 12th thoracic spine to a point 2 cm. laterals to 7th cervical spine.

The places at which pleura descends below costal margin

- Right costoxiphoid angle.
- Right costovertebral angle below 12th rib.
- Left costovertebral angle below 12th rib.

Important Terms

- **Pneumothorax:** A pneumothorax is produced by the presence of air in the pleural cavity.
- **Haemothorax:** It is the blood in the pleural cavity
- **Pleural effusion:** It is the accumulation of free fluid in the pleural cavity
- **Empyema:** It is accumulation of pus in the pleural cavity
- **Paracentesis thoracis and from which site it is done:** It is the process of aspiration of any fluid from the pleural cavity. Done in 6th intercostal space in mid axillary line. **Precaution should be taken during aspiration from pleural cavity.** Needle should be pricked in lower part of intercostal space to avoid injury to intercostal nerves and vessels in costal groove.

Meig's Syndrome

It is a triad of:

1. Ovarian fibroma (benign tumour to ovary)
2. Ascites (fluid in peritoneal cavity) and
3. Right-sided pleural effusion.

LOWER RESPIRATORY TRACT

Trachea

The extent of trachea

Trachea extends from 6th cervical vertebra (lower border of cricoid cartilage) to lower border of 4th thoracic vertebra, where it divides into right and left bronchi.

The relations of cervical part of trachea

Anteriorly:
- Isthmus of thyroid gland
- Inferior thyroid veins below isthmus
- Pretracheal fascia
- Sternohyoid muscle
- Sternothyroid muscle
- Investing layer of deep cervical fascia
- Superficial fascia
- Skin

Posteriorly:
- Oesophagus
- Longus colli
- Recurrent laryngeal nerve

On each side:
- Thyroid gland
- Common carotid artery

The Relations of Thoracic Part of Trachea

Anterior:
- Manubrium sterni
- Sternothyroid muscle
- Thymus
- Left brachiocephalic vein
- Inferior thyroid vein
- Aortic arch
- Brachiocephalic artery
- Left common carotid artery
- Deep cardiac plexus
- Lymph nodes

Posterior:
- Oesophagus
- Vertebral column

Right side:
- Right pleura
- Right lung
- Right vagus
- Azygous vein

3

Thorax

Left side:
- Arch of aorta
- Left common carotid artery
- Left subclavian artery
- Left recurrent laryngeal nerve

The arterial supply of trachea
Inferior thyroid arteries

The nerve supply of trachea
Parasympathetic nerves: Vagus through recurrent laryngeal
It is
1. Sensory to mucous membrane
2. Motor to tracheal muscle
Sympathetic nerves: Through middle cervical ganglion
It is vasomotor.

The lymphatic drainage of trachea
- Pretracheal lymph nodes
- Paratracheal lymph nodes

The variations in the level of bifurcation of trachea with respiration
- Bifurcation of trachea, normally: Between T4 and T5 vertebrae.
- In deep inspiration: T6 vertebra
- In expiration: T4 vertebra

Trachea can be palpated: In suprasternal notch midway between sterna ends of two clavicles.

Tracheal Tug

Arch of aorta lies in close relation to trachea and left bronchus. In aneurysm of aortic arch, a pull or drag is felt on the trachea which is known as tracheal tug.

The tracheal appear in an X-ray
Since trachea is more radiolucent (because of air in it) than neighbouring structures, it appears as a dark area passing downwards, backwards and slightly to the right.
The common causes and effects of tracheal compression
Causes: Pathological enlargement of surrounding structures especially thyroid gland and arch of aorta
Effects: Dyspnoea, cough, husky voice.

Conditions in which tracheostomy is done
1. In laryngeal obstruction
2. For removal of excessive secretions
3. For long continued artificial respiration.

The commonest site for tracheostomy

It is most commonly done in retrothyroid region after cutting the isthmus of thyroid gland.

The tracheotomy is difficult and dangerous in children, because

1. Neck is relatively short and left innominate vein may come up above suprasternal notch.

2. Trachea is softer and more mobile, so it is not readily identified and isolated.

The histological structure of trachea

Trachea consists of following layers from within outwards:

1. Mucosa: Lined by pseudostratified columnar ciliated epithelium. Lamina propria has mainly reticular fibres.

2. Submucosa: Loose areolar tissue

3. Cartilages and muscles: C-shaped hyaline cartilages make the framework of trachea. Posterior gap has transverse fibres of smooth muscles and fibroelastic membrane.

4. Adventitia

The advantage of posterior gap in tracheal cartilage: Posteriorly, the oesophagus lies close to trachea so the oesophagus can dilate into posterior membranous part, during passage of food bolus.

Bronchi

The differences between right and left main bronchus

Right main bronchus

1. Wider shorter (2.5 cm) and more vertical

2. Passes to root of lung at T5

3. Relations:

   1. Azygous vein arches over it from behind to reach superior vena cava

   2. Pulmonary artery lies first below and then anterior to it.

Left main bronchus

1. Narrower, longer (5 cm) and less vertical

2. Passes to root of lung at T6

Relations

1. It passes below the arch of aorta, in front of oesophagus and descending aorta.

2. Pulmonary artery lies first anterior and then above it.

   The foreign bodies and aspirated material tend to pass into right bronchus rather that into left. Because of the greater width and more vertical course of the right bronchus.

LUNGS

Bronchopulmonary segment

- The main bronchus on each side gives off branches to each lobe of the lung, lobar bronchus. Each lobar bronchus then divides into segmental bronchi, each of which supplies a segment of the lung called a bronchopulmonary segment.
- Each segmental bronchus is accompanied by a branch of the pulmonary artery and a tributary of the pulmonary vein.
- Each bronchopulmonary segment is therefore a self-contained, functionally independent respiratory unit of lung tissue.
- These segments are wedge-shaped with their apices at the hilum, and bases at the lung surface. Each is surrounded by connective tissue continuous with that of the visceral pleura. There are also veins which run between the segments and are called intersegmental veins.

The bronchopulmonary segments of the two sides

- Each bronchopulmonary segment receives its name from that of its supplying segmental bronchus
- On the left side, the upper lobe bronchus gives off a combined apicoposterior segmental bronchus whereas on the right they arise separately as apical and posterior segmental bronchi.
- The left upper lobe has a lingular segment which is equivalent to the right middle lobe.
- On the right side there is a medial basal segmental bronchus which is absent on the left.

The knowledge of the bronchial tree and bronchopulmonary segments is important

1. During bronchoscopy
2. For correct interpretation of bronchograms.
3. To determine the appropriate posture for promoting drainage of infected areas of lung
4. For surgical resection of a single or a number of diseased bronchopulmonary segments without affecting the function of the remaining segments.

The differentiating features of the two lungs

1. The right lung has three lobes while the left lung has two lobes.
2. The thin, sharp anterior border of the right lung is vertical while that of the left lung presents a cardiac notch.
3. On the medial surface (mediastinal surface) of the lung, the cardiac impression is much deeper on the left than on the right.
4. The right lung is wider than the left because of the smaller cardiac impression
5. The right lung is shorter than the left because of the higher position of the right dome of the diaphragm.

The structures in root of lungs

- Principle bronchus on left side and eparterial and Hyparterial bronchi on right side.
- One pulmonary artery
- Superior and inferior pulmonary vein
- Bronchial arteries: One on right and two on left side
- Bronchial veins.
- Anterior an posterior pulmonary plexuses nerves
- Lymphatics of lung
- Bronchopulmonary lymph nodes
- Areolar tissue

Level the root of lungs lie: Opposite body of T5–7 vertebra.

The relations of the structures at the root of the lung

From above downwards (differs on two sides)

Right lung	Left lung
• Eparterial bronchus	Pulmonary artery
• Pulmonary artery	Bronchus
• Hyparterial bronchus	Inferior pulmonary vein
• Inferior pulmonary vein	

From before backwards (similar on two sides)

- Superior pulmonary vein
- Pulmonary artery
- Bronchus

The surface marking of the oblique fissure of the lung

It corresponds approximately with the medial border of the scapula when the arm is raised above the shoulder.

The fissure may be presented by a line drawn obliquely from a point 2 cm, lateral to the 4th thoracic spine on the right side and at a slightly higher level on the left side to a point, another point on the 5th rib in the mid axillary line and a third point on the 6th costal cartilage about 7.5 cm from midline.

The breath sound of the apical segment of the lower lobe are heard on auscultation

Posteriorly below the upper end of the oblique fissure

The surface marking of the horizontal fissure of the right lung

It corresponds approximately with a line drawn horizontally at the level of the 4th costal cartilage anteriorly. This line meets that of the oblique fissure in the mid axillary line.

The lingula of the left lung

The upper lobe of the left lung corresponds with the upper and middle lobes of the right lung. The part of it which corresponds to the middle lobe is called the lingula because it projects anteriorly to form the lingula (tongue-shaped structure) below the cardiac notch.

The Azygos Lobe

The azygos vein is occasionally deeply embedded in the apex of the right lung, partly isolating its medial portion. This isolated medial portion of the right lung is referred to as the azygos lobe.

The lymphatic drainage of the lung

The lymphatics of the lung drain centripetally from the pleura towards the hilum into the **bronchopulmonary** lymph nodes. Efferents of these nodes drain into the **trachea-bronchial nodes** which drain into the **paratracheal nodes** and the **mediastinal** lymph trunks. These lymph trunks drain directly into the brachiocephalic vein, or occasionally, indirectly via the right lymphatic duct or the thoracic duct.

MEDIASTINUM

It is a median septum of thorax between two pleural cavities. Strictly speaking, it is septum between two lungs because mediastinal pleurae are also part of it.

The boundaries of mediastinum

- **Superiorly:** Thoracic inlet
- **Inferiorly:** Diaphragm
- **Anteriorly:** Sternum
- **Posteriorly:** Thoracic vertebral column
- **On each side:** Mediastinal pleura

The divisions of mediastinum

Mediastinum is divided by an imaginary plane passing anteriorly through sterna angle and posteriorly through T4 vertebra into:

1. Superior mediastinum
2. Inferior mediastinum: Subdivided by pericardium into:
   1. Anterior mediastinum: In front of pericardium
   2. Middle mediastinum: Pericardium and its contents
   3. Posterior mediastinum: Behind pericardium

The boundaries of superior mediastinum

- **Anteriorly:** Manubrium sterni
- **Posteriorly:** Upper 4 thoracic vertebrae
- **Superiorly:** Plane of thoracic inlet
- **Inferiorly:** Imaginary plane between superior and inferior mediastinum
- **On each side:** Mediastinal pleura.

The contents of superior mediastinum

Arteries:

1. Arch of aorta
2. Brachiocephalic
3. Left common carotid
4. Left subclavian

Veins:

1. Right and left brachiocephalic
2. Upper ½ of superior vena cava
3. Left superior intercostals

Muscles: Origin of

1. Sternothyroid
2. Sternohyoid
3. Longus colli

Nerves:

1. Phrenic
2. Vagus
3. Cardiac
4. Left recurrent laryngeal

Lymph nodes and lymphoid tissue:

1. Thymus
2. Thoracic duct
3. Lymph nodes

Tubes:

1. Trachea and
2. Oesophagus

The contents of anterior mediastinum

1. Superior and inferior sternopericardial ligaments
2. Lymph nodes
3. Mediastinal branches of internal thoracic artery
4. Areolar tissue
5. Thymus

The contents of middle mediastinum

1. Heat with pericardium
2. Ascending aorta
3. Pulmonary trunk
4. Pulmonary arteries
5. Bifurcation of trachea

6. Principal bronchi

7. Lower half of superior vena cava

8. Terminal part of azygous vein

9. Pulmonary veins

10. Phrenic nerve

11. Deep cardiac plexus

12. Tracheobronchial lymph nodes

The contents of posterior mediastinum

1. Descending thoracic aorta

2. Azygous vein

3. Hemiazygous vein

4. Accessory hemiazygous vein

5. Vagus nerves

6. Greater splanchnic nerve

7. Lesser splanchnic nerve

8. Least splanchnic nerve

9. Thoracic duct

10. Posterior mediastinal lymph nodes

11. Oesophagus.

Mediastinal Syndrome

Compression of mediastinal structure by any growth gives rise to a group of symptoms known as mediastinal syndrome.

The pus in posterior mediastinum can enter the thighs

The fascial sheath of psoas major muscle is open by its upper attachment to L2 or L1 Vertebra. This upper edge forms medial lumbocostal arch, from which vertebral part of diaphragm arises. So, psoas sheath opens into posterior mediastinum by a funnel shaped orifice.

Pus in posterior mediastinum enters through funnel shaped orifice and along the psoas sheath extends into thighs.

The infection behind the prevertebral layer of deep cervical fascia cannot extend into posterior mediastinum

The prevertebral layer of deep cervical fascia extends to the superior mediastinum and is attached to the 4th thoracic vertebra, so the neck infections behind this fascia cannot extend down beyond T4.

Infections between which layers of cervical fascia can extend into posterior mediastinum

Posterior mediastinum is continuous through superior mediastinum with the neck between pretracheal and prevertebral layers of cervical fascia. This region includes retrophrayngeal space, spaces on each side of trachea and oesophagus, space between trachea and oesophagus.

PERICARDIUM

It is a fibroserous sac enclosing the heart and roots of great vessels

The sacs of pericardium

The pericardium consists of:

1. **Fibrous pericardium:** Outer, single layered, tough and fibrous.
2. **Serous pericardium:** Inner, double layered and thin

The attachments of fibrous pericardium

Fibrous pericardium is conical in shape.

Apex: Blunt and fused with roots of great vessels and pretracheal fascia

Base: Blends with central tendon of diaphragm.

Anteriorly: By superior and inferior sternopericardial ligaments, attached to body of sternum

The different layers of serous pericardium

1. Parietal pericardium: Outer, fused with fibrous pericardium
2. Visceral pericardium: Inner, fused to heart except where it is separated from heart by blood vessels.

Both layers are continuous at root of great vessels

Pericardial cavity

It is a potential space between parietal and visceral layers. It contains a thin layer of serous fluid.

Oblique sinus of pericardium

It is a space behind heart between the left atrium, anteriorly and parietal pericardium, inferiorly.

Transverse sinus of pericardium

It is a horizontal gap between ascending aorta and pulmonary trunk anteriorly and superior vena cava and atrium posteriorly.

On each side it opens into pericardial cavity.

Surgical importance of transverse sinus

Through this sinus a temporary ligature is given to occlude pulmonary trunk and aorta during cardiac operations.

The developmental origin of sinuses of pericardium

Transverse sinus: Develops due to degeneration of dorsal mesocardium

Oblique sinus: Develops due to absorption of pulmonary veins into left atrium

The nerve supply of pericardium

1. Fibrous and parietal pericardium by phrenic nerve. They are pain sensitive
2. Visceral pericardium: By autonomic nerves of heart.

3

Thorax

The arterial supply of pericardium

1. Visceral layer: by coronary arteries
2. Fibrous and parietal layer: By branches of internal thoracic, musculophrenic and descending thoracic aorta.

The contents of the pericardium

1. Heart with cardiac vessels and nerves
2. Ascending aorta
3. Pulmonary trunk
4. Lower half of superior vena cava
5. Terminal part of inferior vena cava.
6. Terminal part of pulmonary veins.

HEART

The position of heart: It is placed obliquely behind body of sternum and adjoining parts of costal cartilages of ribs.

1/3 of it lies to right and 2/3 of it lies to left of median plane.

The divisions of heart

Heart is composed of four chambers:

1. Two artria, right and left
2. Two ventricles, right and left

The atria are separated from ventricles by coronary sulcus (groove)

The atria are separated by interartrial groove and the ventricles by anterior and posterior interventricular grooves.

- Heart has 4 chambers.
- The upper two are the atria separated from each other by interatrial septum.
- The inter-atrial septum is oblique so that the right atrium lies in front and to the right and the left atrium lies to the left and behind.
- The atria have thin walls about 3 mm.
- The lower chambers are the ventricles separated from each other by inter-ventricular septum.
- The right atrium and the right ventricle are communicated by right atrio-ventricular orfice guarded by the tricuspid orifice.
- The left atrium and the left ventricle are communicated by left atrioventricular orifice guarded by the mitral or bicuspid valve.
- Each atrium has an auricle which is shaped like ear and has rough inner surface.

The structures in anterior and posterior interventricular grooves

In anterior interventricular groove:

1. Interventricular branch of left coronary artery
2. Great cardiac vein

In posterior interventricular groove

1. Interventricular branch of right coronary artery
2. Middle cardiac vein

Chambers form the upper border of heart

Two atria, chiefly left atrium.

Chambers form the left border of heart

Mainly by left ventricle and partly by left auricle.

The chambers forming the surfaces of heart

Anterior surface:

Mainly by right ventricle and right auricle

Partly by left ventricle and left auricle

Inferior surface:

Left 2/3 by left ventricle

Right 1/3 by right ventricle

Left surface:

Mostly by left ventricle and upper end by left auricle.

Right auricular appendage and its characteristic features

It is the upper prolonged end of right atrium, which covers the root of ascending aorta. Externally, it is notched and interior is sponge like.

The clinical importance of structure of right auricular appendage

Its sponge like interior prevents free flow of blood and favour thrombosis which may dislodge to cause pulmonary embolism.

The parts of right atrium and how they are developed

Three parts:

1. Smooth posterior part: Derived from right horn of sinus venosus.
2. Rough anterior part including auricle: Derived from primitive atrial chamber
3. Septal wall: Derived from septum primum and septum secondum.

The veins opening in the right atrium

1. Superior vena cava
2. Inferior vena cava
3. Cardiac sinus
4. Anterior cardiac veins
5. Venae cordis minimi

Eustachian Valve

It is a rudimentary valve guarding the opening of inferior vena cava. During embryonic life it guides the inferior caval blood to left atrium through foramen ovale.

The features of septal wall of right atrium

It has:

1. Fossa ovalis: Saucer shaped depression in lower part, formed by septum primum
2. Limbus fossae ovalis: It is prominent margin of fossa ovalis and represents free edge of septum secundum.

The parts of right ventricle

1. Inflowing part: Rough and has muscular ridges called trabeculae carneae.
2. Outflowing part: Smooth

The two parts are separated by a ridge, supraventricular crest.

The different types of trabeculae carneae

1. Ridges: Fixed elevations
2. Bridges: Fixed at ends but free in middle
3. Papillary muscles: Bases attached to ventricular wall and apex project into ventricular cavity and are connected to chordae tendineae.

The left atrium is developed

1. Greater part is smooth and is derived from absorption of pulmonary vein
2. Auricle develops from primitive atrial chamber.

Fossa Lunata

It is an impression in septal wall of left atrium, corresponding to fossa ovalis of right atrium

The developmental origin of ventricles

The ventricles develop from:

1. Bulbus cordis
2. Primitive ventricle

Interventricular septum develops

1. Muscular part: Upgrowth from apex of heart
2. Membranous part: Downgrowth from interatrial septum

Right Atrium

- Its cavity is partly smooth and partly rough. The anterior part is rough and posterior part is smooth.
- These two parts are separated from each other by a ridge called **crista terminalis** corresponding with a groove externally called **sulcus terminalis.**
- This chamber receives all the venous blood from all parts of the body except the lungs.
- It has the **opening of superior vena cava** above and behind.
- The **opening of inferior vena cava** is guarded by a valve and the opening lies below and behind.

- The valve of the inferior vena cava is continued upwards to form a raised margin called **annulus ovalis** which outlines the front and upper part of the oval depression called **fossa ovalis.**
- In the foetal life there is a passage for the blood to pass from right atrium to left atrium and later closure is represented by fossa ovalis.
- If the foramen ovale remains open in the adult, it will allow the venous blood to flow from right atrium to mix with the arterial blood in the left atrium resulting in blue baby.
- **The fossa ovalis** represents septum primum and limbus fossa ovalis representing septum secundum of foetal life.
- The **opening of coronary sinus** is also guarded by a valve and lies in front and to the left of the opening of inferior vena cava.
- The **tricuspid opening** is in the inferior part.
- Except the tricuspid orfice all other openings are present in the smooth posterior part.
- The tricuspid valve has three cusps namely anterior, posterior and septal.
- The anterior part is rough due to the presence of parallel muscular ridge like comb called **musculi pectinati.**
- The **crista terminalis** is a ridge which separates two embryologically two different parts.
- The rough anterior part is derived from atrium proper and the posterior smooth part is derived from sinus venosus of the embryo.

Left Atrium

- Forms the **posterior surface or the base of the heart.**
- Its wall is smooth and its auricle is the only part which is not smooth.
- It has the "**Opening of 4 pulmonary veins.**"
- It also has one opening for communication with left ventricle.
- The pulmonary veins open in the upper part of the posterior surface
- The mitral opening is in the lower part.
- The mitral/bicuspid valve has two cusps namely anterior and posterior.

Right Ventricle

- Forms 2/3 of the sternocostal surface and 1/3 of the diaphragmatic surface
- The wall of right ventricle is three times thicker than atria.
- It is semilunar on cross section because the ventricular septum is convex to the right
- The wall is thin because it pushes blood only to the lungs.
- Its musculature is rough called **trabeculae carneae** which are fewer in number.
- There are also three papillary muscles namely anterior, posterior and septal.
- The apex of each papillary muscle gives attachment to tendinous cords called **chordae tendinae** which resemble the cords of a parachute, whose ends are attached to the borders and ventricular surfaces of the valves.

- The cusps represent the silk of the parachute.
- The contraction of the muscles tenses the chordae and this prevents the cusps from being turned inside out.
- The upper and anterior parts are called infundibulum and leads to the pulmonary trunk
- Inside lies the **septomarginal trabeculae/moderator band** which stretches from the ventricular septum to the anterior wall of the right ventricle. It carries the right crus of the conducting system with it and perhaps prevents the over distension of heart.

Left Ventricle

- Forms 1/3 of the sternocostal surface and 2/3 of the diaphragmatic surface.
- The wall of the left ventricle is **three times thicker than right ventricle** because it pushes blood to all parts of the body.
- It is circular on cross-section.
- It has many and fine **trabeculae carneae**
- Has only **two papillary muscles** the anterior and posterior. They are larger than those of right ventricle.
- The upper and anterior part of the left ventricle is called the aortic vestibule and leads to aorta.
- The wall of aortic vestibule is made up of fibrous tissue which is non-contractile.

Valves of Heart

Two AV valves direct flow of blood between atria and ventricles.

Two other valves direct flow of blood from the ventricles to the systemic and pulmonary circulation. These are often called as semilunar valves because of the crescent, moon shape of their leaflets.

Tricuspid directs right arterial blood anteriorly and to the left into right ventricle and it has three leaflets of unequal size.

Mitral has two major leaflets and directs blood flow from left atrium into left ventricle.

Aortic is semilunar and directs blood from left ventricle into aorta and has three fibrous leaflets

Pulmonary is also semilunar that directs the blood from right ventricle into pulmonary trunk and this valve has also three leaflets. The pulmonary, Aortic, Mitral lie behind the left border of the sternum as indicated below

- **Pulmonary lies deep to the left third sternocostal junction.**
- **Aortic lies opposite the left third intercostals space.**
- **Mitral lies deep to the left fourth sternocostal junction.**
- **Tricuspid lies behind the center of the sternum opposite the left fourth intercostal space.**

Related to these anatomical sites as indicated above the opening and the closure of all these valves is not heard at these sites but at other places due to the propogation of the sound and clinically speaking the **auscultatory sounds are better heard on the sites indicated below.**

- **Pulmonary at the left second sternocostal junction.**
- **Aortic at right second sternocostal junction.**
- **Mitral at the apex of the heart.**
- **Tricuspid at the xiphisternal junction.**

Valvular endocardium is most commonly involved in rheumatic carditis.

Mitral regurgitation is the most common feature of rheumatic carditis.

Rheumatic vegetations are small, multiple, bead like nodules arranged in arrow along the margin of contact (and not the free margin) of the cusps on their proximal aspects (at the atrial side of the mitral valve).

Valvular lesions heal by fibrosis causing deformity of valves mostly mitral regurgitation. Calcification of the injured cusps is common.

Mitral valve prolapse is mostly of the posterior leaflet or sometimes both in the left atrium. It may be associated with Marfan's syndrome. In this case the mucopolysaccharide replaces the valve fibrosa, associated with thickening of chordae tendinae.

Aortic stenosis may be of three types namely aortic valvular stenosis, subvalvular and supravalvular.

Isolated pulmonary *stenosis* is associated with fusion of valve cusps.

Ebsteins anomaly is associated with the displacement of the tricuspid valve into the right ventricle thus dividing the chamber into upper atrialised and lower functional portion resulting in rheumatic vagetations hypertrophy, arrhythmias and heart failure.

Stenosis of Valve

Narrowing of valve orifice due to fusion of valve cusps.

Incompetence of Valve

The imperfect closure of the valve due to dilatation of valve orifice or stiffening of valve cusps.

The Septal Defects

These are the defects resulting from involvement of interatrial or interventricular septum.

1. **Atrial septal defects** which include osteum secondum and osteum primum defects and osteum secondum defect lies high up in the atrial wall, while the osteum primum defect lies below. These result in communication between left and right atria.

3

Thorax

2. **Inter ventricular septal defects** which consist mainly of failure of development of membranous part. These are often associated with other septal defects.

3. Complete failure of a septum to form, resulting in formation of common atrium or common ventricle or both.

Dextrocardia

This is a congenital anomaly in which the heart position is reversed and it lies on the right side of the thorax. This may be associated with the reversal of all the intra-abdominal organs **(Situs inversus).**

The effect of pulmonary stenosis

There will be right ventricular hypertrophy because heart tries to force blood through the narrowed valve. This will be associated with congestion in the right atrium followed by secondary right atrial hypertrophy.

Fallot's Tetralogy

This is the commonest congenital anomaly of the heart and consists of:

1. Pulmonary stenosis
2. Right ventricular hypertrophy
3. Ventricular septal defect
4. An over-riding of the aorta over the septal defect. So, the aorta receives blood from both ventricles.

Complete Transposition of Great Arteries

It is a condition in which aorta arises from right ventricle and pulmonary trunk from left ventricle.

Blood Supply of Heart

1. The right coronary artery arises from the anterior aortic sinus. It is smaller than left
2. The left coronary artery arises from the left posterior aortic sinus.

The branches of the right coronary artery

1. Marginal branch
2. Posterior (inferior) interventricular branch
3. Nodal branch
4. Right atrial branch
5. Infundibular
6. Terminal branches.

The branches of the left coronary artery

1. Anterior interventricular branch
2. Branch to diaphragmatic surface of left ventricle
3. Left atrial branch

The continuation of the left coronary artery after anterior interventricular branch is called the circumflex artery.

The distribution of the right coronary artery

1. Large part of the right ventricle except area adjoining anterior interventricular groove
2. Most of the right atrium
3. Part of the left ventricle, near interventricular septum.
4. Posterior part of interventricular septum
5. SA node in 60% of the cases
6. AV node and bundle of His except part of left branch of AV bundle.

The distribution of the left coronary artery

1. Large part of the left ventricle
2. Right ventricle adjoining anterior interventricular groove
3. Left atrium
4. Anterior part of interventricular septum
5. SA node in 40% of the cases
6. Part of left branch of AV bundle

Both the interatrial and interventricular septa are supplied by branches of both coronary arteries.

The coronary arteries anastomosis:

They anastomose to a slight extent. The interventricular branches of the two coronary arteries anastomose near the apex of the heart, and in the interventricular septum. Coronary arteries also anastomose with vasa vosorum of aorta, internal thoracic artery and bronchial arteries.

The clinical importance of the anastomosis between the coronary arteries

The anastomosis between the branches of the coronary arteries is inadequate to compensate for the sudden occlusion.

A blockage therefore leads to death (infarction) of the affected cardiac tissue.

Angina Pectoris

It is a clinical condition characterized by pain in front of the chest radiating to the ulnar side of the left arm and forearm. This is due to an incomplete obstruction of the coronary arteries.

CORONARY SINUS

The tributaries of the coronary sinus

1. Great cardiac vein
2. Middle cardiac vein
3. Small cardiac vein

4. Oblique vein of the left atrium

5. Posterior vein of the left ventricle

6. Right marginal vein

The besian veins

These are small veins present in all chambers of heart opening directly into cavity of chambers.

The coronary sinus is developed from the left horn of the sinus venosus.

The coronary sinus opens into the posterior wall of right atrium

Conducting System of the Heart

The functions of conducting system of heart

1. It is responsible for initiating and maintaining normal cardiac rhythm.

2. Ensures proper coordination of atrial and ventricular contractions.

The sinuatrial (SA) node and where is it located

The SA node is the pacemaker of the heart. It is situated in the upper part of the **sulcus terminalis** just to the right of opening of the superior vena cava.

The position of AV node

The AV node lies in the **interatrial septum** near the opening of the coronary sinus. It receives impulse from SA node.

Atrioventricular Bundle—its Divisions

AV bundle forms the connection between atrial and ventricular musculature. It begins at AV node and reaches posterior margin of membranous part of ventricular septum. Here it divides into left and right branches, which descend on left and right side of interventricular septum beneath endocardium. Each branch divides and subdivides to form **Purkinje fibres, which terminate in ventricles.**

The histological differences between fibres of conducting system and cardiac muscle

1. Nodal fibres have more striations and are narrower than cardiac muscle fibres.

2. Purkinje fibres are broader than myocardial fibres

3. These contain fewer organelles

4. Plasma membrane is thin

5. Desmosomes are more numerous.

The moderator band: The moderator band also called the **septomarginal trabecula** (one of the trabeculae carneae) extends from the ventricular septum to the anterior papillary muscle. This is important as it carries the right branch of the atrioventricular bundle. It may assist in preventing over distension of ventricle.

The Nerve Supply of the Heart

Nerve supply of heart is by:

1. Parasympathetic fibres via vagus nerve. These are cardioinhibitory.

2. Sympathetic fibres from T3–5 segments of spinal cord. These are cardioaccelerator and sensory.

Both types of nerves form superficial deep cardiac plexus and supply the heart.

The superficial cardiac plexus formed. Its branches are:
The superficial cardiac plexus formed by:
1. The inferior cervical cardiac branch of the left vagus
2. The cardiac branch of the left superior cervical sympathetic ganglion

It gives branches to deep cardiac plexus, right coronary artery and left pulmonary plexus.

The deep cardiac plexus formed and its distribution is:
The deep cardiac plexus is formed by:
1. Cardiac branches of the vagus
2. Cardiac branches of both recurrent laryngeal nerves
3. The cardiac branches of cervical and thoracic branches of sympathetic ganglia.

It gives branches to coronary and pulmonary plexuses and atria.

Major Blood Vessels of Thorax

Superior Vena Cava

Superior vena cava is formed

By the union of two brachiocephalic veins behind the lower border of first costal cartilage close to sternum.

The tributaries of superior vena cava
1. Azygous vein
2. Mediastinal veins
3. Pericardial veins

The pathway for the collateral circulation in obstruction of superior vena cava
1. If obstructed above opening of azygous vein: Venous blood from upper half of body is returned through azygous vein and superficial veins of chest are dilated up to costal margin.
2. If obstructed below opening of azygous vein: Venous blood is returned through inferior vena cava via femoral vein and superficial veins are dilated on chest and abdomen up to saphenous opening in thigh (thoracoepigastric vein).

Superior vena cava is developed
1. Upper half, up to opening of azygous vein: Right anterior cardinal vein
2. Lower half, below opening of azygous vein: Right common cardinal vein.

Superior vena caval syndrome: Invasive malignant tumors, usually anaplastic lung cancers, are the most common cause of the distinctive superior vena caval syndrome. Occasionally, primary venous thrombosis, a chronic fibrosing mediastinitis, or a granulomatous lesion may be responsible. Depending on the rapidity of the development of vena caval obstruction, there are varying degrees of edema of the neck, head and arms, with evidence of venous stasis.

3

Thorax

Aorta

The parts of aorta in thorax

1. Ascending aorta
2. Arch of aorta
3. Descending thoracic aorta

The course of ascending aorta

It begins at level of lower border of 3rd costal cartilage behind left half of sternum. It runs upwards, forwards and to right and continues as arch of aorta at sternal end of upper border of second right costal cartilage.

Aortic sinus

It is dilatation of vessel wall at root of aorta above each cusp of aortic valve.

The branches of ascending aorta

1. Right coronary artery: From anterior aortic sinus
2. Left coronary artery: From left posterior aortic sinus.

The level of beginning and termination of arch of aorta

It begins behind upper border of 2nd right sternochondral joint (lower border of T4) and ends at lower border of body of 4th thoracic vertebra on left side.

Thus it begins and ends at same level but it begins anteriorly and ends posteriorly.

The Branches of Arch of Aorta

- Brachiocephalic artery: Divides into right common carotid and right subclavian artery.
- Left common carotid
- Left subclavian
- Thyroid ima
- Vertebral artery occasionally.

Branches of descending thoracic aorta.

- Posterior intercostals arteries: for 3rd–11th spaces, on both sides.
- Subcostal arteries: on both sides
- Two left bronchial arteries
- Oesophageal branches
- Pericardial branches
- Mediastinal branches
- Superior phrenic

Aortic aneurysm. It is *localized abnormal dilatation of aorta* which can be dangerous as these aneurysms are liable to expand and rupture.

Coarctation of Aorta

It is the narrowing of aorta, occurring usually immediately beyond the origin of left subclavian artery.

It leads to hypertension above the block, e.g. arms, neck and head and hypotension below the block—lower limb.

The developmental origin of aorta

A. Ascending aorta: From truncus arteriosus

B. Arch of aorta:

1. From ventral part of aortic sac and its left horn

2. Left fourth arch artery.

C. Descending aorta:

1. From left dorsal aorta below attachment of fourth arch artery.

2. Fused median vessel.

Ductus arteriosus: It is a communication present in fetal life connecting left pulmonary artery with aorta just distal to origin of left subclavian artery. After birth, it gets obliterated and forms ligamentum arteriosum. **If ductus arteriosus remains patent:** It causes progressive enlargement of left ventricle and pulmonary hypertension.

Sinus of Valvalsa aneurysms: These are dilatations of the aortic sinuses of Valsalva that may rupture into a cardiac chamber, the pulmonary artery, or the pericardium. These aneurysms occur secondary to acquired or congenital disease.

Rupture aorta: Sudden deceleration of the body at the time of impact, with differential rates of deceleration of the thoracic organs, the thoracic aorta, and the great vessels, can cause a tear involving the intima, the intima and media, or the entire wall. *This tear is usually transverse and may be partial or complete.*

Aneurysm of aorta (dilatation of aorta): The thoracic aorta comprises the ascending thoracic aorta, the aortic arch, and the descending thoracic aorta that ends the diaphragmatic hiatus. The etiology of thoracic aortic aneurysms includes *atherosclerosis, cystic medial degeneration, myxomatous degeneration, dissection, infection, trauma, and post-stenotic dilatation.*

Azygous and Hemizygous Veins

Azygous vein is formed *by the union of right ascending lumbar and right subcostal vein at level of T12 vertebra.*

The tributaries of azygous vein

1. Right posterior intercostal veins

2. Right superior intercostal veins

3. Hemiazygous vein

4. Accessory hemiazygous vein

5. Right bronchial veins

6. Oesophageal veins

7. Mediastinal and pericardial veins

8. Right ascending lumbar vein

9. Right subcostal vein

The tributaries of hemiazygous vein
1. 9th–11th left posterior intercostals veins
2. Left ascending lumbar vein
3. Left subcostal vein

ESOPHAGUS

The length of esophagus is 25 cm.

The extent of esophagus
1. It begins in neck at level of lower border of C5 vertebra, i.e. at lower border of cricoids cartilage.
2. It ends in abdomen at level of lower border of T12 vertebra, at cardiac orifice of stomach.

The curvatures of esophagus
Esophagus shows
A. Two side to side curvature towards left.
   1. At root of neck
   2. Oesophageal opening in diaphragm
B. Anteroposterior curvature: Follows curvature of spine

The sites of oesophageal constrictions
1. At its commencement: **6 inches from incisor teeth**
2. Where it is crossed by aortic arch: **9 inches from incisor teeth**
3. Where it is crossed by left bronchus: **11 inches from incisor teeth**
4. As its termination: **15 inches from incisor teeth.**

The Divisions of Oesophagus

The oesophagus is divided into three parts:
1. Cervical
2. Thoracic
3. Abdominal

The Blood Supply of Esophagus

Arterial supply
1. **Cervical part:** Inferior thyroid artery
2. **Thoracic part:** Oesophageal branches of aorta
3. **Abdominal part:** Oesophageal branches of left gastric artery.

Venous drainage
1. **Cervical part:** Into brachiocephalic vein
2. **Thoracic part:** Into azygous vein
3. **Abdominal part:** Into portal vein through left gastric vein. Lower end is site of porto-systemic anastomosis.

The Nerve Supply of Oesophagus

Parasympathetic nerves:

Sensory Motor and Secretomotor

- Upper ½: Recurrent laryngeal nerve
- Lower ½: Oesophageal plexus formed by two vagus nerves.

Sympathetic Nerves Vasomotor

- Upper ½: Fibres from middle cervical ganglion
- Lower ½: Fibres from upper 04 thoracic ganglia.

Clinical Conditions Effecting Esophagus

Achalasia cardia: It is a condition of neuromuscular inco-ordination in which the lower end of oesophagus fails to dilate when food is swallowed. As a result, food accumulates in the oesophagus.

Oesophagus is developed from

The esophagus is developed from the part of foregut lying between pharynx and stomach. It is at first short but later on elongates with the descent of diaphragm and formation of neck.

The characteristic histological features of oesophagus

From within outwards it is made up of:

- **Mucosa:** Lined by stratified squamous epithelium
- **Submucosa:** Contains mucous glands
- **Muscular layer:** Has external longitudinal and inner circular fibre. The muscle fibres are striated in upper two-thirds and smooth in lower one-third.
- **Connective tissue sheath** of areolar tissue.

The common congenital abnormalities of oesophagus

- Atresia with or without tracheoesophageal fistula.
- Stenosis: Narrowing of lumen of oesophagus.
- Short esophagus.

The clinical importance of constrictions of oesophagus

1. During the endoscopy, these constrictions should be kept in mind.
2. These are also commonly the sites of development of strictures.

Oesophageal varices and their clinical importance: *These are the dilatations of the oesophageal veins in portal hypertension, which form anastomosis between azygos (systemic) and left gastric (portal) veins.* Clinical importance: these may rupture leading to severe haemorrhage.

The effect of enlargement of left atrium on oesophagus: *In Mitral stenosis, enlargement of left atrium causes backward displacement of the oesophagus, which can be seen in a barium swallow.*

3

Thorax

THORACIC DUCT/PECQUET DUCT

- This is 45 cm (18 inches).
- The extent of thoracic duct begins from "cisterna chili" near lower border of T12 vertebra. Ends into angle of junction between left subclavian and left internal jugular vein at level of T2 vertebra.

The relations of thoracic duct in aortic opening of diaphragm
1. Anteriorly: Diaphragm
2. Posteriorly: Vertebral column
3. To the left: Azygous vein
4. To the right: Aorta

The tributaries of thoracic duct
In thorax:
1. Channels from posterior mediastinal and intercostals nodes.
2. Left mediastinal trunk may drain.

At root of neck:
1. Left jugular trunk
2. Left subclavian trunk

Which areas the thoracic duct drains lymph
- **Both halves of body below diaphragm**
- **Left half above diaphragm.**

Sympathetic Trunk

The number of ganglia in thoracic sympathetic trunk is twelve, but may be reduced due to fusion adjacent ganglia with one another.

Stellate ganglion: It is a ganglion formed by fusion of first thoracic ganglion with inferior cervical ganglion.

The branches of thoracic part of sympathetic trunk
Lateral branches:
Each ganglion is connected with corresponding spinal nerve by white (preganglionic) and grey (postganglionic) rami communicates.

Medial branches:
- Pulmonary branches to pulmonary plexus
- Cardiac branches to cardiac plexus
- Aortic branches to aortic plexus
- Oesophageal branches to oesophageal plexus from upper five ganglia.
- **Greater** splanchnic nerve: By **roots from ganglia 5 to 9**
- **Lesser** splanchnic nerve: By **roots from ganglia 10 to 11**
- **Least** splanchnic nerve: By **roots of ganglion 12.**

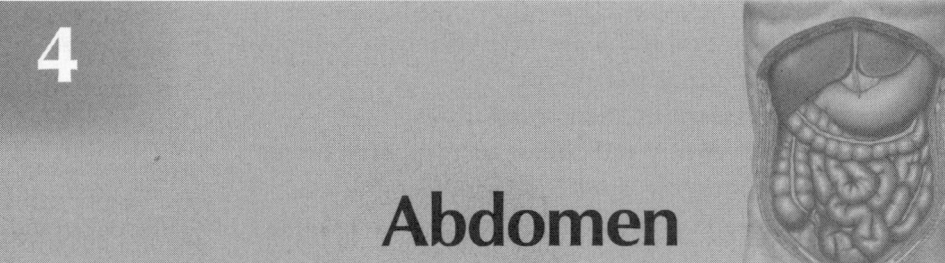

4

Abdomen

ANTERIOR ABDOMINAL WALL

Land Marks
- Xiphoid process at the level of 9th thoracic vertebra.
- Pubic symphysis lies at the level of coccyx.
- Subcostal plane passes through 3rd lumbar vertebra.
- Highest point of iliac crest at the level of 4th lumbar vertebra.
- Anterior superior iliac spine at the level of sacral promontory
- The inter-tubercular plane passes through 5th lumbar vertebra
- The transpyloric plane passes anteriorly through the tip of the 9th costal cartilage.
- The transpyloric plane passes posteriorly through body of 1st lumbar vertebra.

Skin: It is capable of undergoing enormous stretching due to which there may be formation of whitish streaks called **lineae albicantes.**

Umbilicus
The position of umbilicus
1. In anterior median line at level of junction between **L3 and L4 vertebra.**
2. It is lower in infants and those with pendulous abdomen.

Developmental origin of umbilicus: It is a scar formed by the remnants of the root of umbilical cord

Exomphalos: It is the persistence of physiological hernia of midgut loop outside the abdominal cavity.

The importance of umbilicus
Anatomical:
- It marks the **watershed of body.** The lymph and venous blood do not cross the umbilical plane
- Supplied by **T10 segment of spinal cord**
- Site of **portocaval anastomosis. Caput medusae in** portal hypertension is formed around umbilicus.

- **Embryological:** Site of attachment of **umbilical cord. It is the meeting point of four folds of embryonic plate in addition to being a watershed line.**
- It is the site for **umbilical hernia**
- It is a site for **vicarious menstruation.**
- It is the site for **cherry red tumor or raspberry tumor.**
- **Laparoscopic ports are applied through umbilicus.**
- **Sister Mary Josephs node** may be enlarged in relation to umbilicus can indicate gastric cancer.
- **Feces can come out through** umbilicus as a result of fecal fistulae
- **Urine can come out through** umbilicus as a result of urachal fistula
- **Blood can come out through umbilicus** as a result of vicarious menstruation.
- **Omphalitis** is infection of umbilicus as a result of septic cutting of cord during birth.

The remnants of umbilical cord

1. Median umbilical ligament: Remnants of urachus

2. Lateral umbilical ligament: Formed by obliterated umbilical arteries.

3. Ligamenta teres of liver: Remnant of left umbilical vein.

Structures in anterior abdominal wall

The features of superficial fascia of abdominal wall

Below the umbilicus, the superficial fascia is divided into:

1. Superficial fatty layer (fascia of camper)

2. Deep membranous layer (fascia of scarpa)

The attachments of fascia of scarpa

1. It is continuous below with membranous layer of superficial fascia of perineum (Colles' fascia).

2. The line of attachment passes over:
- Along Holden's line (lateral to public tubercle and extends for about 08 cm.
- Pubic tubercle
- Body of pubis
- Deep fascia of adductor and gracilis
- Margins of pubic arch
- Posterior border of perineal membrane

3. Above umbilicus, it merges with fatty layer.

The contents of superficial fascia of abdominal wall

1. Fat

2. Cutaneous nerves

3. Cutaneous vessels

4. Superficial lymphatics

There is no deep fascia in anterior abdominal wall. This absence of deep fascia allows expansion of abdominal wall.

4

Abdomen

The cutaneous nerve supply of anterior abdominal wall

(a) *Anterior cutaneous nerves*
- Lower 5 intercostal nerves (T7–11)
- Subcostal nerve (T12)
- Iliohypogastric (L1)

(b) *Lateral cutaneous nerves*
- 2 intercostal nerves (T10–T11)

The arterial supply of anterior abdominal wall
1. Branches of lower intercostal arteries
2. Branches of internal thoracic artery
   - Superior epigastric
   - Musculophrenic
3. Branches of external iliac artery
   - Inferior epigastric
   - Deep circumflex iliac
4. Branches of femoral artery
   - Superficial epigastric
   - Superficial external pudendal
   - Superficial circumflex iliac
5. Branches of subcostal artery
6. Branches of lumbar arteries.

The lymphatic drainage of anterior abdominal wall
1. Above the umbilicus: Axillary nodes
2. Below the umbilicus: Superficial inguinal lymph nodes

Reasons for non extravasation of urine into thigh in case of injury

The urine will collect in rupture of urethral bulb in perineum. It will be collected in scrotum, perineum and penis and then lower abdomen deep to fibrous fascial plane. It does not extravasate into lower limb, because of attachment of membranous layer to the deep fascia of upper thigh along **Holden's line.**

The drainage of cutaneous veins of anterior abdominal wall
- **Below umbilicus:** Great saphenous vein into femoral vein which drains into inferior vena cava.
- **Above umbilicus:** Lateral thoracic vein to axillary vein which drains into superior vena cava
- **Few paraumbilical veins:** Into left branch of portal vein along ligamentum teres in falciform ligament
- All these veins anastomose with each other.

Caput Medusae
- *Resembling the crown on the head of Greek Goddess.*
- *In portal vein obstruction the superficial abdominal (cutaneous) veins are dilated for collateral circulation around the umbilicus in a radiating pattern.*
- *In caput medusa the blood flows upwards above umbilicus and downwards below umbilicus.*

The clinical importance of thoracoepigastric vein

- It is a subcutaneous vein connecting the great saphenous vein with axillary vein. It becomes dilated and tortuous in vena caval obstructions.
- Clinical importance: In superior caval obstruction, blood in thoracoepigastric vein flows downwards and inferior caval obstruction blood flows upwards.

The muscles of anterior abdominal wall

1. External oblique
2. Internal oblique
3. Transversus abdominis
4. Rectus abdominis
5. Cremaster
6. Pyramidalis

The functions of muscles of anterior abdominal wall

1. Support for abdominal viscera
2. Expulsive acts: Helps in micturition, defaecation, parturition, etc.
3. Forceful expiratory acts: In coughing, sneezing blowing
4. Movements of trunks:
   - Flexion of trunk: Rectus abdominis
   - Lateral flexion: Oblique muscles
   - Rotation of trunk: External oblique with internal oblique of opposite side.
5. Pyramidalis tenses linea alba
6. Cremaster helps to suspend testis and can elevate it.

Cremasteric Reflex—its Clinical Importance

- *On stroking skin of upper part of medial side of thigh there is elevation of testis, due to reflex contraction of cremaster muscle. Reflex is more brisk in children.*
- *Clinical importance: In upper motor neuron lesions above L1 segment the reflex is lost.*

Muscles of Anterior Abdominal Wall

Muscle	Origin	Insertion
External oblique	Lower 8 ribs	Xiphoid process, linea alba, pubic symphysis, pubic crest, pectineal line and anterior two-thirds of outer lip of iliac crest.
Internal oblique	Lateral two-thirds of the inguinal ligament, anterior two-thirds of the inter-mediate lip of the iliac crest, thoracolumbar fascia	Lower three or four ribs and their costal cartilages, xiphoid process, linea alba, pubic crest and pectineal line of the pubis.

Contd...

Abdomen

4

Contd...

Muscle	Origin	Insertion
Transversus abdominis	Lateral one-third of the inguinal ligament, anterior two-thirds of the inner lip of the iliac crest, inner surfaces of the lower six costal cartilages, thoracolumbar fascia.	Xiphoid process, linea alba, pubic crest and pectineal line of pubis (lower fibres of the muscle fuse with the internal oblique to form conjoint tendon and is attached to pubic crest and pectin pubis).
Rectus abdominis	Pubic crest and anterior pubic ligament.	On the front of the wall of the thorax from xiphoid process and 5th, 6th and 7th costal cartilages.
Pyramidalis	Body of the pubis	Linea alba

4

The Inguinal Ligament

Also Known as the **ligament of poupart**. Inguinal ligament is formed by Extension of lower border of external oblique aponeurosis, which is thickened and folded backwards. It extends from anterior superior iliac spine to pubic tubercle.

The attachments of inguinal ligament are:
Upper border:
• **Lateral 2/3: Origin of internal oblique**
• **Medial 1/3: Origin of transverses abdominis**

Lower border: Fascia lata
The extensions of inguinal ligament
• **Pectineal part of inguinal ligament**
• **Pectineal ligament (ligament of Cooper)**
• **Reflected part of inguinal ligament**

Conjoint tendon: It is formed by fusion of lower aponeurotic fibres of *internal oblique and transverses abdominis.* It is attached to pubic crest and medial part of pectin pubis. It guards the weak point of the superficial inguinal ring.

The lumbar triangle of petit:
• **Floor: Internal oblique muscle**
• **Below: Crest of ilium**
• **Laterally: External oblique**
• **Medially: Latissimus dorsi**
It is the site of the primary lumbar hernia.

Rectus Sheath

It is an aponeurotic sheath covering rectus abdominis and pyramidalis muscle with their associated vessels and nerves.

Rectus sheath formed
(a) *Above costal margin:*
   • Anterior wall: External oblique aponeurosis
   • Posterior wall: Deficient, rectus lies on costal cartilages

(b) *Between costal margin and arcuate line:*
- Anterior wall: External oblique aponeurosis

Anterior wall: Anterior lamina of internal oblique

Posterior wall: Posterior lamina of internal oblique, Aponeurosis of transverses abdominis

(c) **Below arcuate line:**
- Anterior wall: Aponeurosis of all three muscles of abdomen
- Posterior wall: Deficient; rectus muscle rests on fascia transversalis.

Arcuate line (fold of Douglas): Represents posterior wall of rectus sheath, at level midway between umbilicus and pubic symphysis.

The tendinous intersections of rectus abdominis
(a) These are transverse fibrous bands which divide the muscle into smaller parts.
(b) *Three in number:* Present
    1. Opposite umbilicus
    2. Opposite free end of xiphoid
    3. In between 1 and 2

Sometimes intersections may be present below umbilicus.
(c) **Traverse only the anterior half of muscle and are adherent to anterior wall of rectus sheath.**

The importance of tendinous intersections of rectus abdominis
- They represent segmental origin of muscle
- Functionally, they make the muscle more powerful by increasing the number of muscle fibres.

The neurovascular plane of abdomen lies between internal oblique and transverses muscle. Various abdominal nerves and vessels run in this plane.

The functions of rectus sheath
- Support the abdominal viscera
- Increases efficiency of rectus muscle by checking bowing during its contraction

The contents of rectus sheath
- **Muscles: Rectus abdominis, pyramidalis**
- **Arteries: Superior epigastric artery, inferior epigastric artery**
- **Veins: Superior epigastric vein, inferior epigastric vein**
- **Nerves: Lower 5-intercostal nerves, subcostal nerve.**

Linea Alba

- It is a raphe formed by interlacing fibres of aponeuroses of three muscles forming rectus sheath
- It extends from xiphoid process to pubic symphysis
- Wider above and narrow below the umbilicus

Divarication of Recti

- Seen in weak children and multipara women
- There is weakness of linea alba, so the fingers can be insinuated between the two recti.

Incisions in Abdomen

Supra umbilical median incisions are given for surgery: The incision through linea alba is given, because it is made of fibrous tissue only, so no blood loss. It also does not cause damage to nerves.

The paramedian incisions of rectus sheath, the rectus muscle is retracted laterally.
• To avoid injury to nerves as they enter the rectus through its lateral border
• On closing the incision, rectus slips back into its place.

The transrectus incisions are not preferred during surgery: Because the rectus receive its nerve supply laterally and muscle medial to incision is deprived of its innervation and hence undergoes atrophy.

Fascia transversalis: It is the part of abdominopelvic fascia lining inner surface of transverses abdominis muscle and is separated from peritoneum by extraperitoneal connective tissue.

The prolongations of fascia transversalis
• Over femoral vessels as anterior wall of femoral sheath.
• At deep inguinal ring, over spermatic cord as internal spermatic fascia.

4

Abdomen

INGUINAL CANAL

The position of inguinal canal: In lower part of anterior abdominal wall, just above the medial half of inguinal ligament. It extends from deep to superficial inguinal ring.

The surface making of deep inguinal ring
• Situated ½ inch above the midpoint between anterior superior iliac spine and pubic symphysis (midinguinal point)
• Oval opening in fascia transversalis
• Larger in males.

The surface making of superficial inguinal ring
• Just above and lateral to pubic crest
• Triangular gap in external oblique aponeurosis
• Medial to ring lie inferior epigastric vessels

The boundaries of inguinal canal
• **Anterior:** Skin, superficial fascia, external oblique aponeurosis, fibres of internal oblique in lateral 1/3
• **Posterior:** Fascia transversalis, extraperitoneal connective tissue, parietal peritoneum, conjoint tendon in medial 2/3, reflected part of inguinal ligament at medial end.
• **Roof:** Arched fibres of internal oblique and transverses abdominis
• **Floor:** Union of inguinal ligament with fascia transversalis, lacunar ligament at medial end.

The structures passing through inguinal canal
- Spermatic cord in males
- Round ligament of uterus in females
- Ilioinguinal nerve in both sexes.

The structures passing through deep inguinal ring
- Same as above except ilioinguinal nerve, which enters between external and internal oblique muscles and passes out through superficial inguinal ring.

The boundaries of Hesselbach's triangle
- **Laterally:** Inferior epigastric artery
- **Medially:** Lateral border of rectus abdominis
- **Inferiorly:** Medial half of inguinal ligament
- It is divided into **two unequal portions** by **obliterated umbilical artery.**

Inguinal Hernia

- *It is the protrusion of the contents of abdomen (usually gut) through an abnormal opening of the body, e.g. femoral canal, inguinal canal, epiploic foramen.*

The different types of inguinal hernia
1. **Indirect (oblique) inguinal hernia:** Herniation occurs through the deep inguinal ring, lateral to inferior epigastric artery.
2. **Direct inguinal hernia:** Occurs through the Hesselbach's triangle. Two types:
   - (a) **Medial direct hernia: Medial to obliterated umbilical artery.**
   - (b) **Lateral direct hernia: Lateral to obliterated umbilical artery.**

Incomplete and complete inguinal hernia
Inguinal hernias are incomplete when it does not pass beyond the superficial inguinal ring. In complete hernia, the herniated gut descends in front of testis into tunica vaginalis.

The differences between direct and indirect inguinal hernia

Direct inguinal hernia	Indirect inguinal hernia
• Less frequent	• More frequent
• Placed over the body of pubic bone	• Placed in the course of inguinal canal
• *Inferior epigastric artery*	
• Medial to the hernial sac	• Lateral to the hernial sac
• *Spermatic cord:*	
• Lies on its posterior	• Lies behind it
• Lateral sides	
• Usually acquired	• Usually congenital

Clinically distinguishing an inguinal hernia from a femoral hernia
An inguinal hernia lies above and medial to the medial end of inguinal ligament at its attachment to pubic tubercle. A femoral hernia lies below and laterals to pubic tubercle.

1. Inguinal hernia common in males because of greater diameter of deep inguinal ring
2. Femoral hernia common in females because of larger femoral ring due to broader pelvis and changes in tissues produced by the pregnancy.

The contents of a hernial sac

- Omentum
- Intestine
- Portion of circumference of intestine
- Portion of bladder
- Fluid

Strangulated hernia: When the blood supply to hernia contents become impaired thus leading to the death of the tissue.

Clinically distinguishing a direct from an indirect inguinal hernia

By deep ring occlusion test in cases of reducible hernia. The hernia is first reduced and deep (internal) inguinal ring is occluded with finger tip and patient is asked to cough while standing. If it is an indirect hernia, as the deep ring is occluded, it prevents hernia contents from descending into scrotum. But a direct hernia will protrude as contents herniate through the posterior wall of inguinal canal.

The Coverings of Inguinal Hernia

Indirect hernia: From without inwards:

1. Skin
2. Fascia of camper
3. Fascia of scarpa
4. External spermatic fascia
5. Cremasteric fascia
6. Internal spermatic fascia
7. Extraperitoneal areolar tissue
8. Parietal peritoneum

The embryological origin of inguinal canal

- It represents the passage of gubernaculum through the abdominal wall.
- It extends from caudal end of developing gonad to labioscrotal swelling.

Classification of Hernia

- **Reducible:** Hernia either reduces itself on lying down or can be reduced by patient/surgeon.
- **Irreducible hernia:** Content cannot be reduced, but there are no complications. It is usually due to adhesions.
- **Obstructed hernia:** Irreducible hernia containing intestine which is obstructed but blood supply is not hampered.

4

Abdomen

- **Strangulated hernia:** Obstruction along with hampering of blood supply of hernial contents.
- **Incarcerated hernia:** When the content of sac is colon which is blocked by faeces. In this case

Mechanism Preventing Inguinal Hernia

- Obliquity of inguinal canal.
- Shutter mechanism of the arched fibers of the internal oblique and transverses abdominus.
- Sphincter action of transverses abdominus and internal oblique muscles at deep inguinal ring.
- Ball valve action of cremaster muscle.
- Presence of strong conjoint tendon in front of Hesselbach's triangle.

MALE EXTERNAL GENITAL ORGANS

The parts of penis
1. Root (attached part): Consist of two crura and one bulb.
2. Body (free part): Consists of two corpora cavernosa and one corpus spongiosum.
Bucks fascia: It is the membranous layer of superficial fascia of the penis

The arterial supply of penis
- Deep artery of penis
- Dorsal artery of penis   } Branches of internal pudendal artery.
- Artery of bulb of penis
- Superficial external pudendal artery: Branch of femoral artery.

The developmental origin of penis
The genital tubercle at cranial end of cloacal membrane, which lengthens to form phallus which enlarges to form penis

Scrotum

It is cutaneous bag containing testis, epididymis and lower part of spermatic cord
The structures forming layers of scrotum.

From without inwards
- Skin
- Dartos muscle
- External spermatic fascia
- Cremasteric fascia
- Internal spermatic fascia

The blood supply of scrotum
- Superficial pudendal
- Deep external pudendal

- Internal pudendal: Scrotal branch
- Inferior epigastric: Cremasteric branch

The nerve supply of scrotum

Anterior 1/3 of scrotum: By L$_1$ segment through

- Ilioinguinal nerve
- Genital branch of genitofemoral nerve.

Posterior 2/3 of scrotum: By S$_3$ segment through

- Posterior scrotal branch of pudendal nerve
- Perineal branch of posterior cutaneous nerve of thigh.
- Dartos is a "subcutaneous muscle" also called "thermostat of testis." It helps in regulation of temperature of testis.
- Scrotum is a common site for edema due to laxity of skin.
- Scrotum is a common site for sebaceous cysts.
- The extravasation of fluid into scrotal sac is bilateral: Because the septum which divides scrotum into right and left compartments, is incomplete superiorly.

The Testis

1. It is suspended in scrotum by spermatic cord
2. It lies obliquely, so that upper pole is tilted forwards and a little laterally and lower pole backwards and medially
3. Left testis is lower than the right.

Sinus of epididymis

It is the extension of the cavity of tunica vaginalis between testis and epididymis from its lateral side, on posterior border.

- Appendix of testis: Remnant of upper end of müllerian duct.
- Minute, oval body at upper pole of testis just beneath the head of epididymis.
- Also called sessile hydatid of Morgagni.

The coverings of testis—From without inwards:

1. Tunica vaginalis
2. Tunica albuginea
3. Tunica vasculosa

The arterial supply of testis

Testicular artery: Branch of abdominal aorta

At posterior border of testis, it divides into branches:

1. Small branches: Enter posterior border
2. Larger branches: Pierce tunica albuginea and run on surface of testis to ramify on tunica vasculosa.

Pampiniform Plexus

- It is a venous plexus emerging from testis
- The anterior part is arranged around testicular artery, middle part around ductus deferens and its artery and posterior part is isolated.

4

Abdomen

- At superficial inguinal ring, plexus condenses into 04 veins.
- Ultimately, one vein is formed which drains into inferior vena cava on right side and left renal vein on left side.

The Lymphatic Drainage of Testis

Pre-aortic and para-aortic lymph nodes at level of L_2 vertebra.

The structure of testis

Testis is divided into 200–300 lobules each containing one to three seminiferous tubules. The tubules anastomose posteriorly into a plexus, rete testis from which efferent ducts arise and pass into head of epididymis.

The developmental origin of testis

Testis arises from mesodermal genital ridge in posterior abdominal wall just medial to developing kidney and links up with epididymis and vas, which develop from mesonephric duct (Wolffian duct)

- **Primordial germ cells: These are endodermal and derived from dorsal wall of yolk sac.**
- **Cells of Sertoli: Derived from coelomic epithelium.**
- **Cells of Leydig: Derived from mesenchymal cells of mesonephros.**

Gubernaculum testis: It is a fibromuscular band attaching the testis to the bottom of scrotum. According to hunter, gubernaculums forms the inguinal canal by its passage through abdominal wall. It develops from a mesenchymal strand.

Processus Vaginalis

- It is a prolongation of peritoneal cavity projecting into scrotum.
- The testis in scrotum slides posterior to this and projects.
- Thus the testis is covered by peritoneum from front and sides.
- About the time of birth it obliterates, leaving the testis covered by tunica vaginalis.

The positions of testis during its descent in foetal life

- **3rd month: Reaches iliac fossa**
- **7th month: Transverses inguinal canal**
- **8th month: Reaches superficial inguinal ring**
- **9th month: Descends into scrotum**
- **Varicocele:** It is the dilatation of pampiniform plexus of veins. It is commoner on left side because of left testicular veins compression by loaded sigmoid colon, left kidney tumor which invade renal veins and obstructs the drainage of left testicular veins, obstruction by angulation at site of entry of left testicular veins into renal vein.
- **Ectopic testis:** The testis descends but is found in an unusual position, e.g. superficial, perineal, femoral, etc. In these cases, the cord is long (unlike the undescended testis).
- **Hydrocele:** It is collection of fluid within the tunica vaginalis.
- **Monorchidism:** Developmental absence of a testicle.
- **Vas aberrans of Haller:** It is blind tube which lies between the tail of epididymis and commencement of vas.

- **The length of epididymis:** When uncoiled 20-feet, but in coiled form the comma shaped body is only 1½ inches long on posterolateral aspect of testis.
- **Developmental origin of appendix of epididymis:** Represents cranial end of mesonephric duct Also known as pedunculated hydatid of Morgagni.
- **Organ of Giraldés (paradidymis):** Free tubules in spermatic cord above head of epididymis. Represent caudal mesonephric tubules.

The Coverings of Spermatic Cord

From within outwards:

1. **Internal spermatic fascia: Derived from fascia transversalis**
2. **Cremasteric fascia: Derived from internal oblique and transverses abdominis muscle.**
3. **External spermatic fascia: Derived from external oblique aponeurosis.**

The constituents of spermatic cord

- Vas deferens
- *Veins:* Pampiniform plexus
- *Arteries:* Testicular, cremasteric, artery of vas
- *Nerves:* Genital branch of genitofemoral testicular plexus of sympathetic nerves (T10). Sympathetic plexus around artery of vas.
- Lymphatics of testis
- Areolar tissue
- Remains of processus vaginalis.

PERITONEUM

Peritoneum is a large serous membrane (sac) lining the abdominal cavity.

The different parts of peritoneum is divided into:

1. **Outer layer, the parietal peritoneum**
2. **Inner layer, the visceral peritoneum**
3. **Folds of peritoneum, which suspend the viscera**
4. **Peritoneal cavity**

The differences between parietal and visceral peritoneum

Features	Parietal peritoneum	Visceral peritoneum
Position	Lines the inner surface of abdominal and pelvic walls (parieties) and lower surface of diaphragm	Lines the outer surface of viscera
Attachment	Loosely attached by extraperitoneal connective tissue	Firmly adherent
Blood and nerve supply	Same as overlying parieties	Same as underlying viscera
Pain sensitivity	Sensitive because of somatic innervations	Insensitive because of autonomic innervation
Development	Derived from somatopleural layer of lateral plate mesoderm	Derived from splanchnopleural layer of lateral plate mesoderm

Abdomen

4

The functions of folds of peritoneum
- These suspend the organs in abdominal cavity
- Provide a degree of mobility to the organs
- Provide media for the passage of vessels, nerves and lymphatics of the suspended organs.

The different types of peritoneal folds
The peritoneal folds are divided into 3 types:
- **Omenta: Folds suspending the stomach**
- **Mesentery: Folds suspending parts of small and large intestine.**
- **Ligaments.**

The peritoneal cavity: It is a potential space lying between the parietal and visceral peritoneum

There are four mesenteries:
1. *Mesentery of small intestine*
2. *Transverse mesocolon*
3. *Pelvic mesocolon*
4. *Mesentery of appendix*

There are four peritoneal folds related to stomach:
1. *Lesser omentum*
2. *Greater omentum*
3. *Gastrosplenic ligament*
4. *Gastrophrenic ligament*

There are four ligaments attached and specific to liver
1. *Falciform ligament*
2. *Coronary ligament*
3. *Right triangular ligament*
4. *Left triangular ligament*

There are four ligaments related to female genital tract
1. *Medial umbilical ligament*
2. *Two lateral umbilical ligaments*
3. Round ligament of liver

The different parts of peritoneal cavity
The peritoneal cavity is divided into two parts:
1. **Greater sac: Larger**
2. **Lesser sac: Smaller situated behind lesser omentum, stomach and liver.**

The two sacs communicate with each other through the epiploic foramen (foramen of Winslow).

Peritoneal fossae (recesses): These are small pockets of peritoneal cavity enclosed by small, inconstant folds of peritoneum. More frequent in newborn babies and most of them become obliterated after birth.

Greater omentum: The policeman of abdomen

It is greater omentum hanging down from the greater curvature of stomach and covering the loops of intestine. It is called policeman of abdomen because it limits the spread of infection by moving to the site of infection and sealing it off from the surrounding areas. The anterior two layers descend and fold upon themselves to form posterior two layers which ascend to the anterior surface of head, anterior border of body of pancreas. The folding is such that 1st layer becomes the 4th layer and the 2nd layer becomes the 3rd layer. The part of the peritoneal cavity (lesser sac) between the 2nd and 3rd layers gets obliterated except a small part below the greater curvature. Contents are the right and left gastroepiploic vessels.

The contents of lesser omentum

The right free margin of lesser omentum contains:

1. Hepatic artery
2. Portal vein
3. Bile duct
4. Hepatic plexus of nerves
5. Lymph nodes and lymphatics

Along the lesser curvature of stomach and upper border of duodenum, it contains:

- Right and left gartric vessels
- Gastric lymph nodes and lymphatics
- Branches of gastric nerves.

Peritoneal ligaments: These are the double layers of peritoneum connecting the viscera to each other or to the diaphragm or the abdominal wall or pelvic wall.

Example:

- **Falciform ligament**
- **Right and left triangular ligaments**
- **Superior and inferior layers of coronary ligaments**
- **Gastrophrenic ligament**
- **Gastrosplenic ligament**
- **Lienorenal ligament**
- **Hepatogastric ligament**
- **Hepatoduodenal ligament**
- **Ligaments of the uterus and urinary bladder.**

Mesentery: It extends from duodenojejunal flexure on left side of L2 vertebra to upper part of right sacroiliac joint.

It crosses:

- Third part of duodenum
- Abdominal aorta
- Inferior vena cava
- Right ureter
- Right psoas major.

4

Abdomen

The contents of mesentery

- Jejunal and ileal branches of superior mesenteric artery and veins
- Autonomic nerve plexus
- Lymphatics
- Lymph nodes
- Fat

Falciform ligament: It is a sickle shaped fold of peritoneum which connects antero-superior surface of liver to anterior abdominal wall and under surface of diaphragm.

The clinical importance of epiploic foramen: Internal hernia can occur into lesser sac through the foramen. If the hernia becomes strangulated then it cannot be reduced by enlarging the foramen because of structures around it. So the gut is first aspirated and then reduced back through the epiploic foramen. It is situated at level of T12 vertebra, behind right free margin of lesser omentum.

The Boundaries of Epiploic Foramen

- Anteriorly: Right free margins of lesser omentum with structures in it
- Posteriorly: Inferior vena cava right suprarenal gland T12 vertebra.
- Superiorly: Caudate process of liver
- Inferiorly: First part of duodenum and horizontal part of hepatic artery.

Mesoappendix: It is a small triangular fold of peritoneum which suspends the appendix and contains the vessels, nerves and lymphatics of the appendix.

Transverse mesocolon: Suspends the transverse colon from the posterior abdominal wall. It is attached to the anterior surface of the head, and the anterior border of the body of the pancreas and the line of attachment is horizontal with an upward inclination to the left. It contains the middle colic vessels.

Sigmoid mesocolon: It is triangular and suspends the sigmoid colon from the pelvic wall. Its root is shaped like a letter V inverted. Its apex lies over the left ureter at the termination of left common iliac artery. The left limb of V is attached along the upper half of external iliac artery and the right limb to the posterior pelvic wall extending downwards and medially from the apex to the median plane at the level of 3 sacral vertebra. It encloses sigmoid and superior rectal branches of inferior mesenteric artery.

Subphrenic Spaces

These are the potential spaces below the diaphragm and are formed by reflections of peritoneum around liver. They are:

1. **Intraperitoneal spaces:**
   - **Left subphrenic space**
   - **Left subhepatic space (lesser sac)**
   - **Right subphrenic space**
   - **Right posterior (subhepatic) space**

2. Extraperitoneal spaces:
   - **Right extraperitoneal space (bare area of liver)**
   - **Left extraperitoneal space around left suprarenal and upper pole of left kidney.**

Morisons Pouch and its Clinical Importance

- Right subhepatic space is also known as morisons pouch or hepatorenal pouch.
- Clinical importance: This is the most dependent part of peritoneal cavity of abdomen proper. This is the commonest site of subphrenic abscess and also fluid effusions tend to accumulate here.

Rectouterine pouch (pouch of Douglas): This is the most dependent part of peritoneal cavity in standing position and of pelvic cavity in supine position.

The boundaries of Rectouterine pouch
- **Anteriorly: Uterus and posterior fornix of vagina**
- **Posteriorly: Rectum**
- **Floor: Rectovaginal fold of peritoneum**

Clinical importance of rectouterine pouch: This being the most dependent part of peritoneal cavity, so the pus tends to collect here and form the pelvic abscess.

The clinical importance of pertioneal fossae: Some of these may persist and may be the site of an internal hernia and strangulation.

Zygosis: Some of the abdominal organs possess mesentery during the embryonic life, e.g. duodenum. Ascending and descending colon, rectum. But due to fusion of their mesentery with peritoneum of posterior abdominal wall (zygosis) these become retroperitoneal.

The different peritoneal fossae:
1. **Lesser sac**
2. **Duodenal fossae**
   - **Superior duodenal fossa**
   - **Inferior duodenal fossa**
   - **Para duodenal fossa**
   - **Duodenojejunal fossa**
   - **Retroduodenal fossa**
   - **Mesentericoparietal fossa of Waldeyer**
3. **Caecal fossae**
   - **Superior ileocaecal fossa**
   - **Inferior ileocaecal fossa**
   - **Retrocaecal fossa**
4. **Intersigmoid fossa**

The developmental origin of peritoneum
1. **Parietal layer: From somatopleural layer of lateral plate mesoderm**
2. **Visceral layer: From splanchnopleural layer of lateral plate mesoderm.**

4

Abdomen

The composition of peritoneal fluid

1. Water electrolytes and solutes derived from interstitial fluid of neighboring tissue and from plasma of adjacent blood vessels

2. Proteins

3. Desquamated mesothelial cells, macrophages, fibroblasts, lymphocytes.

- **Peritonism:** The irritation of peritoneum produces rigidity of abdominal muscles in that region. **The parietal peritoneum** is supplied by somatic spinal nerves which also supply muscle and skin of the parieties, so, when parietal peritoneum is irritated the abdominal muscles are reflexly contracted, thus producing rigidity of abdominal wall in that region.
- **Peritonitis:** Inflammation of peritoneum
- **Ascites:** Collection of free fluid in peritoneal cavity.
- **Pneumoperitoneum:** Gas in peritoneum
- **Hemoperitoneum:** Blood in peritoneum
- **Paracentesis abdominis:** It is the tapping of ascitic fluid: Done with a trochar and cannula by puncturing the abdomen either in median plane midway between umbilicus and pubic symphysis or at a point just above the anterior superior iliac spine.

The functions of peritoneum

- **Absorption:** Fluid and solutes by mesothelium, which acts as a semipermeable membrane. This property of peritoneum is used in dialysis in case of kidney/renal failure in a procedure is **called peritoneal dialysis.**
- **Healing and adhesions:** By transformation of mesothelium into fibroblasts.
- **Movement of viscera:** *Peritoneum* provides a slippery surface for free movement of abdominal viscera.
- **Protection of viscera:** Phagocytic cells of peritoneum guard against infections.
- **Storage of fats:** Especially in peritoneal folds.

The differences between male and female peritoneum

1. In male: Peritoneum is a closed sac lined by mesothelium.

2. In females:
- Peritoneal cavity communicates with exterior through uterine tubes
- Peritoneum covering fimbria is lined by columnar ciliated epithelium.
- Peritoneum covering ovaries is lined by cubical epithelium.

REGIONS OF ABDOMEN

Abdomen is divided into nine regions by:

- **Two vertical planes: Right and left lateral planes.**

  Passing from midinguinal point and crossing tip of ninth costal cartilage (mid-clavicular lines)

- Two horizontal planes:
  1. Subcostal plane: Passes through lower border of 10th costal cartilage and near upper border of body of L3.
  2. Transpyloric plane: Can be used instead of subcostal plane. Passes through tip of ninth costal cartilage and lower border of L1.
  3. Transtubercular plane: Passes through tubercles of iliac crest and body of L5 vertebra near upper border.

The nine regions of abdomen
- *Upper:*
  1. Right hypochondrium
  2. Left epigastrium
  3. Epigastrium
- *Middle:*
  4. Right lumbar
  5. Left lumbar
  6. Umbilical
- *Lower:*
  7. Left iliac
  8. Right Iliac
  9. Hypogastrium.

The structures lying at level of L1 vertebra
- Transpyloric plane
- Pylorus
- Duodenojejunal flexure
- Pancreas
- Hilum of kidneys

The structures lying at level of L5 vertebra
- Inter (trans) tubercular plane
- Common iliac veins end
- Inferior vena cava begins.

The structures lying at level of L2 vertebra
- Spinal cord ends
- Thoracic duct begins
- Azygous vein begins.

Coeliac trunk: The coeliac trunk supplies derivatives of foregut, i.e.

1. Lower end of esophagus
2. Stomach
3. Upper 1½ parts of duodenum up to opening of common bile duct
4. Liver

4

Abdomen

5. Spleen and
6. Greater part of pancreas.

The coeliac trunk develops: from one of the vitelline arteries (C_7 segment).
The branches of coeliac trunk
1. Left gastric
2. Hepatic and
3. Splenic arteries

The branches of hepatic artery
1. Gastroduodenal artery
2. Hepatic artery proper
3. Right gastric artery
4. Supraduodenal artery
5. Cystic artery

The branches of splenic artery
1. Pancreatic branches
2. Short gastric arteries
3. Left gastroepiploic artery

Superior Mesenteric Artery

Supplies the derivatives of midgut, i.e.
1. Lower 2½ of duodenum below opening of common bile duct
2. Jejunum
3. Ileum
4. Appendix
5. Caecum
6. Ascending colon
7. Right 2/3 of transverse colon
8. Lower ½ of head of pancreas

It arises from abdominal aorta at L1 vertebra behind the body of pancreas
The branches of superior mesenteric artery
1. Inferior pancreaticoduodenal
2. Jejunal
3. Ileal
4. Ileocolic
5. Right colic
6. Middle colic

The relations of superior mesenteric artery
A. Above the root of mesentery
   • Anteriorly: Body of pancreas and splenic vein
   • Posteriorly: Aorta, left renal vein, uncinate process of pancreas and third part of duodenum
   • To the right: Superior mesenteric vein

B. Within the root of mesentery

• It crosses: Inferior vena cava, right ureter, right psoas

• To its right: Superior mesenteric vein

The tributaries of superior mesenteric vein

1. Inferior pancreaticoduodenal

2. Jejunal

3. Ileal

4. Ileocolic

5. Right colic

6. Middle colic

7. Right gastroepiploic vein

Occlusion of Superior Mesenteric Artery

When the superior mesenteric artery is completely occluded, then the marginal artery may become significantly dilated as it is required to supply the whole of the midgut loop.

Occlusion of the aorta or common iliac arteries may result in a similar dilatation of the marginal artery, which then becomes an important source of collateral supply to the legs.

Inferior Mesenteric Artery

It supplies the derivatives of hindgut, i.e.

1. Left 1/3 of transverse colon

2. Descending colon

3. Sigmoid colon

4. Rectum

5. Anal canal above the pectinate line

The branches of inferior mesenteric artery

1. Left colic

2. Sigmoid

3. Superior rectal artery

Marginal Artery

• It is an arterial arcade situated along the concavity of colon formed by anastomosis between ileocolic, right colic, middle colic, left colic and sigmoid arteries. Vasa recta arise from the marginal artery and supply the colon.

• The clinical importance of marginal artery: It forms extensive anastomosis, so it is capable of supplying the colon even in absence of one of the main feeding trunks. This fact is utilized in surgery of colon.

Portal Vein

The characteristic feature of portal vein: Portal vein is one vein which begins and also ends in capillaries.

The areas from which the blood is drained by the portal vein

1. Abdominal part of alimentary tract

2. Spleen

3. Gallbladder

4. Pancreas

Portal vein is divided into 3 parts

1. Infraduodenal

2. Retroduodenal

3. Supraduodenal

The relations of different parts of portal vein

A. Infraduodenal part:

- Anteriorly: Neck of pancreas
- Posteriorly: Inferior vena cava

B. Retroduodenal part:

- Anteriorly: First part of duodenum, Gastroduodenal artery, Common bile duct
- Posteriorly: Inferior vena cava

C. Supraduodenal part: Lies in the free margin of lesser omentum

- Anteriorly: Bile duct, hepatic artery
- Posteriorly: Inferior vena cava.

Formation: Portal vein is formed at the level of L2 vertebra behind the neck of pancreas, by union of superior mesenteric and splenic veins.

Termination: It ends at the right end of porta hepatis by dividing into a right branch and a left branch.

The tributaries of portal vein

- Splenic vein
- Superior mesenteric vein
- Left gastric vein
- Right gastric vein
- Superior pancreaticoduodenal vein
- Cystic vein
- Paraumbilical veins

The sites of portal systemic communications, the portal and systemic veins forming these

Sites	Portal vein	Systemic vein
Umbilicus	• Left branch of portal vein through paraumbilical vein	• Veins of anterior abdominal wall
Lower end of esophagus	• Oesophageal tributaries of left gastric	• Oesophageal tributaries of the accessory hemiazygous vein
Anal canal	• Superior rectal vein	• Middle and inferior rectal veins
Bare area of liver	• Hepatic vein	• Phrenic and intercostals veins
Posterior abdominal wall	• Veins of duodenum ascending and descending colon	• Retroperitoneal veins of abdominal wall and renal capsule
Liver	• Rarely ductus venosus remains patent and then connects left branch of portal vein	• Inferior vena cava

The importance of portal systemic communications: These communications form the important pathways of collateral circulation in portal obstruction and portal hypertension.

The developmental origin of portal vein
1. **Infraduodenal part:** Part of left vitelline vein
2. **Retroduodenal part:** Dorsal anastomosis between two vitelline veins.
3. **Supraduodenal part:** Part of right vitelline vein.

SPLEEN

The spleen lies obliquely along the long axis of 10th rib. It lies mainly in **left hypochondrium** but the posterior end extends into epigastrium. It is directed downwards, forwards and laterally.

Harris dictum: The average size and weight of spleen is 01 inch thick, 03 inches broad, 05 inches long, and 07 ounces in weight and aling 9th, 10th and 11th Ribs.

The ends, borders and surfaces of spleen
Ends:
1. **Anterior:** Expanded, directed downwards and forwards
2. **Posterior:** Rounded, directed upwards, backwards and medially

Borders:
1. **Superior:** Notched near anterior end, sharp separates diaphragmatic surface from gastric impression
2. **Inferior:** More rounded and separates renal impression from diaphragmatic surface
3. **Intermediate border:** Rounded and separates gastric and renal impressions.

Surfaces:

1. Diaphragmatic surface: Convex

2. Visceral surface: Concave and has following impressions:
   • Gastric impression: For fundus of stomach
   • Renal impression: For left kidney
   • Colic impression: For splenic flexure of colon
   • Pancreatic impression: For tail of pancreas.

The structures lying at hilum of spleen

The hilum transmits splenic vessels and nerves. It provides attachment to gastrosplenic and lienorenal ligaments.

The peritoneal ligaments attached to spleen

1. Gastrosplenic ligament

2. Lienorenal ligament

3. Phrenicocolic ligament

The structures lying in the gastrosplenic ligament

1. Left gastroepiploic vessels

2. Short gastric vessels

3. Lymphatics

4. Sympathetic nerves

5. Fat

The structure lying in the lienorenal ligament

It contains:

1. Tail of pancreas

2. Splenic vessels

3. Pancreaticosplenic lymph nodes

4. Lymphatics

5. Sympathetic nerves

6. Fat

The tributaries of splenic vein

1. Short gastric

2. Left gastroepiploic

3. Pancreatic

4. Inferior mesenteric vein

The functions of spleen

• Haemopoieses: Important during fetal life. Lymphopoiesis continues throughout life

• Immune responses: Under antigenic stimulation increased lymphopoiesis occurs in spleen.

- **Phagocytosis:** By the reticular cells, free macrophages and endothelial cells. They remove cell debris and old RBCs and other blood cells and micro-organisms.
- **Storage of RBCs**
- **Culling and pitting:** Destruction of worn out and rigid RBCs in red pulp.

The developmental origin of spleen: From left layer of cephalic part of dorsal mesogastrium, into a number of nodules which fuse to form a lobulated mass.

- **The accessory spleen:** These are the splenic nodules which have failed to fuse to form a lobulated mass.
- **Splenosis:** Fragments of splenic tissue after rupture disseminate.
- **Polycystic disease of spleen:** May be associated with cysts in spleen and can be associated with polycystic kidney disease.
- **Wandering spleen:** Occurs with a longer fold of peritoneum attached to spleen and because of that has excess mobility.
- **Torsion of spleen:** Occurs in wandering spleen and as a result of torsion spleen undergoes atrophy.
- **Autosplenectomy:** Can occur as a result of infarction of spleen because of certain anemias like sickle cell anemia due to blockage of blood supply to spleen.
- **Splenomegaly:** It is a feature of variety of diseases, infectious, neoplastic in which spleen enlarges in size. Important causes of splenomegaly are malaria, kala-azar, chronic myeloid leukemia, hairy cell leukemia, etc.
- **Kehr's sign:** Splenic infarction due to obstruction of branches of splenic artery, causes referred pain in left shoulder due irritation of under surface of diaphragm by effused blood.
- **Splenic flexure syndrome:** It is characterized by recurrent pain and abdominal distention in the left upper quadrant of the abdomen. It is caused by a pocket of gas trapped in the large intestine below the spleen at the splenic flexure of colon.
- The symptoms are relieved by defecation or passing flatus.
- **Splenorrhaphy is repair of spleen:** Because spleen has a role in immunogenesis, removal of spleen is not preferred. Repair of Spleen is called splenography.
- **Splenectomy:** It is the *surgical removal of spleen.*
- **OPSI: Overwhelming postsplenectomy infections** is a serious condition which can occur after removal of spleen as a result of which the immune response to infections is decreased and the patient is liable and more prone to develop particular infections.

4

Abdomen

ESOPHAGUS

Important anatomical points
- **The esophagus** is proximal part of GIT about 25 cm (10 inches) in length extending from the pharynx to the stomach.
- **It is divided into four segments: Pharyngoesophageal, cervical, thoracic, and abdominal.**

- It is lined by squamous epithelium except in its terminal part where it is columnar.

The esophagus has three sites of anatomic narrowing

- **The cervical constriction** occurs at the level of the cricopharyngeus sphincter at a distance of 15 cm from incisor teeth.
- **The bronchoaortic constriction** is located at the level of the fourth thoracic vertebra behind the tracheal bifurcation is at a distance of 25 cm from incisor teeth, where the left mainstem bronchus and aortic arch cross the esophagus.
- **The diaphragmatic** constriction is at a distance of 40 cm from incisor teeth, where the esophagus transverses the diaphragm.
- **The esophagus is a mucosal-lined muscular tube that lacks a serosa.**
- Beneath the adventitia is a coat of longitudinal muscle that overlies an inner layer of circular muscle. Between the two muscular layers is a thin intramuscular septum of connective tissue that contains fine blood vessels and ganglion cells of Meissner's and Auerbach's plexuses.
- **Both the longitudinal and circular muscle layers of the upper third of the esophagus are striated, whereas in the lower two-thirds, they are nonstriated and in the middle they are mixed.**

Blood Supply

The cervical esophagus receives blood from the superior thyroid artery as well as the inferior thyroid artery of the thyrocervical trunk.

The major blood supply of the intrathoracic esophagus is from four to six aortic esophageal arteries, supplemented by collateral vessels with the inferior thyroid, intercostal and bronchial, inferior phrenic, and left gastric arteries.

The venous drainage of the esophagus includes the hypopharyngeal, azygos, hemiazygos, intercostal, and gastric veins.

- **Lower end of esophagus** is a site for portosystemic anastomosis and variceal haemmorrhage.
- **Compression of esophagus:** In cases of mediastinal syndrome causes difficulty in swallowing. Referred to as dysphagia.
- Pain during swallowing is referred to as *odynophagia.*
- Failure of esophagus to separate from trachea can result in a condition referred to as **tracheoesophageal fistula.**
- **Mega esophagus** is a clinical condition in which esophagus is massively dilated. It is seen especially in **Chagas' disease.**
- **Barrett's esophagus** is squamocolumnar metaplasia at lower end of esophagus which can progress to **adenocarcinoma of esophagus. It is hence a premalignant condition.**
- **Achalasia cardia** is failure of relaxation of lower end of esophagus due to **neuromuscular incoordination.**
- **Esophagoscopy** is a diagnostic procedure in which an endoscope is used for visualization of interior of esophagus.
- **Rarely** the lower end of esophagus can be involved in e**sophagitis, inflammation of esophagus.**

STOMACH

It lies obliquely in upper and left part of abdomen, occupying epigastric, umbilical and left hypochondriac region.

The normal variations in capacity and shape of stomach
- Capacity: At birth: 30 ml
- At puberty: 1000 ml
- In adults: 1.5–2 litres
- Shape: When empty: j-shaped
- When distended: Pyriform
- In obese: More horizontal (steer horn stomach)

The different parts of stomach
1. Cardiac part: Subdivided into:
   - **Fundus**
   - **Body**
2. Pyloric part: Subdivided into:
   - **Pyloric antrum**
   - **Pyloric canal**

Stomach has:
- **Two orifices: Cardiac and pyloric**
- **Two curvatures: Lesser and greater**
- **Two surfaces: Anterior and posterior**

The pyloric orifice is recognised by a surgeon by
- **Circular groove (pyloric constriction) produced by pyloric sphincter which feels like a firm ring.**
- **Prepyloric vein: Lies anteriorly in pyloric constriction**

The level of orifices of stomach
- **Cardiac orifce (physiological sphincter): T11 vertebra**
- **Pyloric orifice: L1 vertebra**

The bare areas of stomach
1. **Greater and lesser curvatures, along the peritoneal reflections**
2. **Triangular area on posterior surface close to cardiac orifice and related to left crus of diaphragm.**

The structures forming the stomach bed

These structures are related to posterior surface of stomach
1. **Spleen: Related to fundus and is separated by the cavity of greater sac**
2. **Other structures are separated by cavity of lesser sac**
   - **Diaphragm**
   - **Left kidney**

4

Abdomen

- Left suprarenal
- Pancreas
- Splenic artery
- Splenic flexure of colon
- Transverse mesocolon

The blood supply of stomach

Arterial supply:

- Left gastric artery: Branch of coeliac trunk
- Right gastric artery: Branch of common hepatic
- Right gastroepiploic artery: Branch of gastroduodenal
- Left gastroepiploic artery: Branch of splenic
- Short gastric arteries: Branches of splenic

Venous drainage: Into portal, superior mesenteric and splenic veins

The lymphatic drainage of stomach

- Stomach is subdivided by an imaginary line along longitudinal axis of stomach into right 2/3 (superior gastric area) and left 1/3 is subdivided into upper 1/3 (pancreaticolineal area) and lower 2/3 (inferior gastric area)
- Superior gastric area: Coeliac nodes through superior gastric nodes.
- Inferior gastric area: Coeliac nodes through inferior gastric, subpyloric and partly hepatic nodes.
- Pancreaticolineal area: Coeliac nodes through pancreaticolineal nodes.
- Pylorus: Coeliac nodes through subpyloric and partly hepatic nodes.

The nerve supply of stomach

1. Sympathetic nerves: T6–T10 segments.

   These are

   (a) Vasomotor

   (b) Motor to pyloric sphincter

   (c) Chief pathway for pain sensation

2. Parasympathetic nerves: Vagus as

   (a) Anterior gastric nerve (mainly left vagal fibres): Supplies anterior surface of fundus and body of stomach, pylorus and pyloric antrum.

   (b) Posterior gastric nerve (mainly right vagal fibres): Supplies posterior surface of fundus, body and pyloric antrum and gives a branch to coeliac plexus.

These are motor and secretomotor to stomach.

Nerves of latarjet: Anterior and posterior vagi are also known as nerves of Latarjet.

The functions of stomach

- As a reservoir of food
- Digestion: Mainly breakdown of proteins to peptones

- As antiseptic acid barrier: By HCL
- Self protection: From HCL by mucus
- Absorption: Salt, water, alcohol and certain drugs
- Secretion of intrinsic factor of castle

Highly selective vagotomy: It does not cause stomach atony. Branches which supply the acid secreting body of stomach are only cut, thus preserving innervation and function of pyloric antrum.

Part of the stomach X-ray shows gas: Fundus of stomach which appears as a dark shadow below left dome of diaphragm.

Gastric canal and its clinical importance: These are the mucosal folds (rugae) along the lesser curvature which are arranged longitudinally to form a canal. Clinical importance: gastric canal allow rapid passage of fluid along the lesser curvature to lower part before it spreads to other parts to stomach. Thus it is irritated most by the swallowed liquids, and hence it is more vulnerable to peptic ulcer.

The different types of glands in stomach
1. Cardiac glands: Tubular glands
2. Glands of body and fundus: Tubular glands
3. Pyloric glands: Convoluted tubular glands

The cell types present in glands of stomach
1. Mucous cells: Secrete mucous
2. Zymogen cell (chief cells): Present in glands of fundus and body; secrete gastric enzymes.
3. Oxyntic cells (parietal cells): Present in glands of fundus and body; secrete HCL.
4. Mucous neck cells: Present at neck of glands; secrete mucous.
5. Argentaffin cells: Present at bases of gastric glands of fundus; secrete gastrin and secrotonin.

Clinically important points
- **Leather bottle stomach: Also referred to as linitis plastica is a** thickening of stomach wall due to proliferation of fibrous tissue especially in submucosa. The mucous membrane appears normal.
- **Hourglass stomach:** It follows cicatrisation of a saddle shaped lesser curve ulcer.
- **Tea pot deformity:** It is a Radiological finding as a result of healing subsequent to peptic ulcer. It can be due to carcinoma stomach as well.
- **Trichobezoar:** This is presence of a hair ball in stomach and present in people having trichotillomania and absence of hair on head and seen especially in psychiatric patients.
- **Hypertrophic pyloric stenosis:** It is hypertrophy of muscle of pyloric end of stomach and can present with gastric outlet obstruction. In infants it is called as congenital hypertrophic pyloric stenosis but can be present in adults as well as an acquired defect.
- **Peptic ulcers:** These are a common entity and are a breach in gastric mucosa due to hypersecretion of acid.

4

Abdomen

- **Gastric pain** is felt in the epigastrium because the stomach is supplied from segments T6 to T10 of the spinal cord, which also supply the greater part of the abdominal wall. Pain is produced either by spasm of the muscle, or by over distension. The interior of the stomach can be visualized by taking a radiograph after giving a barium sulphate meal. It can also be examined directly by the use of gastroscope, which can be passed into the stomach through the mouth.
- **The dumping syndrome** refers to an abnormally rapid emptying of the stomach contents, usually following partial gastrectomy or vagotomy.
- **The prepyloric vein of Mayo** passes in front of pyloroduodenal junction and is an important landmark.
- **The black shadow seen on CXR** below the diaphragm on left side indicates gas in fundus of stomach.

LIVER

The anatomical lobes of the liver

The liver is divided anatomically into two lobes, a right and a left by falciform ligament anteriorly and superiorly, by the fissure for ligamentum teres inferiorly and by the fissure for ligamentum venosum posteriorly.

Right lobe forms 5/6 part of liver and has two additional lobes:
- Caudate lobe on the posterior surface
- Quadrate lobe on the inferior surface and is rectangular in shape. Left lobe forms 1/6 of liver.

Porta hepatis: It is a deep transverse fissure, 05 cm long, on the inferior surface of right lobe of liver, between quadrate lobe below and front and caudate lobe above. Through it vessels, nerves and ducts pass to and from liver. Lips of portahepatis provide attachment to lesser omentum.

The structures lying in the portahepatis and relations of these within it

Through portahepatis portal vein, hepatic artery and hepatic plexus of nerve center and right and left hepatic ducts and a few lymphatics pass out of the liver.

Within the porta hepatis, from behind forwards lay portal vein, hepatic artery and bile ducts (VAB).

The boundaries of caudate lobe: Caudate lobe is bounded on the right by the groove for inferior vena cava, on left by the fissure for ligamentum venosum and inferiorly by porta hepatis. Above it is continuous with the superior surface.

The bare areas of the liver

These are the parts of the liver not covered by the peritoneum. These include:
- Main bare area: Situated on the posterior surface of the right lobe of liver, limited by coronary and right triangular ligament.
- Groove for inferior vena cava: Situated on the posterior surface of right lobe of liver, between caudate lobe and main bare area.

- Gallbladder fossa: On the inferior surface of the right lobe of the liver; on to the right of the quadrate lobe.
- Portahepatis
- Along the lines of reflection of peritoneum.

The peritoneal ligaments of the liver are:

1. **Falciform ligament:** Connecting anterosuperior surface of liver to the anterior abdominal wall and under surface of diaphragm.
2. **Left triangular ligament:** Connecting superior surface of left lobe of liver to diaphragm.
3. **Right triangular ligament:** Connects lateral part of posterior surface of right lobe of liver to the diaphragm.
4. **Coronary ligament:** Encloses bare area of the liver, with superior and inferior layers.
5. **Lesser omentum:** Attached to lips of porta hepatis.

The relations of quadrate lobe of liver: Quadrate lobe is related to lesser omentum, pylorus and first part of duodenum.

Ligamentum venosum: It is the remanant of ducts venosus of fetal life. It is connected above to left hepatic vein near its entry into inferior vena cava and below to the left branch of portal vein, thus forming a by-pass for blood during fetal life.

The blood supply of the liver: Liver is unique in the fact that it receives most of its blood from a vein (portal vein). Liver receives 20% of its blood from hepatic artery and 80% from portal vein. Before entry, these divide into right and left branches. Within liver they divide to form segmental vessels and redivide into interlobular vessels which run in portal canals. Further divisions open into the hepatic sinusoids. Thus in the hepatic sinusoids both arterial and venous blood mix.

The hepatic sinusoids drain into interlobular veins, which form sublobular veins and inturn form hepatic veins, which drain into inferior vena cava.

Portal triad: The interlobular branches of the hepatic artery and portal vein and interlobular bile ductile together form a portal triad and lie within the portal canal.

The functional lobes of the liver

The liver is divided into two functional (physiological) right and left lobe, on the basis of intrahepatic distribution of hepatic artery, portal vein and biliary ducts. These lobes do not correspond to the anatomical lobes of the liver. The physiological lobers are separated by a plane passing on the anterosuperior surface along a line joining the cystic notch to the groove for inferior vena cava, on the inferior surface the plane passes through gallbladder fossa and on the posterior surface through the middle of caudate lobe.

Each lobe is further divided and subdivided into segments.

Clinical importance of functional segments of liver: The portal canals do not cross from one segment to the other, so the hepatic segments are of surgical importance.

4

Abdomen

Riedel's lobe: Sometimes, the lower border of the right lobe of liver, a little to right of gallbladder, projects down as a tongue like process, this is known as Riedel's lobe.

The gallbladder is rarely involved in the malignancy of liver: Because of the absence of lymphatic pathways from liver to gallbladder.

The developmental origin of liver

From ventral surface of foregut as an outgrowth known as hepatic diverticulum, close to point where it is continuous with yolk stalk. The diverticulum proliferates to form the liver. The connective tissue of liver is formed by the mesoderm of septum transversum.

- **Hepatitis:** It is infection/inflammation of liver mostly as a result of viruses: Hepatitis A, B, C, D, E, G.
- **Hepatomegaly:** Liver may be increased in size in a variety of conditions. A condition referred to as hepatomegaly.
- **Hepatic abscess:** Liver has got a good blood supply and as a result is a common site for abscesses.
- **Fatty liver:** Accumulation of fat in liver is of common occurrence.
- **Non-neoplastic and neoplastic tumors of liver:** Liver is a common site for **hydatid cysts, hemangiomas, hepatic adenomas and metastatic secondaries** from other organs.

Extra-hepatic Biliary Apparatus

The structures forming the extra-hepatic biliary apparatus
It is formed by:
1. Right and left hepatic ducts
2. Common hepatic duct
3. Gall bladder
4. Cystic duct (3–4 cm)
5. Bile duct (8 cm long: 6 mm in diameter)

GALLBLADDER

The parts of the gallbladder are
Gallbladder is divided into three parts:
1. Fundus
2. Body
3. Neck, it becomes continuous with cystic duct.

Hartmann's pouch: It is the dilated posteromedial wall of the neck of gallbladder. It is directed downwards and backwards. Some regard it as pathological feature.

The clinical importance of Hartmann's pouch: The gallstones may become impacted in the pouch and cause obstruction.

The capacity of gallbladder: 30 to 50 cc, but is capable of 50 fold distention.

The common hepatic duct: It is a duct formed by the left and right hepatic duct. It is joined by cystic duct at an acute angle and then forms the common bile duct.

Accessory hepatic ducts and their clinical importance: These are present in 15% subjects and arise usually from right lobe of liver. These terminate into gallbladder or common hepatic duct or bile duct. If undetected, they are responsible for oozing of bile from wound after cholecystectomy, i.e. removal of gallbladder.

Spiral valve of Heister: Spiral valve has 5–10 crescentic folds of mucous membranes in the cystic duct which are arranged spirally to form a valve like structure.

The structures supplied by the cystic artery: The cystic artery (usually a branch of right hepatic artery) supplies blood to gallbladder, cystic duct, hepatic ducts and upper part of the bile duct. The cystic artery is an end artery.

The venous drainage of the gallbladder: The superior surface of the gallbladder drains into hepatic veins through gallbladder fossa. Rest of gallbladder is drained by cystic veins.

Crypts of Luschka: The mucous membrane contains indentations of the mucosa that sink into the muscle coat, these are known as crypts of Luschka.

Caterpillar turn or Moynihan's hump: It is dangerous anomaly when the hepatic artery takes a tortuous course and the cystic artery is short. Thus tortuosity is known as caterpillar turn.

The functions of gallbladder
1. Storage of bile
2. Concentration of bile
3. Regulates pressure in biliary system, to maintain normal choledochoduodenal mechanism
4. Secretion of mucin
5. Changing the reaction of bile: Bile excreted by liver has pH 8.2 and gallbladder changes pH to 7.5–7.2.

Referred pain felt over the right shoulder in acute cholecystitis: The referred pain is felt at some other region having the same segmental innervations as the site of lesion (on right side). **Referred pain of gallbladder** is radiated to right shoulder as well as to inferior angle of right scapula. In acute cholecystitis, the under surface of the diaphragm is also inflammed. The pain sensation from under surface of diaphragm is carried by the phrenic nerve via C4 spinal segment and skin over the shoulder is also supplied by the C4 spinal segment.

Courvoisier's law: According to the Courvoisier's law the dilatation of the gallbladder occurs only in extrinsic obstruction of bile duct, e.g. by carcinoma of head of pancreas. Intrinsic obstruction (e.g. by stones) do not cause any dilatation because of associated fibrosis.

Charcot's triad of cholecystitis
Stone in bile duct causes:
1. Intermittent biliary colic
2. Intermittent jaundice following each colic
3. Intermittent fever

Cholelithiasis: The gallbladder is a common site for stone formation. Gallstones are a common biliary pathology. **The old dictum about gallstones is fatty, fertile, flatulent, female of forty or fifty.**

Calot's triangle: Also known as the cystohepatic triangle is bounded by cystic duct, common hepatic duct and right hemilever. It is an important part for cholecystectomy. It contains cystic artery, cystic lymph node of Lund.

The developmental origin of extrahepatic biliary apparatus

1. Bile duct is formed by the narrowing of connection between hepatic diverticulum and foregut.
2. Another ventral outgrowth from common bile duct forms the cystic duct and gallbladder. Hepatic ducts are formed by lower end of hepatic diverticulum.

The bile duct first opens into ventral wall of duodenum, later it migrates to dorsal (right) surface of duodenum to mesenteric border. This migration occurs due to differing rates of growth of duodenal walls.

In certain cases of maldevelopment the biliary as well as extrahepatic biliary system does not develop, a condition referred to as **biliary atresia.**

Remember: The haemorrhage during cholecystectomy is controlled by compressing the hepatic artery, which gives off cystic branch, between, finger and thumb where it lies in anterior wall of foramen of Winslow. This maneuver is called **Pringle's maneuver.**

The developmental anomalies of gallbladder

1. **Absence of gallbladder**
2. **Gallbladder may be septate**
3. **Double gallbladder with a single or separate cystic ducts**
4. **Floating gallbladder**

The normal variations in bile ducts

Normally: Cystic duct joins the common hepatic duct on right side to form common bile duct near upper border of duodenum.

Variations:
- **Accessory hepatic ducts present.**
- **Common hepatic and cystic ducts lie parallel before forming one duct.**
- **Cystic and common hepatic ducts unite behind pancreas.**
- **Cystic duct may be absent, the common hepatic duct entering gallbladder and common bile duct leaving it.**
- **Cystic duct may join common hepatic duct in front or back of duodenum.**

DUODENUM

The position of duodenum: Duodenum lies above the level of umbilicus against L1–3 vertebrae, extending ½ inch to right and 01 inch to left of median plane.

The length of duodenum and its different parts

Duodenum is a 10 inches long, curved around the head of the pancreas in form of C. It is divided into 04 parts:

1. First (superior) part, 02 inches long
2. Second (descending) part 03 inches long
3. Third (horizontal or inferior) part, 04 inches long
4. Fourth (ascending) part, 01 inch long.

The peritoneal relations of duodenum

- **First part:** The proximal 01 inch is suspended by lesser omentum above and greater omentum below, therefore it is moveable. Distal 01 inch is fixed because it is retroperitoneal and is covered with peritoneum only anteriorly.
- **Second part:** Retroperitoneal and fixed. Anteriorly crossed by peritoneum except in middle where it is related to transverse colon.
- **Third part: Also retroperitoneal and fixed.** Covered by peritoneum anteriorly except where crossed by superior mesenteric vessels and root of mesentery.
- **Fourth part:** Mostly retroperitoneal. Terminal part is moveable due to mesentery.

The relations of first part of duodenum

- **Anteriorly: Quadrate lobe of liver and gallbladder.**
- **Posteriorly: Bile duct, portal vein, gastroduodenal artery**
- **Superiorly: Epiploic foramen**
- **Inferiorly: Head and neck of pancreas.**

The relations of second part of duodenum

- **Medially: Head of pancreas and bile duct**
- **Laterally: Right colic flexure**
- **Anteriorly: Right lobe of liver, transverse colon, small intestine.**
- **Posteriorly:** Anterior surface of right kidney near medial border, right renal vessels, right psoas major, inferior vena cava.

Relations of third part of duodenum

- **Anteriorly: Superior mesenteric vessels and root of mesentery**
- **Posteriorly: Right ureter, right psoas major, right testicular or ovarian vessels, inferior vena cava, and abdominal aorta.**
- **Superiorly: Head of pancreas**
- **Inferiorly: Coils of jejunum**

Structures related to fourth part of duodenum

- **Superiorly: Body of pancreas**
- **To the right: Upper part of root of mesentery**
- **To the left: Left kidney and left ureter**
- **Anteriorly: Transverse colon and mesocolon lesser sac and stomach**
- **Posteriorly: Left sympathetic chain, left psoas major, left renal and testicular vessels and inferior mesenteric vein.**

4

Abdomen

The duodenum develops partly from foregut and partly from midgut. The junction of the two is in the second part of duodenum where the common bile duct opens.

The blood supply of duodenum: Arterial supply: The part above the level of common bile duct opening is supplied by superior pancreaticoduodenal artery and below it by the inferior pancreaticoduodenal artery.

The first part is also supplied by right gastric and gastroepiploic artery and branches of gastroduodenal and hepatic artery.

Venous drainage: The veins drain into splenic, superior mesenteric and portal veins.

Ligament of Treitz

It is a fibromuscular band which supports the duodenojejunal flexure. It arises from right crus of diaphragm and is attached below to posterior surface of flexure and third and fourth parts of duodenum.

It is made up of:
1. Striated muscle fibres in upper part
2. Elastic fibres in middle part
3. Smooth muscle fibres in lower part

The importance of ligament of Treitz
1. It marks the duodenojejunal junction
2. When it is attached only to flexure its contraction narrows duodenojejunal angle thus causing partial obstruction.

Duodenal cap and its clinical importance
- In barium meal X-ray, the first part of duodenum is seen as a triangular homogeneous shadow, known as duodenal cap.
- The duodenal cap is formed due to protrusion of pylorus into proximal half of first part of duodenum which is thus kept patent and filled with barium. Rest of duodenum shows floccular shadow.
- Clinical importance: persistent deformity of duodenal cap indicates chronic duodenal ulcer.

The clinical importance of relations of duodenum
- In barium meal X-ray, widening of duodenal loop, suggests carcinoma of the pancreas.
- In a duodenal ulcer (commonest in first part), liver and gallbladder may be affected if the perforation of ulcer occurs or haemorrhage occurs, if gastroduodenal artery is affected.
- Third part of duodenum may be obstructed by pressure from superior mesenteric artery.

Intestines

Small intestine about 06 m long, is divided into:
1. Upper fixed part: Duodenum 25 cm is length
2. Lower mobile part: Upper 2/5 forms jejunum and lower 3/5 forms ileum.

4

Abdomen

Valves of kerkring: These are circular folds of mucous membrane which begin in second part of duodenum and extend up to proximal half of ileum.

These increase the absorptive surface area and also retard the passage of food.

The different parts of large intestine

The large intestine 1.5 m long is divided into:

1. **Appendix: 09 cm long**
2. **Caecum: 06 cm long**
3. **Transverse colon: 50 cm long**
4. **Ascending colon: 12.5 cm long**
5. **Descending colon: 25 cm long**
6. **Sigmoid colon: 37.5 cm long**
7. **Rectum: 12.5 cm long**
8. **Anal canal: 3.8 cm long**

The differences between small intestine and large intestine

Calibre	Small intestine	Large intestine
Calibre	• Smaller	• Wider
Sacculations	• Absent	• Present
Taeniae coli	• Absent	• Present
Appendices epiploicae	• Absent	• Present
Fixity	• Greater part is freely mobile	• Greater part is fixed
Transverse mucosal folds	• Permanent	• Obliterated when longitudinal muscle coat relaxes
Villi	• Present	• Absent
Peyer's patches	• Present in ileum	• Absent

The differences between jejunum and ileum

Features	Jejunum	Ileum
Location	• Occupies upper and left part of intestinal area	• Occupies lower and right part of intestinal area
Lumen	• Larger	• Narrow
Mesentery	• Windows present • Fat less • Arterial arcades 01 or 02 • Vasa recta longer and fewer	• Windows absent • Fat abundant • Arterial arcades 03 to 06 • Vas recta shorter and more
Circular mucosal folds	• Larger and more closely set	• Smaller and sparse
Villi	• Large thick more	• Shorter thinner and fewer
Peyer's patches	• Absent	• Present
Solitary lymphatic follicles	• Fewer	• More numerous

4

Abdomen

Taenia coli: These are ribbon like bands formed by longitudinal muscle coat, present only in large intestine till terminal part of sigmoid colon.

COLON

The functions of colon are:

1. Lubrication of faeces, by mucus
2. Absorption of salt, water and other solutes
3. Bacterial flora of colon synthesizes vitamin B
4. Mucoid secretion of colon has IgA antibodies which protect it from invasion by micro-organisms.
5. The microvilli of some columnar cells serve a sensory function.

Phrenico-colic ligament: It is a horizontal fold of peritoneum, attaching left colic flexure to the 11th rib. It supports the spleen and forms the partial upper limit of left paracolic gutter.

Characteristic feature of arterial supply of transverse colon

The right 2/3 of transverse colon develops from midgut, so it is supplied by superior mesenteric artery.

The left 1/3 is formed from hindgut, so it is supplied by inferior mesenteric artery.

Remember the Numericals

- Length of esophagus — 25 cm
- Capacity of stomach at birth — 30 ml
- Capacity of stomach in adult — 1500 ml
- Length of duodenum — 10 inches
- First part — 2 inches
- Second part — 3 inches
- Third part — 4 inches
- Fourth part — 1 inch
- Length of small intestine — 6–7 metres
- Length of large gut — 1.5 metres
- Anorectal junction — At tip of coccyx

APPENDIX

The dimensions of appendix: The length of appendix varies from 2 to 20 cm, average about 09 cm it is longer in children.

The different positions of the appendix: The base of the appendix is fixed but its tip can point in any direction. Depending on it following positions of the appendix are described:

4

Abdomen

1. Retrocaecal, commonest
2. Pelvic
3. Paracolic
4. Splenic
5. Promontoric
6. Mid inguinal

Valve of Gerlach: It is an indistinct semilunar fold of mucous membrane guarding the appendicular orifice.

The peritoneal relations of appendix: Appendix is suspended by a small, triangular fold of peritoneum is called mesoappendix. The fold passes upwards behind ileum and is attached to the left layer of mesentery.

The characteristic feature of blood supply of appendix

The appendix is supplied only by appendicular artery, a branch of ileo-colic artery. It runs first in the free edge of appendicular mesentery and then distally along the wall of appendix.

- **McBurney's point:** It is the point of maximum tenderness in acute appendicitis. It lies at the junction of medial 2/3 and lateral 1/3 of a line joining umbilicus to anterior superior iliac spine.

- **Murphy's triad:** Appendicitis first causes pain around umbilicus. Then followed by vomiting and fever. This sequence of symptoms is known as murphys triad.

- **The gangrene of appendix** is common in acute infections: Because appendicular artery supplying the appendix gets thrombosed and it has no collateral circulation.

- **Psoas test and obturator test** are used for appendicitis.

CAECUM

The position of caecum: It is situated in the right iliac fossa above the lateral half of inguinal ligament.

Communications of the Caecum

Caecum communicates:
1. **Superiorly with ascending colon**
2. **Medially with ileum**
3. **Posteromedially with appendix.**

The different shapes of caecum are three types
1. **Conical type**
2. **Ampullary type, commonest**
3. **Intermediate type.**

MECKEL'S DIVERTICULUM

It is persistent proximal part of the vitellointestinal duct, which normally disappears during 6th week of intrauterine life. Position of persistent Meckel's diverticulum: It is situated 02 feet proximal to the ileocaecal valve, attached to antimesenteric border of ileum.

The clinical importance of Meckel's diverticulum:
1. It may cause intestinal obstruction
2. Acute inflammation of diverticulum may resemble appendicitis
3. It is often the site of heterotrophic gastric mucosa with oxyntic cells.

The effect of patent Meckel's diverticulum: Small intestine contents being discharged at the umbilicus.

The infections of Meckel's diverticulum are dangerous

Because:
1. Its walls are thinner so, it perforates more easily
2. It lies in middle of peritoneal cavity, so more chances of widespread peritonitis.

Enterotomata: The vitellointestinal duct is closed at both ends, i.e. umbilical and intestinal end, but remains patent in middle. This may cause cysts behind navel called enterotomata.

Vitellointestinal Duct Persists as a Fibrous Band

1. This fibrous band passes from umbilicus to some part of mesentery or small gut.
2. This band may cause compression of loop of gut under it.
3. If attached to branch of mesenteric artery, which may be torn during abdominal operations.

PANCREAS

- Pancreas is called a double gland because it is partly exocrine and partly endocrine.
- The secretions of the pancreas
- Exocrine part secretes pancreatic juice which has digestive functions.
- Endocrine part secretes hormones, e.g. insulin, glucagon.
- The pancreas lies across the posterior abdominal wall at the level of L1 and L2 vertebra.

The shape and different parts of pancreas
Pancreas is a J-shaped organ. It is divided into parts:
1. Head with the uncinate process
2. Neck
3. Body
4. Tail

The relations of head of pancreas:

- **Anterior surface:** Gastroduodenal artery, transverse colon, jejunum over area covered by peritoneum
- **Posterior surface:** Inferior vena cava, renal veins, right crus of diaphragm, bile duct
- **Superior border:** Superior pancreaticoduodenal artery
- **Inferior border:** Third part of duodenum and inferior pancreaticoduodenal artery
- **Right lateral border:** Second part of duodenum, terminal part of bile duct.
- Uncinate process is related anteriorly to superior mesenteric vessels and posteriorly to aorta.

Relations of neck of pancreas

- **Anterior surface:** Peritoneum, lesser sac, pylorus
- **Posterior surface:** Beginning of portal vein

The relations of body of pancreas

- **Anterior surface:** Lesser sac, stomach
- **Posterior surface:** Aorta with origin of superior mesenteric artery, left crus of diaphragm, left suprarenal, left kidney, left renal vessels, splenic vein.
- **Inferior surface:** Duodenojejunal flexure, coils of jejunum, left colic flexure
- Anterior and inferior surface are covered by the peritoneum
- **Inferior border:** Superior mesenteric vessels
- **Superior border:** Coeliac artery, hepatic artery, splenic artery
- **Anterior border:** Provides attachment to root of transverse mesocolon.

Relations of tail of pancreas

Tail of pancreas lies in lienorenal ligament and is related to gastric surface of spleen.

The arterial supply of pancreas

1. Pancreatic branches of splenic artery
2. Superior pancreaticoduodenal artery, a branch of coeliac trunk.
3. Inferior pancreaticoduodenal artery, a branch of superior mesenteric artery.

The ducts draining the secretions of exocrine part of pancreas

The two ducts carrying the exocrine secretion of pancreas are:

1. **Main pancreatic duct (of Wirsung):** Joins with bile duct to form ampulla of vater and open at major duodenal papilla in 2nd part of duodenum, 8–10 cm distal to pylorus.
2. **Accessory pancreatic duct (of Santorini):** Opens at minor duodenal papilla in 2nd part of duodenum, 6–8 cm distal to pylorus.

Pseudopancreatic cyst: Anterior to the pancreas lies the stomach, separated from it by the lesser sac. The sac may be closed off and distended with fluid either from perforation of posterior gastric ulcer or as a result of acute pancreatitis, thus forming pseudopancreatic cyst.

Carcinoma of head of pancreas is associated with obstructive jaundice.

4

Abdomen

4

Abdomen

The head of pancreas lies in the C-curve of the duodenum in relation to the opening of the common bile duct. Therefore, carcinoma of the head of the pancreas will cause the compression of the common bile duct and causes obstructive jaundice.

The developmental origin of pancreas

1. *From:*

   (a) Dorsal diverticulum from duodenum: Larger.

   (b) Ventral out pouching from side of common bile duct: Smaller

   The ventral pouch rotates posteriorly to fuse with lower aspect of dorsal diverticulum, trapping the superior mesenteric vessels between two parts.

2. Ducts of two segments communicate and that of smaller takes over the main pancreatic flow to form the main duct and the duct of larger portion persist as accessory duct.

The common developmental anomalies of pancreas

- Annular pancreas: Two segments of pancreas completely surround second part of deuodenum.

- Accessory pancreatic tissue, in duodenum (usually, jejunum and ileum).

Acute pancreatitis: Includes a broad-spectrum of pancreatic disease, which varies from mild parenchymal edema to severe hemorrhagic pancreatitis associated with loss of parenchymal viability, with subsequent gangrene and necrosis. The clinical presentation of acute pancreatitis is quite variable, from episodes of mild abdominal discomfort alone to a severe illness associated with hypotension, metabolic derangements, sepsis, fluid sequestration, multiple organ failure, and death.

Chronic pancreatitis: It is a clinical entity that includes recurrent or persistent abdominal pain and evidence of exocrine and endocrine pancreatic insufficiency. It is marked pathologically by irreversible parenchymal destruction of pancreatic tissue.

Annular pancreas: It is a rare condition that results when histologically normal pancreatic tissue completely or partially encircles the second portion of the duodenum. Annular pancreas is thought to arise from failure of normal clockwise rotation of the ventral pancreatic bud.

Suprarenal (Adrenal) Glands

Each adrenal is composed of **two functionally distinct endocrine glands**. The adrenal cortex and the medulla each have distinct embryologic, anatomic, histologic and functional characteristics.

Development: The **adrenal cortex arises from coelomic mesoderm.** The gland then differentiates into a thin outer definitive cortex and a thick inner fetal cortex by the eighth week. The fetal cortex actively produces fetal steroids during gestation but involutes rapidly after birth. The definitive cortex persists and develops into the functional adrenal cortex, which has distinct **zona glomerulosa and fasciculata** at birth. **The zona reticularis** develops later.

The adrenal medulla arises from neural crest

The position of adrenal glands

1. Posterior abdominal wall over the upper pole of kidneys behind the peritoneum.

2. In front of crus of diaphragm opposite vertebral ends of 11th intercostals space and 12th rib.

The parts of adrenal glands seen in cross-section

1. Cortex: Outer; mesodermal origin

2. Medulla: Inner; neural crest origin.

The blood supply of suprarenal glands

Arterial supply:

1. Superior suprarenal artery: Branch of inferior phrenic

2. Middle suprarenal artery: Branch of abdominal aorta

3. Inferior suprarenal artery: Branch of renal artery.

Venous drainage:

Right suprarenal vein: Drains into inferior vena cava.

Left suprarenal vein: Drains into left renal vein.

The structures lying between two suprarenal glands

1. Crura of diaphragm

2. Aorta (abdominal)

3. Coeliac artery plexus

4. Inferior vena cava

The Two Suprarenal Glands

		Left	Right
1.	Shape	Semilunar	Triangular
2.	Size	Larger	Smaller
3.	Position	Upper part of medial border of kidney	Upper part of anterior surface of kidney
4.	Level	Lower	Higher
5.	Hilum	Near lower end	Near upper end
6.	Peritoneal relations	Separated from stomach by peritoneum	Only lower part related to peritoneum

Visceral Relations

• Anterior surface superior: Stomach medial—inferior vena cava
• Inferior: Pancreas lateral—Part of bare area of liver
• Posterior surface medial—Crus of diaphragm inferior—kidney
• Lateral: Kidney superior—crus of diaphragm.

Chromaffin System

• It is made up cells which have an affinity for salts of chromic acid.

- Develop from the neural crest
- Cells secrete adrenaline and noradrenaline.

The components of chromaffin system

- Suprarenal medulla
- Para-aortic bodies
- Paraganglia
- Small masses of cells among ganglia of sympathetic chain, splanchnic nerves and prevertebral autonomic plexus.

4

KIDNEYS

The kidneys are situated retroperitoneally on the posterior abdominal wall on each side of the vertebral column. The right kidney is slightly lower than left and the left kidney is a little nearer to the median plane.

- **The kidneys vertically extend from upper border of T12 vertebra to centre of body of L3 vertebra.**
- **The right kidney is slightly lower than the left.**

The relation of transpyloric plane to kidneys: Transpyloric plane passes through the upper part of hilus of right kidney and through lower part of hilus of the left.

The measurements of normal kidney

Each kidney is:

- 11 cm long
- 6 cm broad
- 3 cm thick

Left kidney is a little longer and narrower

The anterior relations of the kidneys

Right kidney:

- **Right suprarenal**
- **Liver**
- **Second part of duodenum**
- **Hepatic flexure of colon**
- **Small intestine.**
- **Hepatic and intestinal surfaces are covered by peritoneum.**

Left kidney:

- **Left suprarenal**
- **Stomach**
- **Spleen**
- **Pancreas**
- **Jejunum**

Abdomen

- Splenic flexure
- Descending colon
- Splenic vessels.
- The gastric, splenic and jejuna surfaces are covered by peritoneum.

The posterior relations of kidney

Both kidneys are related to:

1. Diaphragm
2. Medial and lateral arcuate ligaments
3. Psoas major
4. Quadratus lumborum
5. Transverses abdominis
6. Subcostal vessels
7. Iliohypogastric, subcostal and ilioinguinal nerves.

The right kidney is also related to 12th rib and the left kidney to 11th and 12th ribs.

The coverings of the kidneys

From within outwards the coverings are:

1. Fibrous capsule: Thin membrane, made up of white and yellow fibres and smooth muscle fibres.
2. Perirenal (perinephric) fat: Outer to the fibrous capsule. It is thickest at the borders of the kidney.
3. Renal fascia (fascia of gerota): Fibroareolar sheath around the perirenal fat.

   Superiorly, two layers of renal fascia first enclose the suprarenal gland in a separate compartment, and then they fuse with each other and become continuous with fascia on undersurface of diaphragm.

   Inferiorly, the two layers remain separate and enclose ureter.

   Laterally, the two layers fuse and become continuous with fascia transversalis.

   Medially, anterior layer passes in front of renal vessels and fuses with connective tissue around aorta and inferior vena cava. The posterior layer, fuses with fascia covering quadrates lumborum and psoas major. At medial border of kidney fascia forms a septum.
4. Pararenal (paranephric) fat: Fat outer to renal fascia is more abundant posteriorly and towards the lower pole of the kidney.

The fascia of Toldt and fascia of Zuckerkandl: The anterior layer of renal fascia is known as fascia of Toldt and posterior layer as fascia of Zuckerkandl.

The arrangement of structures found at the Hilus of kidney

From before backwards (VAP)

- **Renal vein**
- **Renal artery**
- **Pelvis of the ureter**

The Vascular Segments of the Kidney

Each renal artery at the hilus of the kidney divides into an anterior and posterior branch, which in turn divides into segmental arteries which supply a definite part (segment) of the kidney. In each kidney there are five segment, i.e. apical, upper, lower, middle and posterior.

The clinical importance of vascular segments of kidney: Each segmental artery is an end artery, so the vascular segments are independent units. So the intersegmental incisions are given for the removal of a part of the kidney.

Care should be taken in exposure of kidney from behind when 12th rib is to be excised: Push up the pleura which cross the medial half of the 12th rib.

The Development of Kidneys

Kidneys are formed in the sacral region and then ascend upwards. The kidney develops from:

- **Mesonephric duct: Gives rise to pelvis, calyces and collecting tubules.**
- **Metanephros: Develops into glomeruli and proximal part of renal duct system.**

The common congenital abnormalities of kidneys

- Congenital polycystic kidney
- Horseshoe kidney
- Congenital absence of one kidney
- Unilateral fused kidney
- Accessory kidneys
- Pelvic kidneys

Renal angle: The lower border of 12th rib and the outer border of erector spinae form the renal angle. Clinically on palpation the tenderness in this region denotes renal pathology. A surgeon prefers to expose the kidney by starting the incision at the renal angle.

At times the 12th rib may be absent or unusually small and fails to project beyond the lateral border of erector spinae. In such cases 11th rib forming the angle with erector spinae may be mistaken for renal angle. This puts the surgeon at risk of opening up of pleural cavity since the line of pleural reflection passes above the true renal angle.

URETER

These are pair of narrow, thick walled muscular tubes which convey urine from the kidneys to urinary bladder.

The length of the ureter: Each ureter is about 25 cm long, of which upper half lies in abdomen and lower half in pelvis.

The course in the ureter: It is divided into two parts:

Abdomen

4

1. **In the abdomen:** Ureter begins at renal pelvis (funnel-shaped dilatation) from the hilus of the kidney and descends along its medial border. It gradually narrows and becomes ureter proper at the lower pole of the kidney. It descends on psoas muscle and enters pelvis by crossing in front of the termination of common iliac artery.
2. **In the pelvis:** It first runs downwards, backwards and laterally, following the anterior margin of greater sciatic notch. Opposite ischial spine it turns forwards and medially to reach base of urinary bladder.

Ureter enters bladder wall obliquely and opens at the lateral angle of trigone.

The sites at which constrictions are present in ureter

Three sites:

- **Pelvi ureteral junction (related to transverse process of L2 Vertebra).**
- **Brim of lesser pelvis (related to sacroiliac joint)**
- **At its passage through bladder wall (slightly medial to ischial spine).**

The clinical importance of constrictions of ureter: A ureteric calculus is likely to lodge at one of these three levels.

The relations of ureter in its forward course in pelvis

In males:

- **Ductus deferens: Crosses ureter superiorly from lateral to medial side**
- **Seminal vesicle: Below and behind ureter**
- **Vesical veins: Surround terminal part ureter**

In females:

- **Ureter lies in lower and medial part of broad ligament of uterus.**
- **Uterine artery: First above and in front of ureter and then crosses superiorly from lateral to medial side.**
- **Ureter lies 2 cm later to supravaginal parts of cervix.**
- **Ureter lies above lateral fornix of vagina.**
- **Terminal part of ureter lies anterior to vagina.**

The arterial supply of ureter

- *For upper part:* Renal artery, branches of gonadal and colic arteries.
- *For middle part:* Branches from aorta, gonadal and iliac arteries.
- *For lower part:* From vesical, middle rectal or uterine arteries.

The nerve supply of ureter

- **Sympathetic nerves; T10–L1**
- **Parasympathetic nerves: S2–4**

They reach through renal, aortic and both hypogastric plexuses.

Renal colic is wrongly named and should be better termed as ureteric colic: It is the spasm of ureter by a stone. There is sudden, agonizing pain in the loin.

The pain of renal colic is referred to cutaneous area innervated by T_{11}–L_2.

Developmental origin of ureter: From part of ureteric bud that lies between the pelvis of kidney and vesicourethral canal.

The congenital abnormalities of ureter

- Ureter may be duplicated.

- Ureter may end into prostatic urethra, vas deferens, seminal vesicles, vagina and rectum.
- Upper end of ureter may not be connected to kidney.
- Ureter may have diverticula.

Postcaval ureter and its clinical importance

The right ureter instead of lying to right of inferior vena cava may pass behind it.

Clinical importance: May lead to compression of ureter and obstruction to flow of urine.

The reflux of urine from bladder into ureter is prevented: The intravesical oblique course of ureter has a valvular action which prevents the reflux of urine from bladder to ureter.

DIAPHRAGM

The origin of diaphragm

Arise from periphery, in three parts:

- *Sternal:* Back of xiphoid process
- *Costal:* Inner surfaces of cartilages and adjacent parts of lower six ribs.
- *Lumbar:* Medial and lateral lumbocostal arches and from lumbar vertebrae by right and left crura.

Lumbocostal Arches

These are tendinous arches in the fascia covering the muscles in posterior abdominal wall, e.g. medial lumbocostal arch in fascia over upper part of psoas major and lateral lumbocostal arch in fascia over upper part of quadratus lumborum.

The origin of crus of diaphragm

- Right crus: From anterolateral surface of body of L1, 2, 3
- Left crus: From anterolateral surface of body of L1, 2

The insertion of muscle fibres of diaphragm

- Trilobed central tendon, which lies below and is fused to the pericardium.

The nerve supply of diaphragm

- Motor: Phrenic nerve (C3, 4).
- Sensory: Phrenic nerves: Central part
- Lower six thoracic nerves: Peripheral part.

The other structures supplied by phrenic nerve

Sensory fibres to:
1. Pleura: Mediastinal and diaphragmatic.
2. Pericardium: Fibrous and parietal layer of serous pericardium.
3. Peritoneum: Below central part of diaphragm.
4. Through coeliac plexus to falciform and coronary ligaments of liver, gallbladder, suprarenals and inferior vena cava.

4

Abdomen

Functions of diaphragm

- Separates the thoracic and abdominal cavity
- Principal muscle of inspiration
- In all expulsive acts, e.g. sneezing, coughing, vomiting, defaecation, etc., it provides additional power to each effort.

The variations in position of diaphragm with posture

Level of diaphragm is:

- **Highest in supine position**
- **Lowest in sitting position**
- **Midway in standing**

The structures passing through the opening of diaphragm

1. **Caval opening (T3):** Slightly to right of median plane. Transmits inferior vena cava and half of the right phrenic nerve.
2. **Oesophageal opening (T10):** Slightly to left of median plane. Transmits oesophagus, right and left vagi, oesophageal branches of left gastric artery with accompanying veins.
3. **Aortic opening (T12):** Central transmits (from right to left) vena-azygous thoracic duct and aorta.
4. **Smaller orifices in diaphragm:**
   1. Between xiphoid slip and that from 7th cartilage: Superior epigastric vessels.
   2. Between slips from 7th and 8th costal cartilages: Musculophrenic vessels.
   3. Between each pair of remaining slips: One of lower five intercostal nerves and vessels.
   4. Behind lateral lumbocostal arch: Subcostal nerve and vessels.
   5. Behind medial lumbocostal arch: Sympathetic trunk.
   6. Each crus: Greater, lesser and least splanchnic nerves. Left crus in addition is pierced by vena hemiazygous.

   Irritation of diaphragm causes pain in shoulder tip: Because phrenic nerve and supraclavicular nerves have same root valve, i.e.C3, 4.

Eventration of diaphragm: This is congenital defect, in which the high position of diaphragm occurs due to replacement of left half of diaphragm by fibrous membrane.

Foramen of Morgagni: Also called space of larry: it is space between the xiphoid and costal origins of diaphragm. Site of congenital hernia.

Foramen of Bochdalek: This is a commonest site of congenital diaphragmatic defect in periphery of diaphragm in region of 10th and 11th ribs attachment.

The development origin of diaphragm

Diaphragm is developed from:

- Septum transversum
- Pleuro-peritoneal membrane
- Ventral and dorsal mesenteries of oesophagus
- Mesoderm of body wall

4

Abdomen

Posterior Abdominal Wall

The branches of abdominal aorta

Ventral branches:

- Coeliac trunk
- Superior mesenteric artery
- Inferior mesenteric artery.

Dorsal branches:

- Lumbar
- Median sacral

Lateral branches:

- Inferior phrenic
- Middle suprarenal
- Renal
- Testicular or ovarian.

Terminal branches: Common iliac arteries.

The tributaries of inferior vena cava

1. Common iliac veins
2. Third and fourth lumbar veins
3. Right testicular or ovarian vein
4. Renal veins
5. Right suprarenal vein
6. Hepatic vein

Cisterna chili: It is a 5–7 cm long lymphatic sac, situated in front of L1–2 vertebrae, to the right of abdominal aorta. It continues upwards as thoracic duct.

Lumbar Plexus

It is formed by:

- Ventral rami of upper four lumbar nerves
- First lumbar nerve also receives a contribution from subcostal nerve
- L4 nerve gives a contribution to lumbosacral trunk (L4, 5) which forms part of sacral plexus.

The branches of lumbar plexus

1. Femoral nerve (L2, 3, 4)
2. Genitofemoral nerve (L1, L2)
3. Iliohypogastric nerve (L1)
4. Ilioinguinal nerve (L1)
5. Lateral cutaneous nerve of thigh (L2, L3)
6. Lumbosacral trunk (L4, L5)
7. Obturator nerve (L2, 3, 4)

The muscles of posterior abdominal wall

1. Psoas major
2. Psoas minor
3. Iliacus
4. Quadratus lumborum

The actions of psoas major

- Helps in maintaining posture at hip. Balances trunk while sitting.
- With iliacus, flexor of hip joint.
- One psoas, causes lateral flexion of trunk on that side.
- Lateral rotation of hip.

Psoas Abscess

Tuberculous disease of body of any of the thoracic or lumbar vertebrae gives rise to a cold abscess (no signs of inflammation). This abscess trickles under the psoas sheath up to the insertion of psoas major. This painless swelling may be mistaken for a femoral hernia and flexion deformity of hip it due to spasm of psoas.

Internal iliac artery

It is smaller terminal branch of common iliac artery.

It is about one and half inches long (3–3.5 cm).

It begins in front of sacroiliac joint.

It divides into anterior and posterior divisions.

Divisions at upper margin of greater sciatic notch.

Branches from anterior division: Six in males and seven in females.

- Superior vesical artery
- Inferior vesical
- Obturator artery
- Middle rectal
- Inferior gluteal
- Internal pudendal

In females, inferior vesical is replaced by vaginal artery.

Uterine artery is the 7th branch in females.

Branches from posterior division:

- Superior gluteal.
- Ilio-lumbar.
- Lateral sacral.

THE URINARY BLADDER

It is a reservoir for urine

- It varies in size, shape, position and relations, according to its content and the state of neighbouring viscera.

4

Abdomen

- The base (fundus) of the bladder is triangular and posteroinferior. In females it is closely related to the anterior vaginal wall
- In males, it is related to the rectum although it is separated from it above by the rectovesical pouch and below by the seminal vesicle and vas deferens on each side
- The bladder and rectum are separated only by rectovesical fascia, commonly known as **Denonvilliers' fascia.**
- The neck is the lowest region and is also the most fixed. It is 3–4 cm behind the lower part of the symphysis pubis. In males the neck rests on, and is in direct continuity with, the base of the prostate; in females it is related to the pelvic fascia, which surrounds the upper urethra.

Trigone of Bladder

- It is composed of smooth muscle
- **Ureteric orifices:** The slit-like ureteric orifices are placed at the posterolateral trigonal angles
- **Internal urethral orifice:** The internal urethral orifice is sited at the trigonal apex, the lowest part of the bladder. There is often an elevation immediately behind it in adult males which is caused by the median prostatic lobe, sometimes known as the uvula of the bladder.

The peritoneal folds of urinary bladder
- Median umbilical fold
- Medial umbilical fold
- Lateral false ligament
- Posterior false ligament.

The ligaments formed by the pelvic fascia around urinary bladder
- Lateral true ligament
- Median puboprostatic ligament
- Lateral puboprostatic ligament

In females, bands similar to puboprostatic ligaments are known as pubovesical ligaments.
- *Median umbilical ligament:* Remnant of urachus
- Posterior ligament

Blood Supply

The bladder is supplied principally by the superior and inferior vesical arteries, obturator and inferior gluteal arteries. In the female additional branches are derived from the uterine and vaginal arteries.

The veins which drain the bladder form a complicated plexus on its inferolateral surfaces and pass backwards in the lateral ligaments of the bladder to end in the internal iliac veins.

Lymphatics which drain the bladder begin in mucosal, intermuscular and serosal plexuses. There are three sets of collecting vessels, most of which end in the external iliac nodes.

Urinary bladder is developed from:

- *Epithelium of urinary bladder: Endodermal, cranial part of vesicourethral canal*
- *Epithelium of trigone: Mesodermal absorbed mesonephric ducts*
- *Muscular and serous coat: Splanchnopleuric mesoderm.*

Common congenital anomalies of urinary bladder

- Bladder may be duplicated
- **Splincter vesicae** may be absent
- **Hourglass bladder:** Divided into two compartments by a constriction in middle of organ
- Communication with rectum or vagina may exist **(fistulas)**
- **Congenital diverticula** may be present

Ectopica vesicae: *Congenital defect in which lower part of anterior abdominal wall and anterior wall of bladder does not develop. The cavity of bladder may be exposed on surface of body. Usually associated with epispadias (urethra opens on dorsal aspect of penis)*

URETHRA

The male urethra is 18–20 cm long and extends from the internal orifice in the urinary bladder to the external opening, or meatus, at the end of the penis.18–20 cm in length with 3 parts

- **Prostatic (3 cm semilunar)**
- **Membranous (2 cm stellate)**
- **Spongy/penile (15 cm slit shaped)**
- **In males: 18–20 cm**
- **In females: 4 cm long**

The part of urethra in male

The features of floor of prostatic part

- *Urethral crest (veru montanum):* Median longitudinal ridge.
- *Colliculus seminalis:* Elevation in middle part of crest
- *Prostatic sinuses:* On each side of crest. Has an opening of prostatic gland.

Position of bulbourethral gland: These are placed one on each side of membranous urethra. Their ducts open into penile urethra.

The variations in shape of lumen of male urethra

1. *Prostatic part:* **Semilunar**
2. *Membranous part:* **Star shaped**
3. *Spongy part:* **Transverse,** *except external urethral orifice which is vertical slit.*

4

Abdomen

The characteristic features of sphincters of urethra

1. Internal urethral sphincter vesicae:
- Involuntary
- Supplied by sympathetic nerve
- Made up of smooth muscle fibres with elastic and collagenous fibres

2. External urethral sphincter urethrae:
- Voluntary
- Supplied by pudendal nerve
- Made up of striated muscle fibres

Home's tubules: *These are glandular invaginations of transitional epithelium on each side of internal urethral orifice near bladder neck in female.*

Part of male urethra is ruptured during instrumentation: *Membranous part because it is narrowest and least dilatable.*

Commonest cause of urethral stricture: *Gonococcal infection*

The instruments in urethra should be introduced with beak downwards: Because immediately within external meatus, urethra dilates into a terminal fossa, whose roof bears a mucosal fold (lacuna magna) which may catch the tip of catheter.

Urethra is Developed From

The female urethra: Caudal part of vesicourethral canal.

Male urethra:
- From urinary bladder up to opening of ejaculatory ducts: Endodermal (caudal part of vesicourethral canal)
- Rest of prostatic urethra and membranous urethra: Pelvic part of definitive urogenital sinus.
- Penile part except terminal part: Epithelium of phallic part of definitive urogenital sinus.
- Terminal part of penile urethra: From ectoderm.

Hypospadias: *Due to inability of urethral folds to unite anteriorly, the urethra opens on undersurface of penis.*

Epispadias: *The urethral orifice opens on the dorsal aspect of penis.*

PROSTATE

- It is a fibromuscular, glandular organ that surrounds the neck of the urinary bladder and the proximal portion of the male urethra.
- The gland is supported anteriorly by the puboprostatic ligaments, inferiorly by the genitourinary diaphragm (external urinary sphincter), and posteriorly by the rectal wall, which is separated from the prostate by an obliterated pelvic reflection of the peritoneum is called Denonvilliers' fascia

Structural Zones

- There are two well defined zones separated by an ill defined irregular capsule and the zones are absent anteriorly.
- **The outer larger zone** is composed of large branched glands the ducts of which curve backwards and open mainly into prostatic sinuses and this zone is frequently the site of cancer formation.
- **The inner smaller zone** is composed of submucosal glands opening into prostatic sinuses and a small group of short simple mucosal glands surrounding the upper part of the urethra and this zone is typically prone to benign hypertrophy.

Blood Supply

The prostate is supplied by branches from the **inferior vesical, middle rectal and internal pudendal arteries.**

Branches of these form subcapsular and a periurethral plexus.

The veins form a rich plexus around the sides and base of the gland. The plexus receives the deep dorsal vein of the penis and communicates with the vesical plexus and with the internal pudendal vein and drains into the vesical and internal iliac vein. **Valveless communication exists between the prostatic and vertebral venous plexus through which the prostatic carcinoma spreads to the vertebrae and to the skull.**

Lymphatic Drainage

Drain chiefly into the **internal iliac and sacral nodes, and partly into external iliac nodes.**

Nerve Supply

Supplied by both sympathetics and parasympathetics. The gland contains numerous nerve endings, impulses of which are relayed to lower three lumbar and upper sacral segments. The secretions of prostate are produced and discharged after stimulation of both sympathetics and parasympathetics. The prostatic plexus of nerves is derived from lower part of inferior hypogastric plexus.

Age changes

- At birth prostate is small in size, mainly made up of stroma with a simple duct system. Due to stimulation of maternal estrogens during the first 6 weeks the epithelium of ducts undergoes hyperplasia and squamous metaplasia. Between 9 and 14 years the duct system becomes more elaborate and the gland slowly increases in size.
- At puberty, the male hormones bring rapid changes, the gland becomes double in size due to rapid growth of follicles. The stroma is condensed and its relative proportion is reduced.
- From 20 to 30 years there is marked proliferation of the glandular element with infolding of the glandular epithelium into the lumen of the follicles making them irregular.

4

Abdomen

- From 30 to 45 years the size of the prostate remains constant and involution starts. The epithelial infoldings gradually disappear and amyloid bodies increase in number.

- After 45 years the prostate is either enlarged (benign hypertrophy) or reduced (senile atrophy). These changes are progressive till death.

Cave of Retzius: *This is potential retropubic space separating pubic symphysis and anterior surface of prostate. This is filled with fat.*

The pathological capsule of prostate: *In benign tumors of prostate, the normal peripheral part of gland becomes compressed into a capsule around the tumor mass.*

Valveless vertebral veins of Bateson their clinical importance

Some veins of prostatic plexus communicate with plexus of veins lying in front of vertebral bodies and neural canal. These veins are valveless. Clinical importance: Because of these valveless veins, there is a retrograde spread of carcinoma of prostate to pelvis and vertebrae.

Rectal involvement is uncommon in carcinoma of prostate: *Because fascia of Denonvilliers' is rarely penetrated by carcinoma of prostate.*

The Histology of Prostate

- Prostate is composed of glands present in smooth muscle stroma.
- Part of gland in front of urethra has dense muscular tissue and very little glandular tissue. The glands are made up of follicles, lined by columnar cells.

Prostate is developed from:

- It arises from buds arising from prostatic urethra:
- From epithelium: Secretory part
- From mesoderm: Inner glandular zone
- From endoderm: Outer glandular zone
- From mesenchyme: Muscle and connective tissue

The homologous of prostate in female is the urethral glands and paraurethral glands of Skene.

Enucleation of adenoma of prostate: *In enucleating, plane between adenomatous mass and pathological capsule is cleaved, the tumor is removed and peripheral condensed prostatic tissue is left behind. The prostatic venous plexus, lying between true and false capsule, is not disturbed.*

Approaches for prostatectomy

- The enlarged gland is removed, enucleated, leaving behind both the capsules and the venous plexus between them. Prostate can be approached
- Through bladder—**transvesical**
- Through the prostatic capsule—**retropubic**
- Through the perineum/fascia of Denonvilliers'—**perineal approach**

OVARIES

- These are **female gonads.**
- Lie in the **ovarian fossa** bounded in front by obliterated umbilical artery and posteriorly by ureter and internal iliac artery.
- **In nullipara they are vertical and greyish pink in colour** but in **multipara it is horizontal because of the pull by the pregnant uterus.**
- Before ovulation they have a **smooth surface,** but later they become puckered due to scars of ovulation.
- Each ovary has **two ends or poles the upper or tubal and lower or uterine.**
- There are **two borders anterior or mesovarian and posterior or free.**
- The surfaces are medial and lateral. The medial surface is largely covered by the uterine tube. The peritoneal recess between the mesosalpinx and this surface is known as **ovarian bursa.**
- The ovary is covered by peritoneum except along the anterior border where the two layers are reflected on to the posterior layer of broad ligament by a short fold is called **mesovarium.**

Ligaments of Ovary

- There is also a ligament called **the infundibulopelvic/suspensory ligament** which is the lateral part of the broad ligament extending from infundibulum of uterine tube and upper pole of the ovary to the external iliac vessels.
- **The ligament of ovary** is not a peritoneal ligament. It connects the lower pole of ovary to the superolateral angle of uterus.

Arterial supply is by ovarian and uterine arteries.

Veins form the pampiniform plexus which condenses into a single vein on either side and drains into inferior vena cava on the right side and into the left renal vein on the other side.

Lymphatics drain into lateral aortic and preaortic nodes.

Nerve supply by the ovarian plexus contains both sympathetic (T10, T11) and parasympathetic (S2, 3, 4). The sympathetics are for pain and vasomotor and parasympathetics are for vasodilatation.

Applied Aspects

- Ovarian **prolapse**
- *Ovarian carcinoma:* Cancer of ovary can be of different types
- **Teratomas:** These are tumors of ovary having components of all germinal layers
- **Stein leventhal syndrome or polycystic ovarian disease** where ovary can have multiple cysts.
- *Ovarian cysts:* Can be physiological or pathological.

4

Abdomen

UTERUS

- Also called **Womb/Hyster**.
- It is **Pyriform** or pear shaped.
- Length, breadth and thickness is about **3, 2, 1 inches respectively.**
- Weighs about **30–40 gm.**
- Upper expanded part the **body** and lower **cylindrical part cervix.**
- Junction of these parts is marked by a **circular constriction.**
- **Body forms upper 2/3 and cervix forms lower 1/3.**
- Normally the long axis of uterus forms an angle of 90 degrees with long axis of vagina and this angle is open anteriorly called **anteversion.**
- The uterus also is bent on itself forwards and this is **anteflexion** which is about 120 degrees.
- Roughly the long axis of the uterus corresponds with the long axis of the inlet of pelvis.
- The long axis of the vagina to the long axis of the outlet and long axis of the cavity of pelvis.

Superiorly, uterus communicates with the uterine tubes and inferiorly with the vagina.

Fundus is formed by the free upper end of the uterus, is like a dome, covered with peritoneum and is directed forwards when bladder is full. The fertilized ovum is implanted in the posterior wall.

The anterior or vesical surface is covered with peritoneum, is flat and forms the posterior wall of vesicouterine pouch.

The posterior or intestinal surface is convex and related to coils of terminal ileum and sigmoid colon. It is covered with peritoneum and forms the anterior wall of the rectouterine pouch of Douglas.

Each lateral border is convex and round and gives attachment to broad ligament, uterine tube (at the upper end), round ligament of uterus (anteroinferior to tube) and ligament of ovary (posteroinferior to tube). The uterine artery ascends along this border between the two layers of broad ligament.

In coronal section cavity is triangular with apex down. At the apex the cavity becomes continuous with the canal of cervix and the junction is called the **internal os**. The superolateral angles of the cavity receive the openings of uterine tubes.

Cervix of the uterus

- It is about **2.5 cm long.**
- It is **less mobile.**
- Wider in the middle.
- The lower part of the cervix projects into the anterior wall of the vagina which divides it into **supravaginal and vaginal parts.**
- **The supravaginal part** is related anteriorly to the bladder, posteriorly to rectouterine pouch and on each side to the ureter and uterine arteries.

- **The vaginal part** of the cervix projects into the anterior wall of the vagina and the spaces between it and the vaginal wall are called fornices.
- **The cervical canal** opens into vagina by external os which is round and small in nulliparous but in multiparous women there are anterior and posterior lips both of which are in contact with posterior wall of vagina.
- The cervical canal walls show mucosal folds which resemble the branches of tree and
- The folds in the anterior and posterior walls interlock with each other and close the canal.

Arterial supply is by uterine and ovarian arteries. The uterine arteries are tortuous and permit expansion of uterus during pregnancy.

Veins drain finally into internal iliac veins

Lymphatics begin as three intercommunicating networks the endometrial, myometrial and subperitoneal. The upper lymphatics drain into aortic and superficial inguinal nodes. The middle area drains into external iliac nodes and the lower lymphatics go to external iliac, internal iliac and sacral nodes.

Nerve supply is derived from sympathetics (T12–L1) which produces uterine contraction and vasoconstriction. The parasympathetics (S2, 3, 4) produce inhibition and vasodilatation. The pain sensations from the body of uterus pass along the sympathetics and from the cervix along the parasympathetic nerves.

The most important relation of ureter to cervix is worth remembering. Due to close relation of ureter to lateral fornix of cervix, a stone in ureter can be palpated during pervaginal examination.

Lateral extension of tumor from uterus can compress the ureter and cause hydronephrosis and bilateral compression can cause uremia.

Supports of the Uterus

Since uterus is a mobile organ and it is changing shape with reproductive life and because it has to negotiate between two cavities, it needs a good support.

The supports are primary in the form of muscles namely
- **Pelvic diaphragm** if torn during delivery causes later prolapse
- **Perineal body** maintains the integrity of pelvic floor and nine muscles are attached to it.
- **Urogenital diaphragm**

The fibromuscular supports are:
- **Uterine axis**
- **Pubocervical ligaments** connect the cervix to the posterior surface of pubis
- **Transverse cervical ligaments of Mackenrodt's** are condensations of pelvic fascia.
- **Round ligament of uterus** passes through the inguinal canal and is attached to labium majus.

4

Abdomen

The secondary supports are of doubtful value and are formed by:
Broad ligaments, uterovesical fold of peritoneum and rectovaginal fold of peritonem.

Broad Ligament

- These are the folds of peritoneum which attach the uterus to pelvic walls. Various names are given to the parts of broad ligament.
- **Mesovarium** is the attachment between the ovary and posterior layer of the broad ligament.
- **Mesosalpinx** is the part of broad ligament between uterine tube and the ovarian ligament.
- **Mesometrium** is the part of broad ligament below the ligament of ovary.
- **The suspensory ligament** goes to the upper pole of the ovary and infundibulum of the uterine tube to the lateral pelvic wall blending with external iliac artery sheath.

It contains the following structures:
- Uterine tube
- Round ligament of the uterus
- Ligament of the ovary
- Uterine vessels
- Ovarian vessels
- Uterovaginal and ovarian nerve plexuses
- Epoophoron
- Paraoophoron
- Some lymph nodes and lymph vessels
- Dense connective tissue the parametrium.

Applied Anatomy of Uterus

- **Retroverted uterus:** The uterus comes to lie in straight line with the vagina.
- **Intrauterine contraceptive devices** are placed in uterine cavity
- **Caesarean section:** It is operation done for delivery of fetus
- **Hysterectomy:** Removal of uterus
- **Hysterosalpingography:** Method of demonstrating female genital tract (uterus and fallopian tubes)
- **Developmental anomalies of uterus:** *Can be multiple:* Such as septate uterus, bicornuate uterus.

UTERINE TUBE/FALLOPIAN TUBE

The parts of uterine tube
1. **Infundibulum (fimbriated): Opens into peritoneal cavity by abdominal ostium**
2. **Ampulla: Forms lateral 2/3 of tube**

3. **Isthmus:** Forms medial 1/3 of tube

4. **Uterine (interstitial):** Lies within uterine wall and opens into uterine cavity by uterine ostium.

It has two openings **laterally and medially called uterine and abdominal osteum.** The uterine osteum is 1 mm and the abdominal osteum is about 3 mm in diameter.

The lateral end is like a funnel and is called infundibulum and has finger like processes called fimbria. One of the fimbria is long and is attached to the upper pole of the ovary and is known as ovarian fimbria.

The ampulla is thin walled, dilated and tortuous and is about 4 mm in diameter.

The isthmus is narrow, round and cord like.

The Relations of Uterine Tube with Ovary

1. Near lateral pelvic wall, ampulla is related to anterior and posterior borders, upper pole and medial surface of ovary.

2. One of the fimbria is long and is attached to tubal (upper) pole of ovary, it is known as ovarian fimbria.

Mesosalpinx

It is part of broad ligament between mesovarium and uterine tube. The uterine tube lies in the upper free margin of the broad ligament. The part of the broad ligament between the attachment of the mesovarium and the uterine tube is called mesosalpinx.

Blood Supply

Uterine artery supplies the medial 2/3 and the ovarian artery supplies the lateral 1/3. The veins run with the arteries and drain into pampiniform plexus and into the uterine veins.

Lymphatics: Drain into **lateral and preaortic** nodes. From the isthmus they drain into superficial inguinal nodes.

Nerve supply: Sympathetics (T10 to L2) are vasomotor and perhaps stimulate peristalsis. The parasympathetics are derived from vagus and from pelvic splanchnic nerves and produce vasodilatation.

Applied

1. **Salpingitis:** Infection of the tubes. Previously used to be common due to tuberculosis. Nowadays common due to Chlamydia

2. **Sterility:** As a result of scarring of tubes

3. **Tubal pregnancy:** A common form of ectopic which can result in rupture.

4. **Tubal insufflations test or hysterosalpingography** for determining patency of tubes. Used in evaluation of fertility

5. **Tubectomy:** Surgical removal of tubes.

6. **Ectopic pregnancy:** The abnormal implantation of the ovum in uterine tubes instead of uterus can lead to ectopic pregnancy which can cause rupture of fallopian tubes.

VAGINA

- Means a **sheath.**
- It is a **fibromuscular canal.**
- Extends from the **vulva to the uterus.**
- Situated behind the **bladder and the urethra and in front of rectum and anal canal.**
- Closed by a thin annular fold of mucous membrane in the virgins called **hymen** but in married women it is represented by rounded elevations around the vaginal orifice called **carunculae hymenales.**
- The vaginal fornices are four, **one anterior, one posterior and two lateral.**

Relations

- **Anterior wall** is related to base of bladder and urethra.
- **Posterior wall** is related to rectouterine pouch, loose connective tissue. The lower ¼ is separated from the anal canal by perineal body and the muscles attached to it.
- **Laterally** the upper 1/3 is related to transverse cervical ligament, the middle 1/3 is related to pubococcygeus muscle. The lower 1/3 pierces the urogenital diaphragm, be low which it is related to the bulb of the vestibule, bulbospongiosus and greater vestibular glands of Bartholin.

Arterial Supply

It is highly vascular and is supplied by branches from:
1. Vaginal branch of internal iliac artery
2. Cervicovaginal branch of the uterine artery
3. Middle rectal artery
4. Internal pudendal artery

The branches from these arteries anastomose freely and form anterior and posterior midline arteries called **vaginal azygos arteries.**

Veins drain into internal iliac veins

Lymphatics drain into the external iliac, internal iliac and superficial inguinal nodes from the upper, middle and lower parts respectively.

Nerve Supply

Lower 1/3 is pain sensitive and is supplied by the pudendal nerves. The upper 2/3 is pain insensitive and is supplied by sympathetics (L1, L2) and parasympathetics (S2, S3). The sympathetics are vasoconstrictor.

Applied Anatomy

1. **Per vaginal exam**
   - Anteriorly urethra, bladder, pubic symphysis.
   - Posteriorly rectum and pouch of Douglas.
   - Laterally ovary, uterine tube, lateral pelvic walls and ureters.
   - Superiorly the cervix.

2. **Nonmedical abortionists** are not aware of normal anatomy and while doing illegal abortions push their instruments directly backwards through the posterior fornix of vagina instead of cervix and **enter Pouch of Douglas and hence open the peritoneum which can result in severe peritonitis.**

4

Abdomen

RECTUM

- It is the **distal part of large gut**
- It is placed between **the sigmoid colon and anal canal.**
- It is not straight as name indicates and is **curved both anteroposteriorly and from side to side.**
- The three cardinal features of large intestine are absent here like
  - ✓ **No taenia**
  - ✓ **No appendices epiploicae**
  - ✓ **No sacculations.**
- It begins at the level of **S3 vertebra and ends by becoming continuous at the anorectal junction** which in males corresponds to the apex of the prostate and is 2–3 cm in front of and a little below the tip of the coccyx.
- In the lower part it has a dilatation called as the **ampulla.**
- The lateral curves are **three, the upper lateral curve is convex to the right.**
- The middle lateral curve is convex to the left.
- The lower lateral curve is convex to the right

The mucosal folds are longitudinal and transverse.

The arterial supply is from **superior, middle and inferior rectal arteries** and also by the median sacral artery.

The veins drain into the superior and inferior mesenteric veins.

Lymphatics from the upper part pass along the superior rectal vessels to the inferior mesenteric nodes after passing through the pararectal and sigmoid nodes. From the lower half pass along the middle rectal vessels to the internal iliac nodes.

Nerve supply it is from sympathetic L1 and L2 and parasympathetic S2, 3, 4. The parasympathetic nerves are motor to the muscles of the rectum but inhibitory to the internal anal sphincter.

Supports of the rectum are in the form of fascia of Waldeyer, lateral ligament of the rectum, rectovesical fascia and pelvic peritoneum.

- **Prolapse of the rectum, or procidentia:** *It is sagging of* rectum. It is an uncommon problem of obscure etiology characterized by full-thickness eversion of the rectal wall through the anus and its external protrusion as a series of concentric rings.

Dentate Line (White Line of Hilton)

Features	Above	Below
Appearance	Pink colour	Skin colour
Mucosal lining	Cubical epithelium	Squamous epithelium
Nerve supply	Autonomic nerves	Spinal nerves
Venous drainage	Portal venous	Systemic venous system
Embryology	Develop from post allantoic duct	Develop from proctodeum
Lymphatics	Lymphatics to paraortic nodes	Superficial and deep inguinal nodes
Blood supply	Supplied by superior rectal artery	Inferior rectal artery

Anal Canal

- The anal canal begins at the **anorectal junction and ends at the anal verge.**
- It is angulated in relation to the rectum because the pull of the sling-like **puborectalis produces the anorectal angle.**
- It lies 2–3 cm in front of and slightly below the tip of the coccyx, which is opposite the apex of the prostate in males.
- The anal canal is attached posteriorly to the coccyx by the anococcygeal ligament
- The anus is surrounded laterally and posteriorly by loose adipose tissue within the ischioanal fossae, a potential pathway for the spread of perianal sepsis from one side to the other
- Anteriorly the perineal body separates the anal canal from the membranous urethra and penile bulb in males or from the lower vagina in females.
- **Haemorrhoids: Represent** abnormal enlargement of the anal cushions. Are as a result of obstruction of the venous flow during prolonged straining and defaecation.
- **Anal fissures:** These are vertical breaks in the anal epithelium.They are more likely to develop in the anterior of the anus, possibly because stress within the anal canal is concentrated in these regions by the arrangement of the external sphincter fibers. The relative paucity of the arterial supply in these regions probably contributes to poor healing.
- **Imperforate anus and anorectal anomalies:** Imperforate anus occurs approximately once in every 5000 newborn infants and is more common in males. Most anorectal anomalies result from abnormal development of the urorectal septum, resulting in incomplete separation of the cloaca into urogenital and anorectal portions. There is normally a temporary communication between the rectum and anal canal dorsally from the bladder and urethra ventrally but it closes when the urorectal septum fuses with the cloacal membrane.

- **Anal agenesis, with or without a fistula:** The anal canal may end blindly or there may be an ectopic anus or an anoperineal fistula that opens into the perineum. The abnormal canal may, however, open into the vagina in females or the urethra in males.
- **Anal stenosis:** The anus is in the normal position, but the anus and anal canal are narrow.The lumen of the anal canal is reduced.
- **Hemorrhoids/Piles:** These can be:
    - External—External to anal orifice
    - Internal—Internal to anal orifice

Internal Hemorrhoids

- They are **more common and includes interoecternal hemorrhoids**
- Mostly occur at **3 o' clock, 7 o' clock and 11 o' clock** position with patient in lithotomy position
- It has 3 parts
    - Pedicle at anorectal ring
    - Internal hemorrhoid just below anorectal ring
    - External associated hemorrhoid lies between dentate line anal margins.
- Clinical features
    - **Bright red painless bleeding (earliest symptoms)**
    - Mucus discharge
    - Prolapses
    - Pain indicates prolapsed and strangulation
- Investigation
    - On digital examination, they cannot be felt Unless they are thromboses
    - On proctoscopy they bulge into lumen just below anorectal ring.

Perineum

The boundaries of perineum
Superficial:
- **Anterior:** Scrotum in male, mons pubis in female
- **Posterior:** Buttocks
- **Lateral:** Upper part of medial side of thigh

Deep
- **Anterior:** Upper part of pubic arch, arcuate pubic ligament
- **Posterior:** Tip of coccyx
- **Lateral:** Conjoined ischiopubic rami, ischial tuberosity and sacrotuberous ligament.

The Divisions of Perineum

A transverse line joining the anterior parts of ischial tuberosities divide perineum into two triangular regions:

- **Urogenital region:** Anterior
- **Anal region:** Posterior

Perineal body: *Fibromuscular structure in median plane about 1.25 cm in front of anal margin. Support pelvic organs in females.*

The muscles forming perineal body or attached to perineal body

Nine muscles:

1. Unpaired:
- External and sphincter
- Bulbospongiosus
- Fibres of longitudinal muscle coat of rectal ampulla and anal canal.

2. Paired:
- Deep transverses perinei
- Levator ani
- Superficial transverses perinei

The clinical importance of perineal body: It may rupture during child birth, which if unrepaired may lead to prolapse of urinary bladder, uterus and rectum in females.

The boundaries of ischiorectal fossa
- It is a wedge shaped space on each side of anal canal below pelvic diaphragm.
- Base: Skin
- Apex: Meeting of obturator fascia with inferior layer of the pelvic fascia
- Anterior: Posterior border of perineal membrane.
- Posterior: Lower border of gluteus maximus and sacrotuberous ligament.
- Lateral wall: Obturator internus with fascia, medial surface of ischial tuberosity.
- Medial wall: External and sphincter, in lower part; levator ani, in upper part.

The contents of ischiorectal fossa
- Ischiorectal pad of fat
- Inferior rectal nerve and vessels
- Posterior scrotal (or labial in females) nerves and vessels.
- Perineal branch of S4 nerve.
- Perforating cutaneous branches of S2–3 nerves
- Pudendal canal with internal pudendal vessels and pudendal nerve.

The infections perianal space are very painful but those of ischiorectal space are very painful *as the Fat in perianal space is tightly arranged in small loculi formed by complete septa therefore little swelling due to infections cause increased tension and pain, but in ischiorectal space fat is loosely arranged therefore swelling can occur without tension.*

The unilateral ischiorectal abscess if not drained becomes *bilateral because of extension of infection through the horseshoe recess behind anal canal which connects the fossa of both sides.*

The structures piercing the perineal membrane

In males:
- Urethra
- Branches of perineal nerve to superficial perineal muscles.

4

Abdomen

- Ducts of bulbourethral glands.
- Artery and nerve to the bulb (bilateral).
- Urethral artery (bilateral).
- Deep artery of penis (bilateral)
- Dorsal artery of penis (bilateral)
- Posterior scrotal nerves and vessels (bilateral)

In females:
- Urethra
- Vagina
- Artery and nerve to bulb of vestibule
- Deep artery of clitoris
- Dorsal artery of clitoris
- Posterior labial arteries and nerves

The structures forming urogenital diaphragm (old concept)
1. **Deep perineal muscles**
2. **Superior fascia of urogenital diaphragm**
3. **Inferior fascia of urogenital diaphragm**

The Female External Genital Organs

1. **Mons pubis**
2. **Labia majora**
3. **Labia minora**
4. **Clitoris**
5. **Vestibule of vagina having various openings**
6. **Bulb of vestibule**
7. **Greater vestibular glands (of Bartholin)**

The boundaries of gynecological perineum
The area between posterior commissure (skin connecting prominent posterior ends of labia majora) and anus, constitutes gynecological perineum. The position of glands of Bartholin these are homologous with bulbourethral glands (of Cowper) in males. Lie in the superficial perineal space at vaginal orifice. Duct of each gland opens at side of hymen, between hymen and labium minora.

Pudendal Canal

It is formed
1. **By splitting of fascia lunata**
2. **Fascial wall of canal is fused with:**
   - Laterally: Obturator fascia
   - Medially: Perineal fascia
   - Inferiorly: Falciform process of sacrotuberous ligament
   - Superiorly: Arches over ischiorectal fat and fused with inferior fascia of pelvic diaphragm.

4

The contents of Pudendal canal (Alcocks canal)

1. Pudendal nerve (S2, 3, 4)
2. Internal pudendal vessels

The structures supplied by pudendal nerve

By inferior rectal nerve: Supplies external anal sphincter, skin around anus and anal canal below pectinate line.

3. Perineal nerve:
   (a) Posterior scrotal nerves: Posterior 2/3 of scrotum in males and posterior labial nerves (sensory) in females to lower one inch of vagina.
   (b) Muscular branches: To urogenital muscles, anterior parts of external anal sphincter and levator ani. Nerve to bulbospongiosus supplies corpus spongiosum penis and urethra.

4. Dorsal nerve of penis: Supplies skin of body of penis and glans.

The pudendal nerve block given in vaginal operations: Near the ischial spine by a needle passed through vaginal wall and then guided by a finger.

The Branches of Internal Pudendal Artery

- Inferior rectal artery
- Artery of penis
- Perineal artery

The Branches of Internal Iliac Artery

(a) Branches of anterior division:

In males:

1. Superior vesical
2. Obturator
3. Middle rectal
4. Inferior vesical
5. Inferior gluteal
6. Internal pudendal

   In females: Same as above except inferior vesical is replaced by vaginal artery. Also uterine artery.

(b) Branches of posterior division:

1. Iliolumbar
2. Lateral sacral
3. Superior gluteal

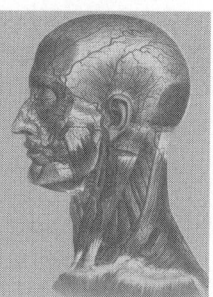

5

Head and Neck

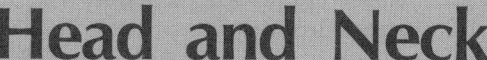

SCALP

S	Skin
C	Connective tissue
A	Aponeurosis
L	Loose areolar tissue

The extent of scalp is:
- Anterior: Supraorbital margins.
- Posterior: External occipital protuberance and superior nuchal lines.
- On each side: Superior temporal lines.

The layers of "SCALP" are:

S: Skin
C: Connective tissue (superficial fascia)
A: Aponeurosis with occipitofrontalis muscle.
L: Loose areolar tissue
P: Pericranium (Periosteum).

The wounds of scalp bleed profusely because of:
- Rich blood supply of scalp and
- The torn vessels fail to retract because of attachment to fibrous fascia.

The wound of scalp heal rapidly because: More vascular the area, the more rapid is healing. The infections of superficial fascia of scalp cause much pain because it is dense and fibrous, so, little swelling causes much increase in tension.

The "dangerous area of scalp": It is the subaponeurotic space (loose areolar tissue). Because:
- Emissary veins which open here may transmit the infection from scalp to cranial venous sinuses.
- Bleeding in this space causes generalized swelling of the scalp and may extend anteriorly into root of nose and eyelids, causing black eye.

The bleeding or pus collection beneath the periosteum is not extensive: Because the periosteum adheres to the suture lines of skull bones, so the collection of blood or pus outlines the affected bone (cephalhaematoma).

Safety valve haematoma: In children, duramater and pericranium are more intimately attached to skull. So, in fractures of vault of skull tearing of both dura and pericranium occurs and the intracranial hemorrhage may make its way through line of fracture and collect in subaponeurotic space of scalp. No signs of compression of brain develop until subaponeurotic space is full of blood; such a collection of blood is termed safety valve haematoma.

The hemorrhage from blood vessels of scalp is arrested by pressing with the fingers firmly down on to the skull on either side of the wound, thus compressing the vessels.

Emissary veins: The veins of the scalp are connected to intracranial venous sinuses by emissary veins which pierce the skull. These emissary veins also connect the scalp with diploic veins of vault of skull. Hence a mode of spread of infections across.

Black eye: It is due to local blow to the eye causing blackish discoloration of both eyelids simultaneously within two hours. This is due to subcutaneous hemorrhage.

It may also be due to grievous injury causing haemorrhage in the subaponeurotic layer. The haemorrhage fills subaponeurotic space up to highest nuchal line posterior; superior temporal line laterally and slowly gravitates under frontalis to the upper eyelid first, followed by lower eyelid causing their discoloration. This usually takes one to two days to appear.

Cephalhaematoma: Pericranium is loosely attached to the bone surface. At sutural lines it dips and blends with endosteum. Any collection of fluid beneath the pericranium results in a swelling resembling the shape of the bone.

This swelling is caused by subcutaneous bleeding and accumulation of blood. It forms in the scalp of a foetus during difficult labour. It enlarges slowly in the first few days after birth.

It usually results from trauma or following forceps delivery. Large cephalhematoma may become infected which requires surgical drainage.

Caput succedaneum: It is a localized pitting edema in the scalp of a fetus that may overlie sutures of the skull. It is usually formed during labour as a result of the circular pressure of the cervix on the fetal occiput. At birth the baby's head may appear markedly deformed. The swelling starts resolving immediately and in few days it disappears.

Moulding: This is the natural process by which a baby's head is shaped during labour as it is squeezed into the birth canal during labour. The head often becomes quite elongated. The skull bones may overlap slightly at the suture lines. The biparietal diameter of the head may be compressed as much as 0.5 cm without intracranial damage. The changes caused by molding resolve during the first few days of life.

Craniosynostosis: It is the premature fusion of one or more of the sutures of the skull causing a limitation in cranial growth characteristic for each suture involved. When a suture is prematurely fused, compensatory growth occurs parallel to the long axis of the suture. Craniosynostosis implies limitation of cranial vault growth. If cranial vault growth does not keep pace with brain growth, this may result in increased intracranial pressure. This may be manifested by optic nerve atrophy, mental retardation, and death. Hydrocephalus may be secondary to a generalized stenosis of the cranial base and can be seen with craniosynostosis.

FACE

5

- **Sensory nerve: Trigeminal**
- **Motor nerve: Facial**

- The wounds of face **bleed profusely** because of its rich vascularity.
- The **edema** in nephrotic syndrome appears first on face and eyelids because, here the skin is very lax, which facilitates rapid spread of oedema fluid.
- The wounds of face **tend to gap** because the facial muscles are inserted into skin making it thick and elastic.
- The facial muscles are called muscles of expression as they are **subcutaneous muscles** and they work under a fine control to bring about different shades of facial expressions.
- **Panniculosus carnosus:** It is a continuous muscular sheath present in lower animals from which facial muscles are derived.
- **The developmental** origin of facial muscles is from **second branchial arch and the motor nerve supply of facial muscles is facial (VII cranial) nerve (nerve of second arch).**

The Facial Artery

The face is highly vascular and the facial artery is a tortuous artery.

In the neck:
- Ascending palatine
- Glandular
- Submental
- Tonsillar

In the face:
- Inferior labial
- Lateral nasal
- Superior labial

The Veins of the Face

They accompany the arteries. The **facial vein** is the largest vein of the face.

Head and Neck

The **supratrochlear** and the **supraorbital veins** join at the medial canthus of the eye to form the **angular vein** which continues as the facial vein. Ultimately draining into the **internal jugular vein.**

Dangerous Area of Face

- Upper lip
- Lower part of nose.

Because infections of these sites are very common which may spread in retrograde direction in facial vein and cause infection and thrombosis of the cavernous sinus through deep connections of the facial vein. Following factors facilitate the spread of infection:

- It is difficult to immobilize this part of the face.
- Absence of deep fascia fails to restrict infection
- Veins here do not have valves.

Once the infection enters the anterior facial vein it incites thrombus formation, which may occlude the facial vein and open up alternative passage of venous return, namely:

- *Via superior ophthalmic vein draining in the cavernous sinus*
- *Via infraorbital vein which joins inferior ophthalmic vein to drain in cavernous sinus.*
- *Via deep facial vein to join pterygoid venous plexus which is connected to cavernous sinus by emissary vein.*

Along these alternative pathways the infection may enter cavernous sinus. Since the flow of blood is sluggish in cavernous sinus the infection can grow. The cavernous sinus is close to pituitary and cranial nerves II, III, IV, V-1 and V-2 of V CN and VI CN will be affected. **The patient may present with ophthalmoplegia along with pituitary dysfunctions. It may prove fatal.**

Lymphatic Drainage of Face

Face is divided into three lymphatic territories

- **Upper:** Drains into **Pre auricular nodes**
- **Middle:** Drains into **Submandibular nodes**
- **Lower:** Drains into **Submental nodes**

Facial fractures: Commonly result from vehicular accidents, assaults, and other blunt trauma to the face. Maxillary fractures often occur in a characteristic pattern first described by Le Fort.

- **The Le Fort I fracture** extends from the pyriform aperture to the pterygom axillary fissure. This fracture presents as a mobile upper jaw and lower midface.
- **The Le Fort II fracture** extends from the pterygom axillary fissure through the anterior maxilla to the nasofrontal junction. When examined as described previously, this fracture presents as a mobile midface and nose.

- **The Le Fort III fracture** separates the entire facial skeleton from the cranium. This fracture extends from the pterygom axillary fissure through the zygomatic frontal sutures across the floor of the orbit to the nasofrontal junction.

Rhytidectomy: It is facial face lift: The pathogenesis of wrinkles is related to the underlying histologic changes seen primarily in the dermis of aging and sun-damaged skin. The total amount of ground substance (glycosaminoglycans and proteoglycans) diminishes with age. The elastic fibers responsible for the physiologic recoil of skin become altered, and there is noted laxity.

ORBIT

The different layers of eyelid.
- Skin
- Superficial fascia (has no fat).
- Palpebral fascia (forms orbital septum)
- Conjunctiva.

The glands found in eyelid
- **Zeis's glands: Large sebaceous glands of cilia. Found at lid margin**
- **Moll's glands: Sweat glands. Present at lid margin.**
- **Meibomian glands (tarsal glands): Sebaceous glands. Present in posterior surface of tarsi.**

The modifications of palpebral fascia
- Tarsal plates, in the lids and
- Palpebral ligament, at the angles.

Nerve Supply of Eyelids

- Upper eyelid and whole of bulbar conjunctiva supratrochlear and supraorbital nerves (branches of ophthalmic nerve).
- Lower eyelid: Infraorbital nerve (branch of maxillary nerve).
- **Chalazion: It is chronic inflammation of tarsal gland, causing a localized swelling.**
- **Stye: It is infection of Zeis's gland. The lid margin is oedematous and gland is swollen and painful.**

The constituents of lacrimal apparatus

- Lacrimal gland and its ducts
- Conjunctival sac
- Lacrimal puncta and lacrimal canaliculi
- Lacrimal sac and
- Nasolacrimal duct

Nature of lacrimal gland: Exocrine and serous.

Parts of Lacrimal Gland

- **Orbital part:** Larger, in lacrimal fossa in roof of orbit.
- **Palpebral part:** Smaller, in upper eyelid.
  - **The removal of palpebral part of gland is equivalent to functional removal of whole gland:** Because the ducts of orbital part also pass through the palpebral part so, when palpebral part is removed the secretions of orbital part cannot be drained.
  - **The advantage of blinking of lids:** It helps to spread the lacrimal fluid in front of eye and deep surface of lids, thus keep the conjunctiva moist.
  - **Valve of Hasner:** It is a fold of mucous membrane at the lower end of nasolacrimal duct.
  - **Epiphora:** It is leakage of tears down the face, due to the blockade of nasolacrimal duct.

Eyeball

Tenon's sheath: It is a thin membranous sheath around the eyeball. Extends from optic nerve to sclerocorneal junction. Eyeball can move freely within it.

Structures piercing fascial sheath of eyeball:
- **Tendons of extraocular muscles**
- **Ciliary vessels.**
- **Ciliary nerves.**

Suspensory Ligament of Lockwood

- It is thickened Tenon's capsule in lower part.
- Formed by union of margins of sheath of inferior rectus and inferior oblique with medial and lateral check ligaments.

The extraocular muscles

Voluntary muscles
Rectus:
✓ Superior rectus
✓ Inferior rectus
✓ Medial rectus
✓ Lateral rectus
Oblique:
✓ Superior oblique
✓ Inferior oblique
Levator palpebrae superioris involuntary muscles:
✓ Superior tarsal
✓ Inferior tarsal
✓ Orbitalis

Nerve Supply of Extra-ocular Muscles

✓ Superior oblique: Trochlear nerve
✓ Lateral rectus: Abducent nerve
✓ Superior, inferior and medial rectus, inferior oblique and levator: Oculomotor nerve (LR_6SO_4).

Conjugate movements of eye: The normal co-ordinated movements of both eyes are called conjugate movements. These are usually horizontal and vertical.

Nystagmus: It is involuntary rhythmical oscillatory movements of eye due to inco-ordination of ocular muscles.

Squint: It is the abnormal deviation of eye due to weakness or paralysis of a muscle.

Nose and Paranasal Air Sinuses

The skeleton of the nose consists of the nasal bones, the ascending processes of the maxilla, the upper lateral cartilages, the lower lateral cartilages, and the septal cartilage. The nasal septum is the medial wall of each nasal cavity. The lateral wall of each nasal cavity provides the attachment for the **three turbinates.**

Structures Forming Nasal Cavity

Roof: From anterior to posterior
✓ Nasal part of frontal bone
✓ Nasal bone
✓ Nasal cartilages
✓ Cribriform plate of ethmoid
✓ Inferior surface of body of sphenoid bone.
Floor: Palatine process of maxilla, horizontal plate of palatine.

Structures Forming Nasal Septum

Bones:
• Vomer
• Perpendicular plate of ethmoid
• Margins by nasal spine of frontal, rostrum of sphenoid and nasal, palatine and maxilla

Cartilage:
• Septal cartilage
• Inferior nasal cartilage.
Cuticular part: Lower end, formed by skin.

The Arteries Forming the Little's Area

• It is the anteroinferior part of nasal septum containing anastomosis between:
  Superior labial branch of facial artery and sphenopalatine artery. Large capillary network. The clinical importance of little's area: It is the commonest site of bleeding from the nose.

The bones forming the lateral wall of nose
- Nasal
- Frontal process of maxilla
- Lacrimal
- Labyrinth of ethmoid with superior and middle conchae
- Inferior nasal conchae
- Perpendicular plate of palatine bone
- Medial pterygoid plate.

Nasal conchae: These are shelf like bony projections from lateral wall of nose directed downwards and medially. They are three in number:
- Superior
- Middle
- Inferior

The meatuses of nose: These are the passages beneath the overhanging conchae.

> **Opening in middle meatus**
> ✓ Opening of frontal air sinus.
> ✓ Opening of maxillary air sinus.
> ✓ Opening of middle ethmoidal air sinus.
> **Openings in superior meatus**
> ✓ Opening of posterior ethmoidal air sinus.
> **Openings in inferior meatus**
> ✓ Nasolacrimal duct.
> **Sphenoidal air sinus opens into:** Sphenoethmoidal recess above the superior concha.

Nasal fracture: The nose is a vulnerable leading part. Fractures of the nasal bones are the most common fractures of the facial bones. Fractures of the nose may involve the ascending processes of the maxillae and the nasal processes of the frontal bones as well as the nasal bones. A fracture of the nose is usually an open fracture.

Septal hematomas: Lie between the quadrangular cartilage and the perichondrium. Septal hematomas frequently become infected, and abscess formation produces avascular and septic necrosis of the septal cartilage, which causes a saddle deformity of the nose.

Septal abscesses: These are located between the cartilage and the perichondrium. They may involve both sides of the cartilage.

Deviations of the nasal septum. Deviations of the nasal septum may be caused by trauma or may occur as developmental abnormalities, particularly in individuals with highly arched palates. Deviations of the nasal septum produce varying degrees of nasal obstruction. Deviations of the septum are corrected by septoplasty or submucous resection of the nasal septum. In these procedures, the muco-perichondrium is elevated from the cartilage. The deviated cartilage and bone are resected or remodeled to straighten the septum.

Perforations of the nasal septum: It may be secondary to nasal surgery or repeated trauma, as in picking the nose. In the past, perforations due to syphilis and tuberculosis were common.

Rhinoplasty: It is performed for physiologic as well as cosmetic purposes. A deformed nose is usually associated with airway obstruction. The aims of rhinoplasty are to eliminate the airway obstruction and to correct the external deformity of the nose.

Foreign bodies: Children put objects in their noses. Erasers, beans, buttons, pebbles, wool nap, paper, and sponge rubber are common foreign bodies. A foreign body in the nasal cavity produces a severe inflammatory reaction and causes a foul-smelling, bloody, unilateral discharge.

Bleeding from the nose: It is a common clinical problem. Ninety per cent of the time, epistaxis occurs from a plexus of vessels in the anteroinferior part of the septum.

Choanal atresia: It is a malformation in which the opening of the nasal cavity into the nasopharynx is obstructed by a partition of mucous membrane and bone. The malformation may occur unilaterally or bilaterally. If it occurs bilaterally, it produces respiratory distress in the neonate.

The Paranasal Air Sinuses

- **Frontal**
- **Maxillary**
- **Sphenoidal**
- **Ethmoidal**

Frontal Sinus

- The paired frontal sinuses, situated posterior to the superciliary arches, lie between the outer and inner tables of the frontal bone.
- The arterial supply of the frontal sinuses is from the supraorbital and anterior ethmoidal arteries.
- The veins drain into the anastomotic vein in the supraorbital notch connecting the supraorbital and superior ophthalmic veins.
- Lymphatic drainage is to the submandibular nodes.
- The sinuses are innervated by branches from the supraorbital branch of the ophthalmic nerve.

Sphenoid Sinus

- The paired sphenoidal sinuses lie posterior to the upper part of the nasal cavity, within the body of the sphenoid bone. As the sphenoidal septum often deviates from the midline, the sinuses are often unequal in size.
- The sphenoidal sinuses are related above to the optic chiasma and hypophysis cerebri and on each side to the internal carotid artery and cavernous sinus.
- The arterial supply of the sphenoidal sinus is via the posterior ethmoidal branch of the ophthalmic artery and nasal branch of the sphenopalatine artery.
- Venous drainage is through the posterior ethmoidal vein draining into the superior ophthalmic vein.
- Lymph drainage is to the retropharyngeal nodes.

- The sensory nerve supply arises from the posterior ethmoidal nerves, while parasympathetic secretomotor fibres are derived from orbital branches of the pterygopalatine ganglion.

Ethmoidal Sinuses

- These are small, thin-walled cavities in the ethmoidal labyrinth, completed by the frontal, maxillary, lacrimal, sphenoid and palatine bones.
- They range from 3 large to 18 small sinuses on each side, and their openings into the nasal cavity are also very variable in position.
- They are divided into anterior, middle and posterior ethmoidal air cells.
- The ethmoidal sinuses receive their arterial supply from nasal branches of the sphenopalatine artery and the anterior and posterior ethmoidal branches of the ophthalmic artery.
- Venous drainage is by the corresponding veins.
- The lymphatics of the anterior group drain to the submandibular nodes, and those of the posterior group to the retropharyngeal nodes.
- The sensory innervation is from the anterior and posterior ethmoidal branches of the ophthalmic nerve, and the orbital branch of the pterygopalatine ganglion supplies parasympathetic secretomotor fibres.

The Maxillary Sinus

- **It is the largest of the paranasal sinuses and is situated in the body of the maxilla.**
- **It is** pyramidal in shape and its thin walls correspond to the orbital (roof), alveolar (floor), facial (anterior) and infratemporal (posterior) aspects of the maxilla.
- All of the openings are nearer the roof than the floor of the sinus which means that the natural drainage of the maxillary sinus is reliant on an intact mucociliary clearance system.
- The arterial supply of the maxillary sinus is derived mainly from the maxillary artery via anterior, middle and superior posterior alveolar branches, and infraorbital and greater palatine arteries.
- Veins corresponding to the arteries drain into the facial vein or pterygoid venous plexus. Lymph drainage is to the submandibular nodes.
- The nerve supply is derived from the maxillary nerve via the infraorbital and anterior, middle and posterior superior alveolar nerves.

Osteomeatal Complex

The term osteomeatal complex or osteomeatal unit, refers to the **maxillary sinus ostium, ethmoid infundibulum, hiatus semilunaris and frontal recess.**

It is the final common pathway for drainage of secretions from the maxillary, frontal, anterior and middle ethmoid sinuses into the middle meatus, and obstruction plays a pivotal role in the development and persistence of sinusitis.

CSF Rhinorrhea: A fracture of frontal bone, tearing the dura and piameter, causes communication between nasal cavity and subarachnoid space and CSF, may trickle through nostril on the affected side.

Antrum of highmore: Maxillary sinus is also called as the antrum of Highmore.

TRIANGLES OF NECK

The deep fascia in the neck: Fascia colli
is divided into an
- **Carotid sheath**
- **Investing layer**
- **Pretracheal layer**
- **Prevertebral layer**

Investing Layer

Investing layer lies deep to the platysma, and surrounds the neck like a collar. It splits to enclose
- **Muscles**—trapezius and sternocleidomastoid;
- **Salivary glands**—parotid and submandibular.
- **Spaces**—suprasternal supraclavicular
- **Forms pulleys for** digastric and omohyoid

Pretracheal Fascia

Its importance is that it encloses and suspends the thyroid gland and forms its false capsule on either side forms "**Ligament of Berry**"

Prevertebral Fascia

It covers the anterior vertebral muscles and forms the floor of the posterior triangle of the neck.

The cervical and brachial plexuses lie behind the prevertebral fascia. As the subclavian artery and the brachial plexus emerge from behind scalenus anterior, they carry the prevertebral fascia downwards and laterally as the **axillary sheath.**

Carotid Sheath

It is a condensation of deep cervical fascia around the
- **Common and internal carotid arteries**
- **Internal jugular vein**
- **Vagus nerve.**

The external carotid artery lies outside the sheath.

The structures palpable anteriorly in the midline of the neck
- **Body of hyoid bone**
- **Adam's apple (thyroid cartilage)**
- **Arch of cricoids cartilage**

- Tracheal ring
- Isthmus of thyroid gland
- Suprasternal notch

Platysma: It is a **subcutaneous muscle** forming a thin fleshy sheath running upwards and medially on the neck from deltoid and pectoral fasciae to the base of mandible. Functions: (a) Helps in releasing pressure of the skin on superficial veins and (b) pulls the angle of mouth downwards.

Jugular arch: A transverse channel in the suprasternal space connecting the two anterior jugular veins.

Position of subhyoid bursa—its function.

Position: Between posterior surface of body of hyoid bone and thyrohyoid membrane.

Function: Lessens friction between above two structures during swallowing.

The contents of suprasternal space of Burns are:

- Sternal head of sternomastoid
- Jugular venous arch
- Interclavicular ligament
- Lymph node.

The structures traversing supraclavicular space are:

- External jugular vein
- Supraclavicular nerves
- Cutaneous vessels
- Lymphatics.

The contents of carotid sheath are:

- Common carotid artery
- Internal carotid artery
- Internal jugular vein
- Vagus nerve.

The boundaries of anterior triangle of neck

- Anterior: Anterior median line of neck
- Posterior: Anterior border of sternomastoid
- Base: Base of mandible and a line joining angle of mandible to mastoid process.
- Apex: Manubrium sterni.

The subdivisions of anterior triangle

✓ Submental
✓ Digastrics
✓ Carotid
✓ Muscular triangle.

The boundaries of digastric triangle

✓ Anteroinferiorly: Anterior belly of digastrics

✓ Posteroinferiorly: Posterior belly of digastrics stylohyoid.
✓ Base: Base of mandible and a line joining angle of mandible to mastoid process.
✓ Roof: Skin
✓ Superficial facia: It has platysma and cervical branch of facial nerve.
✓ Deep fascia: Splits to enclose submandibular gland.
✓ Floor: Mylohyoid, hyoglossus and Middle constrictor muscle.

Areas drained by submental lymph nodes
✓ Superficial tissues below the chin.
✓ Central part of lower tip and the adjoining gum.
✓ Anterior part of floor of mouth
✓ Tip of tongue.

Areas drained by submandibular lymph nodes
✓ Centre of forehead
✓ Nose with frontal maxillary and ethmoidal air sinuses.
✓ Inner canthus of eye.
✓ Upper lip and anterior part of cheek with underlying gum and teeth.
✓ Outer part of lower lip with lower gum and teeth.
✓ Anterior 2/3 of tongue (excluding tip)
✓ Floor of mouth
✓ Efferents from submental nodes

The structures passing between external and internal carotid arteries.
✓ Styloglossus
✓ Stylopharyngeus
✓ Glossopharyngeal nerve
✓ Pharyngeal branch of vagus nerve
✓ Styloid process
✓ Part of parotid gland.

The Carotid Triangle
Superiorly: Posterior belly of digastrics, stylohyoid
Anteroinferiorly: Superior belly of omohyoid
Posteriorly: Anterior border if sternomastoid.

Roof:
• Skin
• Superficial fascia having
• Platysma
• Cervical branch of facial nerve
• Transverse cutaneous nerve of neck.
• Investing layer **of deep fascia.**

Floor:

- Thyrohyoid
- Middle constrictor
- Inferior constrictor.

The contents of carotid triangle

(a) Arteries:

- Common carotid
- Internal carotid
- External carotid.

(b) Veins:

- Internal jugular
- Common facial
- Pharyngeal
- Lingual
- Superior thyroid.

(c) Nerves:

- Vagus
- Superior laryngeal
- Hypoglossal
- Sympathetic chain.

(d) Carotid sheath with its contents

(e) Deep cervical lymph nodes.

Carotid Sinus

- Position: At termination of common carotid artery as slight dilatation.
- Characteristics: Media thin, Adventitia thick,
- Rich innervations by gloss pharyngeal and sympathetic.
- Function: as a baroreceptor helps to regulate blood pressure.

Carotid Body

- It is a 3 to 4 mm pinkish gray structure located near the common carotid bifurcation.
- Normally, the cells of the carotid body sense changes in pCO_2, and pH.

External Carotid Artery (Branches)

It is a branch of common carotid artery. Named so as it lies external to carotid sheath. Branches are:

✓ Anteriorly: Superior thyroid, lingual and facial

✓ Posteriorly: Occipital and posterior auricular

✓ Medial: Ascending pharyngeal

✓ Terminal: Maxillary and superficial temporal.

Ansa Cervicalis

It is a thin loop if nerves formed by C1, 2, 3 that lies embedded in the anterior wall if carotid sheath.

It supplies infrahyoid muscles.

Infrahyoid muscles are:

- ✓ Sternohyoid
- ✓ Sternothyroid
- ✓ Thyrohyoid
- ✓ Omohyoid

Suprahyoid muscles

- ✓ Mylohyoid
- ✓ Digastrics
- ✓ Stylohyoid
- ✓ Geniohyoid

Suboccipital Triangle

The boundaries of suboccipital triangle are:

- Superomedially: Rectus capitis posterior major, rectus capitis posterior minor
- Superolaterally: Superior oblique
- Inferiorly: Inferior oblique.

Roof:
Medially: Fibrous tissue
Laterally: Longissimus capitis.

Floor:
Posterior arch of atlas,
Posterior atlanto-occipital membrane.

The Contents of Suboccipital Triangle

- Third part of vertebral artery
- Dorsal ramus of C1
- Suboccipital plexus of veins.

The boundaries of posterior triangle

- ✓ Anterior: Posterior border of sternomastoid.
- ✓ Posterior: Anterior border of trapezius.
- ✓ Base: Middle 1/3 of clavicle.
- ✓ Apex: Point where trapezius and sternomastoid meet.
- ✓ Roof: Investing layer of deep cervical fascia.
- ✓ Floor: Prevertebral layer of deep cervical fascia covering the muscles.

Structures present in floor of posterior triangle below deep cervical fascia
- Semispinalis capitis
- Splenius capitis
- Levator scapulae
- Scalenus posterior
- Scalenus medius
- First rib
- First digitation of serratus anterior.

Thyroid Gland

The situation of thyroid lies in front and sides of lower part of neck.

The Extent of Thyroid

1. C5, 6, 7 T1 verbebrae
2. Middle of thyroid cartilage to fourth tracheal ring.

The Capsules of Thyroid

True capsule: Condensation of connective tissue of gland
False capsule: From pretracheal fascia.

The thyroid is removed along with true capsule to avoid haemorrhage because the capillary plexus is present deep to true capsule.

Isthmus and its Relations

It is part of thyroid gland connecting two thyroid lobes in lower part.
Extent: Lies against II and III tracheal ring.
Relations:
Anterior surface:
- Strenothyroid
- Sternohyoids
- Anterior jugular veins
- Fascia
- Skin

Posterior surface: II and III tracheal ring
Upper border: Anastomosis between superior thyroid arteries
Lower border: Inferior thyroid veins leave gland

The Arterial Supply of Thyroid: Very Vascular

- Superior thyroid artery: Supplies upper 1/3 of lobes and upper ½ of isthmus.
- Inferior thyroid artery: Supplies lower 2/3 of lobes and lower ½ of isthmus.
- Sometimes, lowest thyroid artery.
- Accessory thyroid arteries: From vessels to oesophagus and trachea

The venous drainage of thyroid
- Superior thyroid vein
- Middle thyroid vein
- Inferior thyroid vein
- Sometimes, fourth thyroid vein (of Kocher)

Goitre: It is any enlargement of the thyroid gland

In partial thyroidectomy the posterior part of lobes are left behind

(a) To avoid risk of removal of parathyroids

(b) To avoid postoperative myxoedema

Thyroid moves with deglutition. Because thyroid is attached to the larynx (cricoid cartilage) by the suspensory ligament of Berry.

The precautions to the taken during thyroidectomy

1. Ligate superior thyroid artery near gland to avoid injury to external laryngeal nerve
2. Ligate inferior thyroid artery away from gland to save recurrent laryngeal nerve

Thyroid Development

Immediately behind tuberculum impar (a midline swelling in mandibular arches) in floor of pharynx a diverticulum called thyroglossal duct develops, which grows down into neck and its tip bifurcates and proliferates to form thyroid gland.

The developing thyroid also fuses with caudal pharyngeal complex.

The common anomalies of thyroid
- Pyramidal lobe present
- Isthmus may be absent
- One of the lobes may be absent
- Thyroid gland may be found in abnormal position, i.e. any where in its path of descent, e.g. in tongue, above or below hyoid.
- Thyroglossal duct may persist and lead to the formation of thyroglossal cysts and fistula.

Parathyroid Glands

- **The number of parathyroid glands—four:** Two superior and two inferior
- **The position** of parathyroid glands: Superior parathyroids: usually lies at middle of posterior border of lobe of thyroid above the level at which inferior thyroid artery crosses recurrent laryngeal nerve.
- Inferior parathyroids: Usually below inferior thyroid artery near lower pole of thyroid lobe.
- **Parathyroids are developed:**
- Superior parathyroids: From endoderm of fourth pharyngeal pouch.
- Inferior parathyroids: From endoderm of third pharyngeal pouch.

- The inferior parathyroids are carried down by the descending thymus, while superior parathyroids are prevented from going down because of its close relationship to thyroid.

The Pituitary Gland

- The average adult pituitary measures $10 \times 15 \times 5$ mm and weighs between 0.4 and 0.9 gm.
- The gland is **oval, bilaterally symmetrical, and brownish red.**
- Lies within the **sella turcica of Pituitary fossa.**
- This fossa is bordered anteriorly, posteriorly, and inferiorly by the sphenoid bone and laterally by the cavernous sinus.
- The floor of the sella forms the roof of the sphenoidal sinus. The diaphragma sellae, a thick reflection of dura mater, covers the roof of the sella.

Blood Supply

- **The inferior hypophyseal artery**
- **The superior hypophyseal artery**

Pituitary apoplexy. Pituitary apoplexy follows sudden hemorrhage into or infarction of a pituitary tumor.

Sheehan's syndrome. Pituitary necrosis may occur rarely after postpartum hemorrhage and hypovolemia. The degree of subsequent hypopituitarism reflects the extent of pituitary necrosis.

Sternocleidomastoid

The origin of sternomastoid
(a) Sterna head: From superolateral part of front of manubrium sterni
(b) Clavicular head: Medial 1/3 of superior surface of clavicle.

The nerve supply of sternomastoid
- **Motor: Spinal accessory nerve**
- **Sensory: Ventral rami of C2, 3.**

Torticollis: Also known as **Wryneck.** The head is bent to one side and chin points to the other side. It occurs due to **spasm of muscles supplied by spinal accessory nerve.** Sternomastoid and trapezius. Torticollis occurs more commonly following **breech delivery and may be associated with eventration of the diaphragm and Erb's palsy** on the same side. The clinical presentation includes a **hard mass within the sternocleidomastoid muscle, ipsilateral facial hemihypoplasia,** head turned away from the side of the mass, and, occasionally, ipsilateral trapezius atrophy.

Mouth
The divisions of oral cavity
1. Vestibule
2. Oral cavity proper.

The boundaries of vestibule

External: Lips and cheeks

Internal: Teeth and gums

Frenulum of lip is formed: It is formed by a median fold of mucous membrane between lips and gums.

The lymphatic drainage of lips: Central part of lower lip drains into submental nodes and rest of lip to submandibular nodes.

The boundaries of oropharyngeal isthmus (isthmus of fauces)

Superior: Soft palate

Inferior: Tongue

On each side: Palatoglossal arches.

Diphyodont teeth: Two sets of teeth are present

First dentition: Milk or deciduous teeth

Second set: Permanent teeth.

The dental formula for deciduous teeth: Incisor 2/2, canine 1/1, premolar 2/2

Total no 20.

The dental formula for permanent teeth: Incisor 2/2, canine 1/1, premolar 2/2, molar 3/3

Total no. 32

The parts of a tooth

• Crown: Projecting above gum.

• Root: Embedded in jaw beneath the gum.

• Neck: Between crown and root.

Salivary Glands

1. Parotid
2. Submandibular
3. Sublingual
4. Small glands in tongue, palate, cheeks and lips.

Parotid Gland

The position of parotid glands: Between ramus of mandible and sternomastoid below the external acoustic meatus.

The attachments of parotid capsule:

✓ It is formed by splitting of investing layer of deep cervical fascia between angle of mandible and mastoid process.

✓ Superficial lamina: Attached above to zygomatic arch.

✓ Deep lamina: To styloid process, mandible and tympanic plate.

✓ Also forms stylomandibular ligament.

The structure within the parotid gland

- Facial nerve: Enters through posteromedial surface and divides into branches which emerge from anteromedial surface.
- External carotid artery: Enters through posteromedial surface and divide into branches.
- Retromandibular vein: Formed within parotid gland by superficial temporal and maxillary veins.

The branches of external carotid artery within the parotid gland.

✓ Posterior auricular artery

✓ Superficial temporal

✓ Maxillary.

The structures pierced by parotid duct

- Buccal pad of fat
- Buccopharyngeal fascia
- Buccinators muscle.

The parotid duct opens: In vestibule of mouth opposite the crown of upper second molar tooth.

The nerves supplying the parotid gland

- Parasympathetic nerve through auriculotemporal nerve: Secretomotor.
- Sympathetic nerved from plexus around ECA: Vasomotor.
- Auriculotemporal nerve: Sensory.
- Greater auricular nerve (C2 fibres): Sensory for parotid fascia.

The parotid swellings are painful: Because the parotid fascia is very dense and unyielding. Therefore, it cannot stretch on parotid swelling and causes increased tension beneath fascia.

Parotid gland is removed surgically: In two parts—superficial and deep, in order to preserve the facial nerve.

Frey syndrome/Baillarger's syndrome: is due to abnormal and inappropriate regeneration auriculotemporal branch of trigeminal nerve there is rednesss, sweating especially on cheeks while eating, talking (gustatory sweating).

Submandibular and Sublingual Glands

The position of submandibular gland: Anterior parts of digastric triangle

The parts of submandibular gland

- Superficial part: Large and superficial to mylohyoid
- Deep part: Small and deep to mylohyoid
- The two parts are continuous round the posterior border of mylohyoid.

The opening of submandibular duct: In the floor of mouth, on the summit of sublingual papilla, at the side of frenulum of tongue.

The nerve supply of submandibular gland.
- Secretomotor: Chorda tympani.
- Sensory: Lingual nerve.
- Vasomotor: Sympathetic fibres from plexus on facial artery.

The nature of submandibular gland: Mixed, but predominantly serous.

The nature of sublingual gland: Mixed, but predominantly mucous.

The ducts of sublingual gland upon: About 15 ducts which open on summit of sublingual fold in floor of mouth.

The developmental origin of salivary glands: Arise as an ectodermal outgrowth from buccal epithelium in relation to line along which maxillary and mandibular processes fuse, i.e. just lateral to angle of mouth to form cheek.

Sublingual and submandibular glands are endodermal in origin, arising in relation to linguo-gingival sulcus.

TEMPOROMANDIBULAR JOINT (JAW JOINT)

Type of joint: Condylar variety of synovial joint.

The Ligaments of TM Joint
- Fibrous capsule
- Articular disc
- Lateral ligament
- Sphenomandibular ligament
- Stylomandibular ligament

The characteristic features of articular disc
- It divides joint into an upper and a lower compartment.
- It has a concavoconvex superior surface and a concave inferior surface
- It has five parts:
  1. Anterior extension
  2. Anterior band
  3. Intermediate thin zone
  4. Thick posterior band
  5. Posterior bilaminar region

The developmental origin of sphenomandibular ligament: It is remnant of dorsal (cephalic) end of Meckel's cartilage

The structures piercing sphenomandibular ligament: Mylohyoid nerve and vessels.

The nerve supply of TM joint
- Auriculotemporal nerve
- Masseteric nerve

The muscles of TM joint (muscles of mastication)
• Masseter
• Temporalis
• Lateral pterygoid
• Medial pterygoid

The developmental origin of muscles of mastication: **Mesoderm of first branchial arch**

The structures passing between two heads of lateral pterygoid
1. Maxillary artery
2. Buccal branch of mandibular nerve

The movements of TM joints
1. Depression of jaw (opening of mouth)
2. Elevation of jaw
3. Protrusion
4. Retraction
5. Rotatory movements (chewing)

Muscles Producing Movements of TM Joint

• Depression: Lateral pterygoid of both sides.
• Elevation: Masseter, temporalis and medial pterygoid of both sides
• Protrusion: Lateral and medial pterygoids
• Retraction: Posterior fibres of temporalis
• Chewing: Medial and lateral pterygoids of each side acting alternately.

The Styloid Apparatus

Consists of the styloid process and the attachments on it
Muscles:
• Styloglossus
• Stylohyoid
• Stylopharyngeus

Ligaments
• Stylohyoid
• Stylomandibular

The relations of styloid process:
• Laterally: Parotid gland
• Medially: Internal jugular vein
• Base: Ensheathed by tympanic plate
• Related to facial nerve
• Apex: Posterior border of ramus of mandible laterally.

An abnormally elongated styloid process causes **Eagle's syndrome**

TONGUE

The parts of tongue
- Anterior 2/3: Oral part
- Posterior 2/3: Pharyngeal part. At junction is a V-shaped groove, sulcus terminalis, with a median pit, foramen caecum.

Papillae and their types: Papillae are projections of mucous membrane situated in anterior 2/3 of tongue.

Types:
- Vallate papillae: 8–12 in number.
  - o Situated immediately in front of sulcus terminalis. Each is a cylindrical projection surrounded by a circular sulcus.
- Fungiform papillae: Numerous
  - o Near tip and margins of tongue.
  - o Each has a narrow pedicle and large rounded head.
- Filiform papillae: Most numerous.
  - o Covers presulcul area of dorsum of tongue pointed and covered with keratin.

The muscles of tongue: Tongue is divided into two halves by a midline fibrous septum. Each half has:

Four intrinsic muscles.
1. Superior longitudinal
2. Inferior longitudinal
3. Transverse
4. Vertical

Four extrinsic muscles.
1. Genioglossus
2. Hyoglossus
3. Styloglossus
4. Palatoglossus.

The lymphatic drainage of tongue
- Tip of tongue: Submental nodes
- Rest of anterior 2/3: Submandibular nodes.
- Posterior 1/3: jugulo-omohyoid node.

Jugulo-omohyoid node is called lymph node of tongue: Because it drains most of the lymph from the tongue.

The Nerve Supply of Tongue

Motor nerves:
- All muscles except palatoglossus: Hypoglossal nerve.
- Palatoglossus: Cranial part of accessory nerve.

5

Sensory:
- Anterior 2/3: (i) Lingual nerve: General sensory. Chorda tympani: Special sensory.
- Posterior 1/3: Glossopharyngeal nerve: General and special sensory.
- Posterior most part: Vagus (internal laryngeal).

The functions of tongue
- Taste
- Speech
- Mastication
- Deglutition.

The taste buds are situated
1. Vallate papillae: Most numerous on sides of papillae.
2. Foliate papillae
3. Posterior 1/3 of tongue.

The tongue is developed
- Anterior 2/3: First branchial arch: Two lingual swellings and one tuberculum impar.
- Posterior 1/3: Third arch: Cranial half of hypobranchial eminence.
- Posterior part: Fourth arch.
- Muscles: Occipital myotomes.
- Connective tissue: Local mesenchyme.

Foramen caecum represents: The site of down growth of thyroglossal duct

The clinical importance of attachment of genioglossus to the genial tubercles of mandible: In unconscious patient or during general anaesthesia, the tongue may fall back and obstruct the respiratory passage. So, the advantage of this attachment is taken by pulling the mandible forwards which prevents the falling back of tongue.

The developmental anomalies of tongue
- Macroglossia: Large tongue.
- Microglossia: Small tongue.
- Bifid tongue: Non fusion of two lingual swellings.
- Surface of the tongue may be fissured.
- Ankyloglossia or Tie tongue.

PALATE

The muscles of soft palate
- Tensor palate
- Levator palate
- Musculus uvulae

- Palatoglossus
- Palatopharyngeus

The arterial supply of soft palate
- Greater palatine branch of maxillary
- Ascending palatine branch of maxillary
- Palatine branch of ascending pharyngeal

The nerve supply of soft palate

Motor nerves:
- Tensor palate: Mandibular nerve
- Other muscles: Pharyngeal plexus (cranial part of accessory through vagus).

General sensory nerves:
- Middle and lesser palatine nerves
- Glossopharyngeal nerve.
  - Lesser palatine nerve.
  - Secretomotor:
  - Lesser palatine nerve.

The functions of soft palate: It controls the opening of the pharyngeal and oropharyngeal isthmus, during chewing, coughing, sneezing, speech and swallowing.

Passavant's muscle: It consists of horizontal fibres of palatopharyngeus at the level of hard palate, which meet with those of opposite side. These contract and form a passavant's ridge.

Palate develops By
✓ Two palatal processes of maxillary process
✓ Frontonasal process, which fuse.

The mesoderm of palate undergoes intra-membranous ossification to form the hard palate. But, the ossification does not extend into posterior most portion, which remains as soft palate.

Cleft palate: This results from defective fusion of various components of palate. It results in communication between mouth and nose.

Otic ganglion: This is a small, oval, flat reddish-grey ganglion situated just below the foramen ovale. It is a peripheral parasympathetic ganglion related topographically to the mandibular nerve, but connected functionally with the glossopharyngeal nerve.

The ciliary ganglion: It is a parasympathetic ganglion which is concerned functionally with the motor innervation of certain intraocular muscles. It is a small, flat, reddish-grey swelling, 1–2 mm in diameter, connected to the nasociliary nerve, and located near the apex of the orbit in loose fat. It lies between the optic nerve and lateral rectus, usually lateral to the ophthalmic artery.

Pterygopalatine ganglion: The pterygopalatine ganglion is the largest of the peripheral parasympathetic ganglia. It is placed deeply in the pterygopalatine fossa, near the sphenopalatine foramen, and anterior to the pterygoid canal and foramen rotundum. It is flattened, reddish-grey in colour, and lies just below the maxillary nerve as it crosses the pterygopalatine fossa. The majority of the 'branches' of the ganglion are connected with it morphologically, but not functionally, because they are primarily sensory branches of the maxillary nerve.

PHARYNX

Length of pharynx: 12 cm
The extent of pharynx
Superiorly: Base of skull including posterior part of body of sphenoid and basilar part of occipital bone.
Inferiorly: C6 vertebra or lower border of cricoids cartilage.

The Attachments of Pharynx on Each Side

✓ Medial pterygoid plate
✓ Pterygomandibular raphe
✓ Mandible
✓ Tongue
✓ Hyoid bone
✓ Thyroid and cricoids cartilages

The parts of pharynx
• Nasopharynx
• Oropharynx
• Laryngopharynx

The characteristic features of nasopharynx
1. Respiratory in function
2. Walls are rigid and non-collapsible.
3. Lined by columnar ciliated epithelium.

The features of lateral wall of nasopharynx
• Pharyngeal opening of auditory tube
• Tubal elevation around the opening
• Salpingopharyngeal fold
• Levator palati fold
• Pharyngeal recess

The clinical importance of pharyngeal recess (fossa of Rosenmüller): It forms a flat pocket. A catheter missing the bubal opening may enter recess and perforate the pharyngobasilar fascia and enter the ICA (internal carotid artery).

Tornwaldt's cyst: Cysts occasionally form in the region of the medial recess of the nasopharynx. These cysts become symptomatic when they become infected. There may be persistent purulent drainage that has a foul taste and odor.

Juvenile angiofibromas: These are vascular neoplasms that occur in pubescent males. They develop in the vault of the nasopharynx from the area of the basis sphenoid and grow to a large size. Angiofibromas may extend into and obstruct the nasal cavity

Malignant neoplasms of the nasopharynx: Malignant neoplasms of the nasopharynx include squamous cell carcinomas, adenocarcinomas, adenoid cystic carcinomas, mucoepidermoid carcinomas

Structures form the junction of nasopharynx
1. Lower border of soft palate
2. Passavant's muscle.

Isthmus of fauces: Also known as oropharyngeal isthmus and it represents the junction of oropharynx and oral cavity.

The junction of oropharynx and laryngopharynx lie at upper border of epiglottis

The position of Piriform fossa: It is present on each side of inlet of larynx. The fossa is bounded medially by aryepiglottic fold and laterally by thyroid cartilage and thyrohyoid membrane.

Beneath mucosa of fossa lie internal laryngeal nerve.

The Clinical Importance of Piriform Fossa

A foreign body may lodge here. If removed damage to internal laryngeal nerve may occur leading to anaesthesia in supraglottic part of larynx. Thus, leading to aspiration pneumonia.

The Different Layers Forming Wall of Pharynx

- Mucosa: lined by squamous epithelium except nasopharynx.
- Submucosa
- Pharyngobasilar fascia: Fibrous sheath
- Muscular coat: It has outer circular layer and inner longitudinal layer.
- Buccopharyngeal fascia.

The muscles of pharynx
Longitudinal layer:
- Stylopharyngeus
- Salpingopharyngeus
- Palatopharyngeus

Circular layer:
- Superior constrictor
- Middle constrictor
- Inferior constrictor

The nerve supply of the pharynx

Motor fibres:

(a) Stylopharyngeus: Glossopharyngeal, nerve.

(b) Other muscles: Cranial accessory through vagus.

(c) Inferior constrictor: Also by external and recurrent laryngeal nerves.

Sensory:

  Glossopharyngeal and vagus

  Nasopharynx: Maxillary nerve.

Taste: Internal laryngeal branch of vagus.

Secretomotor: Greater petrosal nerve.

Pharyngeal Plexus

It is a plexus of nerve, present beneath the buccopharyngeal fascia.
Formed by:

✓ Pharyngeal branch of vagus (cranial accessory fibres)

✓ Pharyngeal branches of glossopharyngeal

✓ Pharyngeal branches of superior cervical sympathetic ganglion.

The Arrangement of Constrictors of Pharynx

These are arranged like three flower pots one above the other, the lower constrictor overlapping the upper one.

Sinus of Morgagni

It is a semilunar gap between base of skull and upper border of superior constrictor.

The structures passing through sinus of Morgagni

1. Auditory tube
2. Levator palate muscle
3. Ascending palatine artery

The structures passing through gap of superior and middle constrictor

1. Glossopharyngeal nerve
2. Stylopharyngeus

The structures passing between middle and inferior constrictor

1. Internal laryngeal nerve
2. Superior laryngeal vessels

The structures passing through gap between inferior constrictor and oesophagus

1. Recurrent laryngeal nerve
2. Inferior laryngeal vessels.

Parapharyngeal abscess: Parapharyngeal abscess may occur in infants and young children as well as in adults. The abscess is usually secondary to streptococcal pharyngitis or tonsillitis. Pus forms in the parapharyngeal space secondarily from the breakdown of lymphadenitis. The pus is located lateral to the superior constrictor of the pharynx and adjacent to the carotid sheath.

5

Head and Neck

Retropharyngeal abscess: Retropharyngeal abscess occurs in infants and young children. These infections are located between the constrictors of the pharynx and the prevertebral fascia. They are secondary to pharyngitis and are due to the breakdown of retropharyngeal lymphadenitis. Infants with retropharyngeal abscesses usually present with stridor and hyperextension of the neck.

Killians dehiscence: This is a weak part in posterior wall of pharynx, just below the level of vocal cords. It is formed because lower part of thyropharyngeus is not overlapped internally by upper and middle constrictors.

The clinical importance of Killians dehiscence: Pharyngeal diverticula may be formed due to out-pouching of dehiscence.

Petrosal Nerves

- **Greater petrosal nerve** is a branch of facial nerve and is parasympathetic to lacrimal glands, glands of pharynx and nose (injury causes absence of lacrimation).
- **Lesser petrosal nerve** is a branch of glossophayngeal nerve and is parasympathetic to parotid gland.
- **Deep petrosal nerve** is a branch of plexus around internal carotid artery and joins greater petrosal nerve to form nerve of pterygoid canal (vidian nerve)
- **External petrosal nerve** is a branch of sympathetic plexus around middle meningeal artery.
- **Greater petrosal nerve + Deep petrosal nerve = Nerve of pterygoid canal (vidian nerve)**
- Parasympathetic secretomotor fibres to parotid traverse through: **Tympanic plexus/Lesser petrosal nerve.**

5

TONSIL

Tonsil occupies tonsillar fossa between diverging palatoglossal and palatopharyngeal arches.

The structures forming tonsillar bed
- Pharyngobasilar fascia
- Superior constrictor and palatopharyngeus muscle
- Buccopharyngeal fascia
- In lower part, styloglossus and 9th cranial nerve.

Waldeyer's ring
It is a lymphatic ring which guards entry to digestive and respiratory passages.
It is formed by four masses of lymphoid tissue
- 2 palatine tonsils
- 1 pharyngeal tonsil
- 1 lingual tonsil.

These are connected together by scattered lymphoid tissue

Adenoid

Pathological enlargement of nasopharyngeal tonsil.

The arterial supply of tonsil
- Tonsillar branch of facial
- Ascending palatine branch of lingual
- Dorsal lingual branch of external carotid
- Ascending pharyngeal branch of external carotid
- Greater palatine branch of maxillary

The Lymphatic Drainage of Tonsils: Jugulodigastric Node

How haemorrhage after tosnsillectomy is checked: By removal of clot from the raw bed

Tonsillitis causes referred pain in the ear: Because of the common nerve supply, i.e. by glossopharyngeal (IX Cranial) nerve.

Peritonsillar abscess: Peritonsillar cellulitis and abscess are complications of acute tonsillitis in which the infection has spread deep to the tonsillar capsule. Pus forms between the tonsillar capsule and the superior constrictor of the pharynx, and the tonsil is displaced medially. The uvula becomes tremendously edematous and is displaced to the opposite side. The soft palate is very red and displaced forward. There is marked trismus due to irritation of the pterygoid muscles, and the head is held tilted toward the side of the abscess

Palatine tonsil develops: These develop in relation to lateral part of second pharyngeal pouch by endodermal proliferation and lymphocyte collection.

LARYNX

The skeleton of the larynx consists of the thyroid cartilage, the cricoid cartilage, the arytenoid cartilages with corniculate and cuneiform cartilages, and the epiglottis.

From root of tongue to trachea. In front of C 3–5 vertebra.

The cartilages forming the skeletal framework of larynx
Unpaired:
- Thyroid
- Cricoids
- Epiglottic

Paired:
- Arytenoids
- Corniculate
- Cuneiform.

Adam's apple: Also called laryngeal prominence. It is formed by fusion of anterior borders of lamina of thyroid cartilage.

It is more prominent in males.

The structures attached to oblique line of thyroid cartilage

- Sternohyoid
- Thyrohyoid
- Inferior constrictor

The histological type of laryngeal cartilages: thyroid, cricoids and bases of arytenoids: Hyaline. Ossify after 25 years of age.

Rest: Fibrocartilage. Never ossify.

Different Laryngeal Joints and what are their Movements

- Cricothyroid joint: Synovial joint.
  - o Between inferior cornu of thyroid cartilage and side of cricoids.
  - o Rotatory movements around transverse axis and gliding movements.
- Cricoarytenoid joint: Synovial joint.
  - o Between base of arytenoids and upper border of cricoids. Rotatory movements around a vertical axis and gliding movements.

Laryngeal ligaments and membranes

- Extrinsic; thyrohyoid membrane
- Hyoepiglottic ligament
- Cricotracheal ligament.
- Intrinsic: Quadrate membrane and conus elasticus.

The Boundaries of Inlet of Larynx

- Anterior; epiglottis
- Posterior: inter-arytenoid fold of mucous membrane
- On each side: Aryepiglottic fold.

The parts of larynx

1. Vestibule of larynx
2. Sinus of larynx
3. Infraglottic part.

The characteristic feature of laryngeal mucous membrane

- Anterior surface and upper ½ of the posterior surface of epiglottis, upper parts of aryepiglottic folds and vocal folds are lined by stratified squamous epithelium. Rest of laryngeal mucosus membrane is covered with columnar ciliated epithelium.
- Mucous membrane is loosely attached except to vocal ligament and posterior surface of epiglottis
- Mucous glands are absent over vocal cord.

The intrinsic muscles of larynx

- Cricothyroid

- Posterior cricoarytenoid
- Lateral cricoarytenoid
- Transverse arytenoids
- Oblique arytenoids
- Epiglottic
- Thyroarytenoid
- Vocalis
- Thyroepiglottic

The nerve supply of larynx

(a) Motor:
- Cricothyroid: External laryngeal nerve
- Other intrinsic muscles: Recurrent laryngeal nerve

(b) Sensory:
- Mucous membrane up to vocal cord : Internal laryngeal nerve.
- Mucous membrane below vocal cord: Recurrent laryngeal nerve.

The effect of lesion of external laryngeal nerve: Weakness of phonation due to loss of tightening effect of cricothyroid on vocal cord.

The effect of lesion of internal laryngeal nerve: Anaesthesia of the mucous membrane in supraglottic part of larynx, so the foreign bodies can readily enter larynx.

The effect of lesion of recurrent laryngeal nerve

(a) When bilateral: Complete loss of phonation difficulty in breathing. Vocal cords lie in between adduction and abduction.

(b) When unilateral: Phonation possible because opposite vocal cord compensates.

The larynx serves as the sounding source for speech. A fundamental tone is produced by the movement of the vocal cords, which is brought about by the flow of exhaled air past lightly approximated vocal cords.

- The internal laryngeal nerve is sensory to larynx above vocal cords.
- The recurrent laryngeal nerve is sensory to larynx below vocal cords.
- All muscles of larynx except cricothyroid are supplied by Recurrent laryngeal nerve.
- Cricothyroid is supplied by external laryngeal nerve.

Muscles and their Actions

- **Abductor of vocal cords:** Posterior cricoarytenoid
- **Adductor of vocal cords:** Lateral cricoarytenoid, Transverse arytenoids, Cricothyroid thyroarytenoid
- **Tensor of vocal cords:**   Cricothyroid
- **Relaxor of vocal cords:**   Thyroarytenoids, vocalis

Semon's law: In progressive lesions of recurrent laryngeal nerve, abductors of vocal cord are first to be paralysed and last to recover, as compared to adductors. But in functional paralysis of larynx, adductors are first paralysed.

Oedema of larynx causes suffocation: Because tissue fluid cannot move downwards due to firm attachment of mucous membrane to vocal ligament and thus, causing obstruction.

The primary function of the larynx is that of a sphincter. During deglutition, both the true vocal cord sphincter and the false vocal cord sphincter are closed, and the epiglottis is drawn posteriorly over the closed sphincter and serves as a watershed, deflecting food and fluid into the pyriform sinuses. The larynx also serves as a sphincter during parturition, coughing, and defecation.

Laryngoceles: These are epithelium-lined diverticula of the laryngeal ventricle and may be located internal or external to the laryngeal skeleton. An internal laryngocele may displace and enlarge the false vocal cord and may cause hoarseness and airway obstruction. External laryngoceles pass through the thyrohyoid membrane and present as a mass in the neck over the thyrohyoid membrane

Vocal nodules: Vocal nodules are caused by using a fundamental frequency that is unnaturally low and using the voice too loudly and too long.

Vocal cord paralysis: follows traumatic, infectious, and neoplastic involvement of the vagus and recurrent laryngeal nerves and degenerative neurologic disorders. Unilateral vocal cord paralysis produces hoarseness and aspiration. Bilateral vocal cord paralysis causes upper airway obstruction with little adverse effect on the voice

Foreign bodies: These are retained in the larynx because they are sharp and stick into the mucous membrane or are irregular and soft and are caught between the two vocal cords in laryngospasm. A frequently fatal laryngeal foreign body is a bolus of meat. The resulting laryngospasm completely occludes the larynx and makes a choking person mute.

EAR

The parts of external ear
- **Auricle (pinna)**
- **External acoustic meatus**

The nerve supply of auricle

Lateral surface:
- **Upper 2/3: Auriculotemporal (branch of mandibular division of trigeminal nerve)**
- **Lower 1/3: Greater auricular (C2, 3)**

Medial surface:
- **Upper 2/3: Lesser occipital (C2)**
- **Lower 1/3: Greater auricular (C2, 3)**

Root: Auricular branch of vagus.

(ii) Motor:

To auricular muscles: Facial nerve.

The Parts of External Acoustic Meatus

(a) Pars externa

(b) Pars media

(c) Pars interna

Ceruminous glands: These are modified sweat glands in skin of external acoustic meatus. Secrete yellow-brown ear wax.

Sometimes syringing of ear produces sudden death

Due to irritation of auricular branch of vagus, reflex cardiac inhibition occurs leading to death.

The pain of external ear radiate to temporomandibular joint and teeth of lower jaw: Because all these structures are supplied by the branches of mandibular nerve (branch of trigeminal nerve)

Tympanic membrane: It is a thin membranous partition between external and middle ear.

The parts of tympanic membrane
- Pars flaccida: Small triangular area above malleolar folds.
- Pars tensa: Greater part of membrane below malleolar folds.

The infections of external ear are very painful: Because the skin is firmly adherent to the underlying bone and cartilage, so the little swelling due to infection causes pain.

Umbo: It is point of maximum convexity on inner surface of tympanic membrane, at the tip of handle of malleus.

The position of middle ear: It is narrow air space situated in the petrous part of temporal bone between the external and internal ears.

The Communications of Middle Ear

Anterior: Nasopharynx through auditory tube

Posterior: Mastoid antrum through aditus antrum.

The contents of middle ear

(a) Ear ossicles: Malleus, incus and stapes

(b) Ligaments of ear ossicles

(c) Muscles: Tensor tympani and stapedius

(d) vessels: Supplying and draining the middle ear

(e) Nerves: Chorda tympani and tympanic plexus.

(f) Air.

(**Remember: Chorda tympani lies** medial to spine of sphenoid. The auriculotemporal nerve also lies close to spine of sphenoid and both these nerves can get damaged in injury to spine of sphenoid.**)**

The arterial supply of middle ear

Mainly by:

(a) Anterior tympanic branch of maxillary

(b) Posterior tympanic branch of posterior auricular

Also by:

(a) Superior tympanic branch of middle meningeal

(b) Inferior tympanic from ascending pharyngeal

(c) Tympanic branch from artery of pterygoid canal.

The throat infections spread to the middle ear: Through the auditory tube

The function of auditory tube: It maintains atmospheric pressure in the middle ear cavity, thus the air pressure on the two sides of tympanic membrane are equalized

Meningitis is common in children suffering from middle ear infection

In children, roof of middle ear presents a gap at unossified petro-squamous suture where middle ear is in direct contact with the meninges.

The functions of middle ear

1. Transmission of sound waves from external to the internal ear by ear ossicles.

2. The intensity of sound waves is increased by ossicles, without any change in frequency.

The nerve supply of muscles of middle ear

(a) Tensor tympani: Mandibular nerve (branch of trigeminal nerve)

(b) Stapedius: Facial nerve

The function of muscles of middle ear

They help to damp down the intensity of high pitched sound waves and thus protect the internal ear.

The types of joints between ear ossicles

  (a) Between incus and malleus: Incudomalleolar joint: Saddle joint

  (b) Between incus and stapes: Incudostapedial joint—ball and socket joint. Both are synovial joints

The Parts of Internal Ear

The cochlea makes two and three-quarter turns in the human. A cross-section through the modiolus, or central bony framework, demonstrates in each turn the **scala vestibuli, the scala media, and the scala tympani.** The scala vestibuli is separated from the scala media by **Reissner's membrane**. The scala media is separated from the scala tympani by the **basilar membrane.** The organ of Corti, with its hair cells and their supporting cells, rests on the basilar membrane.

(a) Bony labyrinth: consists of
- Cochlea
- Vestibule
- Semicircular canals.

(b) Membranous labyrinth: consists of
- Duct of cochlea
- Utricle and saccule
- Semicircular ducts

Membranous labyrinth is filled with endolymph and is separated from bony labyrinth by perilymph.

The Functions of Internal Ear

Cochlear portion: Hearing

Vestibular part: Equilibrium

Semicircular canals act as kinetic labyrinth while utricle and saccule as static labyrinth.

The receptor cells for hearing and where they are located: The receptors are neuroepithelial hair cells situated on the organ of Corti in duct of cochlea

The receptors for equilibrium and where they are located: Receptor cells are hair cells located on macula of utricle and saccule (for static balance) and on crista of ampulla of semicircular ducts (for kinetic balance).

Blunt trauma to the pinna causes a subperichondrial hematoma: When bleeding occurs between the cartilage and the perichondrium, the pinna becomes a reddish-purple shapeless mass. Because the perichondrium carries the blood supply to the cartilage, the cartilage undergoes avascular necrosis if the hematoma is present on both sides of the cartilage, and with time the pinna becomes shriveled.

A hematoma may become organized and calcify, which produces the **cauliflower ear characteristic of wrestlers and boxers.**

Perichondritis of the pinna: Causes accumulation of pus between the perichondrium and the cartilage and leads to avascular and septic necrosis of the cartilage.

Foreign bodies in the external auditory canal: These are a common problem. Beads, erasers, beans, and other objects may be inserted by children and their siblings into their ears.

External otitis: It is infection of the ear canal.

Acute otitis media: Acute otitis media is an infectious inflammatory process in the middle ear, usually secondary to an upper respiratory tract infection. It is the most common localized infection in children.

Acute mastoiditis: In acute otitis media, the infection almost invariably extends through the mastoid antrum into the mastoid cells.

Meniere's disease: It is characterized by hearing loss, tinnitus, and recurrent prostrating vertigo. The pathologic change in the inner ear is generalized dilation of the membranous labyrinth, or endolymphatic hydrops.

Bell's palsy: It is a unilateral facial paralysis that develops suddenly and is accompanied by pain in the postauricular area. It is thought to be of viral etiology. The lesion is in the internal auditory meatus or the intratemporal course of the nerve. The initial pathologic changes are hyperemia and edema. The edema compresses the blood supply to the nerve.

Chemodectomas: Arise in the middle ear. These nonchromaffin paragangliomas are termed **glomus jugulare or glomus tympanicus tumors**, depending on their site of origin. The **glomus tympanicus tumor** arises from the area of Jacobson's nerve in the tympanic plexus on the promontory of the middle ear. **The glomus jugulare tumor** arises from the glomus jugulare body in the jugular bulb.

Acoustic neurinomas: arise from the vestibular division of the eighth nerve as from the auditory division. These neoplasms are derived from Schwann cells. Initially, they produce tinnitus and a neural hearing loss. The patient complains of unsteadiness or imbalance.

EYE

• Anteroposterior length of eyeball	• 24 mm
• Height of eyeball	• 23 mm
• Vertical length of eyeball	• 23 mm
• Circumference of eyeball	• 70 mm
• Depth of anterior chamber	• 2–3 mm
• Volume of eyeball	• 6.5 ml
• Volume of vitreous	• 4 ml
• Volume of orbit	• 30 cc.
• Diameter of macula	• 5.5 mm
• Diameter of fovea	• 1.5 mm
• Diameter of optic disc	• 1.5 mm
• Diameter of foveola	• 0.35 mm

The different layers of eye are:
• Outer or "Fibrous coat" consists of sclera and cornea
• Middle or "Vascular coat" comprises choroid, ciliary body and iris
• Inner or "Nervous coat", retina

The refractive media of eye is formed by:
From before backwards:
• Cornea
• Aqueous humour

- Lens
- Vitreous body.

Lamina fusca of sclera: It is a thin layer of delicate tissue between choroid and sclera

The structures piercing Sclera

- Optic nerve
- Ciliary nerves and arteries
- Anterior ciliary arteries
- Venae verticosae

The layers of cornea seen histologically (from before backwards)

- Corneal epithelium (stratified squamous)
- Bowman's membrane
- Substantia propria
- Descemet's membrane
- Mesothelium

The types of muscle fibres in ciliary body and their function

- **Radial fibres: Function: Relax the suspensory ligament of lens, so the lens bulges and becomes more convex for near vision**
- **Circular fibres: Function: Also relax suspensory ligament of lens.**

The nerve supply of ciliary muscle: Parasympathetic nerves through third cranial nerve

The muscles of iris

- **Sphincter papillae**
- **Dilator papillae**

The nerve supply of iris: Sympathetic nerves supply dilator papillae and parasympathetic nerves supply constrictor (sphincter) papillae.

Fovea centralis: This is the centre of macula. This is thinnest part of retina containing only cones and is the site of maximum acuity of vision.

Blind spot: It is a part of optic disc that contains no rods or cones. This is insensitive to light.

The Layers of Retina

From without inwards:

1. **Outer pigmented layer**
2. **Layer of rods and cones**
3. **External limiting membrane**
4. **Outer nuclear layer**
5. **Outer molecular layer**
6. **Inner nuclear layer (bipolar cells)**
7. **Inner molecular layer**

8. Ganglion cell layer
9. Nerve fibre layer
10. **Inner limiting membrane.**

The arterial supply of retina: Retina is supplied by an end artery, **central artery of retina.** In optic disc, it divides into branches which supplies deeper layer of retina up to bipolar cells. Rods and cones with nuclei are supplied by diffusion from capillaries.

Central retinal artery occlusion (CRAO). The central retinal artery is a branch of the ophthalmic artery, in turn a branch of the internal carotid artery. Occlusion of the central retinal artery causes sudden, usually nearly complete visual loss in one eye. Ophthalmoscopy reveals arteriolar narrowing and vascular stasis.

Central retinal vein occlusion (CRVO). The ophthalmoscopic findings of dilated, tortuous veins, extensive retinal hemorrhages, and disc swelling in one eye have classically been called a central retinal vein occlusion.

Optic atrophy: Results from death of the axons in the retina and optic nerve. A lesion anywhere from the retina through the optic tract can cause optic atrophy.

Glaucoma: It is characterized by elevated intraocular pressure damages the optic nerve. The major types of glaucoma are open-angle, angle-closure, congenital, and secondary. There is increased intraocular pressure.

Cataract: It is a lens opacity. The cataracts characteristically produce painless, gradual loss of vision. Cataracts are described according to their location, e.g. nuclear (deep in the lens), cortical (more superficial), and capsular or subcapsular (on or immediately beneath the capsule).

Important Blood Vessels of Head and Neck

The branches of subclavian vein

- **External jugular**
- **Dorsal scapular**
- **Thoracic duct on left**
- **Right lymphatic duct on right**
- **Sometimes, anterior jugular vein.**

The Branches of Internal Jugular Vein

- **Inferior petrosal sinus**
- **Common facial vein**
- **Lingual vein**
- **Pharyngeal vein**
- **Superior thyroid vein**
- **Middle thyroid vein**
- **Sometimes, occipital vein**

The branches of brachiocephalic vein

Right brachiocephalic:
- Vertebral
- Internal thoracic
- Inferior thyroid
- First posterior intercostals

Left brachiocephalic:
- Vertebral
- Internal thoracic
- Inferior thyroid
- First posterior intercostals
- Left superior intercostals
- Thymic veins
- Pericardial veins

The branches of subclavian artery
- Vertebral artery
- Internal thoracic
- Thyrocervical trunk
- Costocervical trunk
- Dorsal scapular. In 1/3 cases it arises with superficial cervical from thyrocervical trunk.

The branches of internal carotid artery

(a) Cervical part: No branches

(b) Petrous part:
- Caroticotympanic.
- Pterygoid branch.

(c) Cavernous part:
- Cavernous branches to trigeminal ganglion
- Superior hypophyseal
- Inferior hypophyseal.

(d) Cerebral part:
- Ophthalmic
- Anterior cerebral
- Middle cerebral
- Posterior communicating
- Anterior choroidal

The branches of vertebral artery

(a) Cervical branches:
- Spinal
- Muscular

(b) Cranial branches:
* Meningeal
* Posterior spinal
* Anterior spinal
* Posterior inferior cerebellar
* Medullary

The branches of maxillary artery

First part:
* Deep auricular
* Anterior tympanic
* Middle meningeal
* Accessory meningeal
* Inferior alveolar

Second part:
* Deep temporal
* Pterygoid
* Masseteric
* Buccal

Third part:
* Posterior superior alveolar
* Infraorbital
* Greater palatine
* Pharyngeal
* Artery of pterygoid canal
* Sphenopalatine

Remember Important Points about these Blood Vessels

Acute epidural hematoma: Usually follows arterial hemorrhage between the skull and the dura. At the time of impact, a dural artery is torn, and the inbending of the skull initiates the stripping of the dura from the bone. Occasionally, an epidural hematoma follows a torn venous sinus. Most frequently, acute epidural hematomas occur in the temporal or temporoparietal region as a consequence of hemorrhage from one of the branches of the **middle meningeal artery.**

Temporal arteritis: It is seen as a thick cord along the temporal region in which there is inflammation of temporal artery associated with high ESR Levels. Distinct tenderness, redness, and a palpable but nonpulsatile temporal artery are important clues to the presence of arteritis.

Lateral medullary syndrome: It is due to infarction of posterior inferior cerebellar artery. Also termed as Wallenburgs syndrome. It consisting of severe vertigo, nausea, vomiting, nystagmus, ipsilateral ataxia, and ipsilateral Horner's syndrome.

There is an ipsilateral loss of facial pain and temperature sense and a contralateral loss of the same sensory modalities in trunk and limb

Medial medullary syndrome: It is due to infarction of **vertebral artery.**

Remember

The structures passing through internal acoustic meatus
• **7th and 8th cranial nerves**
• **Labyrinthine vessels**

The structures are transmitted through optic canal
• **Optic nerve**
• **Meningeal sheath of optic nerve**
• **Ophthalmic artery**

The structures passing through superior orbital fissure

It is divided into three parts by a common tendinous ring of Zinn. It transmits:

1. **Lateral part:**
   • Lacrimal nerve
   • Frontal nerve
   • Trochlear nerve
   • Meningeal branch of lacrimal artery, and
   • Superior ophthalmic vein

2. **Middle part:**
   • Upper and lower division of oculomotor nerve
   • Nasociliary nerve
   • Abducent nerve

3. **Medial part:**
   • Inferior ophthalmic vein
   • Sympathetic from plexus around internal carotid artery.

The structures passes through foramen rotundum
• Maxillary nerve.

The structures passes through foramen ovale
• Mandibular nerve
• Lesser petrosal nerve
• Accessory meningeal artery
• Emissary vein

The structures passing through foramen spinosum
• Middle meningeal artery
• Meningeal branch of mandibular nerve
• Posterior trunk of middle meningeal vein.

The structures passing through foramen magnum

(A) Through wider posterior part:
- Lower part of medulla
- Tonsils of cerebellum
- Meninges

(B) Through narrow anterior part:
- Apical ligament of dens
- Membrane tectoria

(C) Through subarachnoid space:
- Spinal accessory nerve
- Vertebral arteries
- Sympathetic plexus
- Posterior spinal arteries
- Anterior spinal arteries

The contents of hypoglossal canal
- Hypoglossal nerve
- Meningeal branch of ascending pharyngeal artery.
- Emissary vein

The structures passing through Jugular foramen

(A) Through the anterior part:
- Inferior petrosal sinus
- Meningeal branch of ascending pharyngeal artery

(B) Through the middle part:
- IX, X and XI cranial nerves

(C) Through the posterior part:
- Internal jugular vein
- Meningeal branch of occipital artery.

The structures transmitted by carotid canal
- Internal carotid artery (ICA)
- Venous and sympathetic plexuses around ICA

The structures transmitted by inferior orbital fissure
- Maxillary nerve
- Zygomatic nerve
- Emissary vein
- Infraorbital vessels
- Orbital branches of pterygopalatine ganglion.

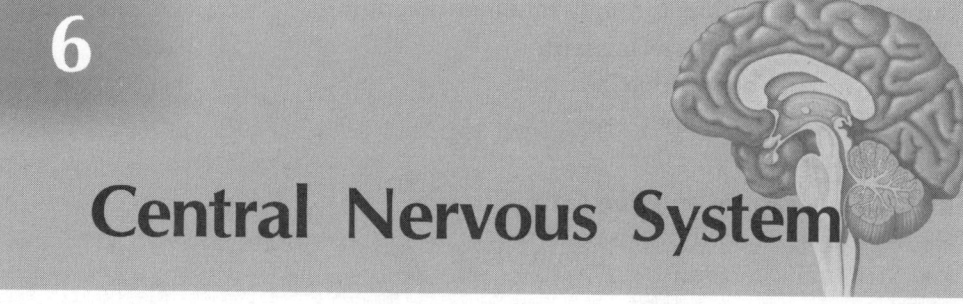

6

Central Nervous System

The divisions of the nervous system

Anatomically the nervous system is made up to:

Central nervous system (CNS): Consisting of
- Brain
- Spinal cord

Peripheral nervous system (PNS): Consisting of
- Somatic (cerebrospinal) nervous system
- Autonomic (splanchnic) nervous system

The constituents of the somatic nervous system: It consists of 12 pairs of cranial nerves and 31 pairs of spinal nerves. The functions of somatic nervous system: It is concerned with the response of body to external environment.

The constituents of autonomic nervous system: It consists of sympathetic and parasympathetic nervous system. The functions of autonomic nervous system: It is mainly concerned with control of internal environment of body, e.g. regulation of heart, bronchial tree, gut and glands of alimentary tract.

The main difference between somatic and autonomic nervous system: The efferent fibers of somatic nervous system reach the effectors without interruption while the efferent fibres of ANS first relays in a ganglion and then post-ganglionic fibers pass to the effectors.

PARTS OF BRAIN

- Forebrain
- Midbrain
- Hindbrain

The Coverings of Brain and Spinal Cord

The coverings of spinal cord
- Spinal dura mater: Represents meningeal layer of cerebral dura mater
- Arachnoid mater
- Spinal pia mater

The folds of cranial dura mater: These are formed by the meningeal layer of the dura mater around brain. These projects inwards and divide the cranial cavity into different compartments.

These are:

1. Falx cerebri
2. Tentorium cerebelli
3. Falx cerebelli
4. Diaphragma sellae.

Meninges and cerebrospinal fluid (CSF)

Meninges

These are the layers of connective tissue covering the brain and spinal cord

The Layers or the Meninges

The meninges consist of three membranous layers.

- **Dura mater: Outer most**
- **Arachnoid: Middle layer**
- **Pia mater: Inner most**

The dura mater is also known as **Pachymeninges.**

The arachnoid and pia mater are together known as **Leptomeninges.**

The Developmental Origin of Meninges

- **Leptomeninges: From neural crest.**
- **Pachymeninges: From mesoderm surrounding neural tube.**

The Layers of the Dura Mater

Dura mater is the thickest and toughest membrane covering the brain and consists of two layers.

- **Endosteal layer: Outer—serves as internal periosteum (endocranium)**
- **Meningeal layer: Inner—provides the protective membrane to brain.**

These two layers are fused to each other except where venous sinuses are enclosed between them.

Structures of the Endosteal Layer

It is attached to:

- Inner surface of cranial bones by fibrous and vascular processes
- To pericranium through sutures and foramina
- To periosteal lining of orbit through the superior orbital fissure

The structures covered by the endosteal layer other than brain

It provides sheaths for:

1. Cranial nerves and fuses with epineurium.
2. Optic nerve, and becomes continuous with sclera

The Coverings of Spinal Cord

- Spinal dura mater: Represents meningeal layer of cerebral dura mater
- Arachnoid mater
- Spinal pia mater

The folds of dura mater: These are formed by the meningeal layer of the dura mater around brain. These projects inwards and divide the cranial cavity into different compartments.

These are:

- Falx cerebri
- Tentorium cerebelli
- Falx cerebelli
- Diaphragma sellae.

The falx cerebri: It is a fold of dura mater, which is sickle shaped and occupies the median longitudinal fissure between two cerebral hemispheres.

The venous sinuses enclosed by the falx cerebri

1. The upper convex margin encloses the, superior sagittal sinus
2. The lower concave free margin encloses, inferior sagittal sinus

Tentorium cerebelli: It is a tent shaped fold of dura mater, forming roof of the posterior cranial fossa. It separates cerebellum from the occipital lobes of the cerebrum.

The sinuses enclosed by the tentorium cerebelli: The attached margin encloses the transverse and superior petrosal sinuses

Trigeminal cave: Trigeminal or meckel's cave is recess of dura mater, formed by the inferior layer of tentorium cerebella, over the trigeminal impression.

Falx cerebelli: It is a small sickle-shaped folds projecting forwards into posterior cerebellar notch.

Diaphragma sellae: It is circular horizontal fold of dura mater forming the roof of hypophyseal fossa.

The structure transmitted by central aperture of diaphragma sellae: Pituitary stalk (infundibulum).

The Cranial Venous Sinuses

The characteristics of venous sinuses of the skull

1. The lie between 02 layers of the dura mater
2. They are lined by endothelium only. Muscular coat is absent.
3. The receive:
   - Venous blood
   - CSF
4. No valves are present.
5. Blood flow is regulated by the emissary veins.

The different venous sinuses of the skull
The venous sinuses of skull can be divided into two broad groups:

Paired

- Cavernous
- Superior petrosal
- Inferior petrosal
- Transverse
- Sigmoid
- Sphenoparietal
- Petrosquamous
- Middle meningeal veins

Unpaired

- Superior sagittal
- Inferior sagittal
- Straight
- Occipital
- Anterior intercavernous
- Posterior intercavernous
- Basilar plexus of veins

The Cavernous Sinus

It is a very important venous sinus.
The relations of cavernous sinus: The relations can be divided into subdivisions:
Structures in lateral wall of sinus:

- Maxillary nerve
- Oculomotor nerve
- Ophthalmic nerve
- Trigeminal ganglion
- Trochlear nerve

Structures lying outside the sinus
- **Superiorly:** Optic tract, internal carotid artery, anterior perforated substance.
- **Inferiorly:** Foramen lacerum, junction of body and greater wing of sphenoid
- **Medially:** Hypophysis (pituitary gland) sphenoidal air sinus.
- **Laterally:** Temporal lobe with uncus.
- **Anteriorly:** Superior orbital fissure, apex of orbit.
- **Posteriorly:** Apex of petrous temporal crus cerebri of midbrain.

Structures passing through the centre of sinus
- Internal carotid artery
- Abducent nerve.

The important communications of cavernous sinus are:

- Into transverse sinus through superior petrosal sinus.
- Into internal jugular vein through inferior petrosal sinus and venous plexus around internal carotid artery
- Into pterygoid plexus of veins through emissary veins.
- Into facial vein through superior ophthalmic vein
- Communication between two sinuses by anterior and posterior intercavernous sinuses and basilar plexus of veins.

The tributaries of cavernous sinus are:

- From meninges: Sphenoparietal sinus, frontal trunk of middle meningeal vein
- From brain: Superficial middle cerebral vein inferior cerebral veins
- From orbit: Superior ophthalmic vein, inferior ophthalmic vein, central vein of retina.

The commonest cause of thrombosis of cavernous sinus: Infection of the danger area of face, nasal cavities and paranasal air sinuses.

Confluence of the sinuses: This is the posterior dilated end of sagittal sinus lying on right side of internal occipital protuberance. It continues as corresponding transverse sinus and it is connected to opposite transverse sinus and drains the occipital sinus.

Arachnoid villi: These are the finger like processes of the arachnoid tissue which project into cranial venous sinuses. Their function is to absorb CSF.

Pacchionian bodies: Also called arachnoid granulations. These are aggregations of arachnoid villi clumped together. Found in adults.

Tela chroidea: These are folds of pia mater enclosing the choroid plexuses.

Cisterns and their functions: These are communicating pools formed by the subarachnoid space at base of brain and around the brainstem.

Function: These reinforce the protective effect on the vital centres in the medulla

The Communications of Subarachnoid Space

It communicates with ventricular system of brain by:

✓ **Foramen of Magendie: Median, single**

✓ **Foramen of Luschka: Lateral, two**

CSF: It is a clear fluid found in subarachnoid space of brain and spinal cord, ventricular system of brain and central canal of spinal cord.

It is formed by choroid plexuses of ventricles of brain

The pathway of circulation of CSF.

> **Lateral ventricles → Interventricular foramina of Munro → Third ventricle → Cerebral aqueduct of Silvius → Fourth ventricle absorbed by arachnoid Villi, perineural lymphatics around cranial nerves → Subarachnoid space around brain and spinal cord → Foramen of Magendie and foramina of Luschka.**

A Sample of CSF Obtained by

✓ Lumbar puncture
✓ Cisternal puncture
✓ Ventricular puncture

The functions of CSF: It is protective and nutritive to the CNS

Hydrocephalous: It is the dilatation of the ventricular system and enlargement of head due to obstruction to flow of CSF within ventricular system in children.

Queckenstedt's test: Done to detect whether there is a blockade to the circulation of CSF in subarachnoid space of spinal cord. Anatomical basis of test: any increase in intracranial pressure, raises the pressure of CSF. This increase is transmitted to CSF. in spinal sub-arachnoid space. Compression of both internal jugular veins above the sternal ends of clavicles dams back blood in skull and so raises the intracranial pressure. Should a part of spinal subarachnoid space be completely cut off from above by a tumor, this increase of pressure will not be transmitted to the part of subarachnoid space below tumor.

Vertebral Column and Spinal Cord

Consists of **33 vertebrae.**

Development

- The vertebral column is formed from the **Sclerotomes of the somites**.
- The cells of the sclerotome become converted into **loose mesenchyme.**
- This mesenchyme migrates medially and surrounds the **notochord.**
- The mesenchyme then **extends back on either side of the neural tube and surrounds it.**
- The extensions of this mesenchyme also take place laterally in the position to be occupied by the **transverse processes** and ventrally in the **body wall**, in the position to be occupied by the **ribs.**
- The mesenchyme derived from each somite is seen as a distinct segment and the cells are distributed uniformly.
- Then the cells soon become condensed in a region that runs transversely across the middle of the segment and this is called **perichordal disc.**
- Above and below it there are less condensed parts.
- The mesenchymal basis of the body (centrum) of each vertebra is formed by fusion of the adjoining, less denser parts of two segments.
- The perichordal disc becomes the intervertebral disc.
- The neural arch, the transverse processes and the costal elements are formed in the same way as body.
- The inter-spinous and inter-transverse ligaments are formed like the inter-vertebral disc.
- **The notochord disappears in the region of the vertebral bodies, but in the region of the intervertebral discs it becomes expanded to form nucleus pulposus.**

- Hence, vertebrae are intersegmental.
- The transverse processes and ribs are also intersegmental.
- The spinal nerves are segmental, therefore, they emerge between the two adjacent vertebrae and lie between two adjacent ribs.
- The blood vessels supplying structures derived from myotome like intercostals vessels are intersegmental like the vertebrae.

In the adult four distinct anteroposterior curves are seen.

- **Primary curves** retain their original posterior convexity and are found in the **thoracic and sacral regions.**
- **Secondary curves** are convex anteriorly are found in cervical and lumbar regions.

The cervical curve appears when the infant holds its head up after the third month.

The lumbar curve develops when the child begins to walk and holds his trunk upright.

Structure of a typical vertebra

- Cylindrical vertebral body
- Linked posteriorly to lamina
- Connected by pedicle
- Spinal canal transmits spinal cord, coverings, roots of nerves
- Spinous process
- Transverse processes
- Superior articular facets
- Inferior articular facets
- Intervertebral foramina for exit of segmental nerves

In the adult male, the average length of the vertebral column is about 28 inches, but in adult female is about 24 inches.

Cervical vertebrae are seven in number. There is a foramen in the transverse process called foramen transversarium and the vertebral artery passes through C1–C6 but not that of C7.

- C1 has no body and it is fused with C2 and is called odontoid process.
- The spine of C7 is the longest and is called vertebra prominens.
- C1, C2, C7 are atypical and the rest are typical.

Thoracic vertebrae are twelve in number. There is one or more articular facets on each side of the body for articulation with the head of the rib. These are called **rib bearing vertebrae.** T1, T9, T10, T11, T12 are atypical and others are typical thoracic vertebrae.

Lumbar vertebrae are five in number: These have larger vertebral bodies, but have no articular facets for the ribs. L5 is atypical but all others are typical lumbar vertebrae.

Sacrum: It is formed by the union of five sacral vertebrae and forms an angle of 210 degrees with the rest of vertebral column called as **sacrovertebral angle.** Sacrum has a base, apex, three surfaces the pelvic, dorsal and lateral. It has also a lateral mass and a sacral canal.

The base has sacral promontary and ala on either side. The sacral index is the ratio between the length and the breadth of the sacrum.

Coccyx: It is the union of four coccygeal vertebrae and is fused with the sacrum to form a single sacrococcygeal mass.

- Between the bodies of two adjacent vertebrae lies the inter vertebral disc.
- They act as buffer in absorbing shock and prevent injuries to column and to the spinal cord. They also contribute ¼ of the total length of the column.
- They also bind the two vertebrae together and are composed of a central part called nucleus pulposus and a peripheral part the annulus fibrosus.
- The discs are thicker in front than behind in the cervical and lumbar regions and are responsible for cervical and lumbar convexity of the vertebral column.

Ossification: There are three primary centers, one in the body and one each for vertebral arch. The body often has two centers which may fail to unite and result in hemi-vertebrae.

There are 5 secondary centers. They appear at puberty and the epiphyses join the rest of the bone at 25 years. There is one center for the spine, one for the tip of each transverse process and one each in the cartilage on the upper and lower surfaces of the body. By the age of 25 years the ring is fused with the vertebrae. The lines of junction between the parts derived from the centrum and the neural arches forms the neuro-central joints.

Applied Anatomy

1. One or more vertebrae may be **absent.**
2. **Additional vertebrae** may be present.
3. **Spondylolisthesis**: The 5th lumbar vertebra together with whole vertebral column on the top of it is displaced on the sacrum.
4. **Lumbarization:** The first sacral vertebra fails to fuse with the rest of the sacrum.
5. Accentuation of forward bending is **Kyphosis.**
6. Accentuation of lateral bending is **Scoliosis**
7. **Lumbar rib:** The first lumbar transverse process may grow out to form the rib
8. **Cervical rib**: Exaggeration of the costal element of C7 or C6
9. **Sacralization of lumbar vertebra:** One or both transverse processes of L5 may develop sufficiently to fuse with sacrum.
10. **Spina bifida** leads to meningocoele, myelocoele, etc.

Relation of vertebrae to spinal segments

The segments of the spinal cord **are not in line with the vertebrae** which correspond to them in number and the differences increase as we go downwards.

- Spine of C6 correspond to C8 spinal cord segment.

- Spine of T3 corresponds to T6 spinal segment
- Spine of T9 corresponds to T12 spinal segment

Spinal Cord

The extent of spinal cord: It extends from the upper border of atlas vertebra to the lower border of L1.

18 inches or 45 cm long

Gives rise to 31 pairs of spinal nerves.

The spinal cord develops: It develops from caudal tubular part of neural tube, which gradually increases in length.

The age changes in the length of the spinal cord:
- Up to 3rd month of fetal life: Spinal cord occupies full extent of vertebral canal.
- At birth: At level of L3 vertebra
- At adolescence; at level of intervertebral disc between L1 and L2 vertebra

The arteries supplying spinal cord

1. Anterior spinal artery—one

2. Posterior spinal arteries—two

Arteries of Adamkiewicz: These are the anastomotic arteries between anterior and posterior spinal arteries at the level of T1 and T11.

The descending and ascending tracts of spinal cord

Descending tracts: Motor in function.
- Anterior corticospinal
- Lateral corticospinal
- Olivospinal
- Reticulospinal
- Rubrospinal
- Tectospinal
- Vestibulospinal

Ascending tracts: Sensory in functions:
- Anterior spinocerebellar
- Anterior spinothalamic
- Fasciculus gracilis
- Fasciculus cuneatus
- Lateral spinothalamic
- Posterior spinocerebellar

Pyramidal Tract

- Arises mainly from area 4 in the **Precentral gyrus.**
- The left area controls the right side and vice versa.
- The representation is upside down.

- The larynx and the tongue occupy a large area due to the delicate movements executed by them.
- The fibers descend in the corona radiata.
- Pass through the posterior limb of the **internal capsule**.
- Then pass in the intermediate 3/5 of the **basis pedunculi**.
- Pass through pons and there are scattered by nuclei points and then clump and pass through **pyramid of medulla**.
- **90–95% of the fibers** cross to the opposite side in the pyramidal decussation to form crossed pyramidal tract and ends in AHC of the spinal cord.
- Remaining fibers descend in the spinal cord as the direct pyramidal tracts which cross in the spinal cord to end on the **Anterior Horn Cells** of the opposite side, but a few fibers end on AHC of the same side.

Laminar Organization in Spinal Cord (Rexed's Lamina)

In spinal cord the neurons have a layered arrangement and ten layers have been recognized. These are numbered by roman numerals, starting at the tip of dorsal horn and moving ventrally into ventral horn.

- **Lamina I corresponds to posteromarginal nucleus.**
- **Lamina II to substantia gelatinosa.**
- **Lamina III and IV to nucleus proprius.**
- **Lamina V and VI to base of dorsal column.**
- **Lamina VII occupies the territory between dorsal and ventral horns.**
- **Lamina VIII corresponds to ventral horn in thoracic segments but at the level of limb enlargements it lies on the medial aspect of ventral horn.**
- **Lamina IX includes the lateral group of the nuclei of the ventral horn.**
- **Lamina X surrounds the central canal.**

Important Terms in Relation to Spinal Cord

Ligamenta denticulata and their functions: These are toothed processes extending from pia to dura, pushing the arachnoid before them. They leave the pia midway between anterior and posterior nerve roots and serve to suspend the spinal cord in midline.

Linea splendens: It is a thickening seen at the anteromedian sulcus.

Filum terminale: It is a fold of piamater which is almost 18–20 cm long and gets attached to the coccyx.

Conus medullaris: It is the lower end of spinal cord which is conical. The apex of conus continues downward as filum terminale, up to first coccygeal space.

Cauda equina: The spinal cord gives rise to spinal nerves which pass out through intervertebral foramina. Below L1 vertebra, nerve roots become more and more oblique to reach respective intervertebral foramina. The bundle of lumbar and sacral nerve roots below termination of spinal cord is termed cauda equina.

Cauda Equina Syndrome

Compression of cauda equina gives rise to Flaccid paraplegia, saddle anaesthesia, which is known as cauda equine syndrome.

Lumbar, sacral and coccygeal nerves roots together with filum terminate resemble tail of a horse-cauda equina.

Compression of cauda equina within the vertebral canal presents a set of features termed as Cauda Equina syndrome. **Features are:**

- *Sensory loss along the distribution of affected spinal nerves*
- *Lower motor neuron paralysis*
- *Bladder and bowel involvement is late.*

Conus Medullaris Syndrome

The terminal part of spinal cord is termed Conus Medullaris. In Conus Medullaris Syndrome there is involvement of S-2, S-3 and S-4 spinal segments. It is essential features are:

Early bladder and bowel involvement

Loss of sensations along the distribution of S-2, S-3 and S-4 spinal nerves (saddle shaped anesthesia).

The effects of complete transection of spinal cord: In the region below section, there is complete loss of sensation with flaccid muscle paralysis

Tabes dorsalis: It is degenerative disease of posterior columns and posterior nerve roots, which is characterized by loss of proprioception (position sense)

Brown-Séquard syndrome: It occurs in hemisection of spinal cord. It is characterized by:

- *Paralysis of affected side below the lesion (corticospinal tract)*
- *Loss of proprioception and fine discrimination on affected side below lesion (fasciculus cuneatus and gracilis)*
- *Loss of pain and temperature senses on opposite side below lesion (spinothalamic tract)*

Site lumbar puncture is done: Lumbar puncture is done to withdraw CSF from subarachnoid space at level between l3 and l4 vertebra.

Syringomyelia: Dilatation of central canal of spinal cord. This is characterized by degeneration of ependymal cells of central canal, which may expand all around leading to involvement of:

- **Crossing fibers of spinothalamic tract**: Bilateral loss of pain and temperature within the segment of lesion. No changes seen above and below the lesion.
- **Anterior horn cells**: Ipsilateral lower motor neuron paralysis at the level of lesion.
- **Preganglionic sympathetic fibers**: Ipsilateral Horners' syndrome.

"Anterior" Cord Syndrome

Most commonly results from occlusion of the anterior spinal artery. The anterior two-thirds of the spinal cord is supplied by the anterior spinal artery. Thus this syndrome has been correlated anatomically with damage to the corticospinal and lateral spin thalamic tracts with relative sparing of the posterior columns.

Clinical Features

Loss of motor function below the level of lesion
Loss of pain and temperature sensation below the level of lesion
Relative preservation of vibration and position sense.

"Central" Cord Syndrome

It usually follows an acute cervical injury. It is characterized by patients with cervical spondylosis/stenosis are predisposed to central cord injuries.

The proposed mechanism of injury suggests that the spinal cord is pinched between a dorsally displaced vertebral body and a buckled ligamentum flavum during hyperextension.

THE MEDULLA

- It is about 3 cm long and is continuous above with the lower border of the pons.
- It is continuous below with the spinal cord at the foramen magnum; and the central canal of the spinal cord extends upwards in the lower
- Half of the medulla.
- The medulla is connected with the cerebellum by means of the inferior cerebellar peduncles.

External Features of the Medulla

A.The anterior surface:

- The anterior surface is grooved in the middle line by an anterior median fissure.
- The most important feature is the presence of a pyramid on either side of the anterior median fissure.
- In the lower part of the medulla the pyramidal decussation can be seen, obliterating the lower end of the anterior median fissure.

The lateral surface

- The most prominent feature is the olive which lies between (the anterolateral and the posterolateral sulci).
- The anterolateral sulcus separates the olive from the pyramid and the rootlets of the hypoglossal nerve come out along this sulcus.
- The posterolateral sulcus separates the olive from the inferior cerebellar peduncle (ICP) and the roolets of the 9, 10 and 11th cranial nerves are attached in line along this sulcus.

The Brainstem

The brainstem is the part of the brain which remains after the cerebral hemispheres and the cerebellum are removed. It consists of:

The Midbrain
The Pons
The Medulla
The Diencephalon

Midbrain

It is the shortest part of the brainstem and lies between the pons (below) and the diencephalons (above) occupying the notch in the tentorium cerebelli. It is largely hidden by the surrounding structures.

The anterior surface has (4 structures)

- Two cerebral peduncles: Which are ropelike bundles of fibers that pass directly into the anterior part of the pons (below) and seem to
- Disappear in the substance of the cerebral hemisphere (above). As the cerebral peduncle passes into the cerebral hemisphere it is overlapped
- By the uncus and the hippocampal gyrus.
- Two oculomotor nerves: Which emerge just medial to the cerebral peduncles in the interpeduncular fossa.

The lateral surface: It consists of:
- **Basis pedunculi: Anteriorly**
- **Tectum: Posterior**
- **Tegmentum: In the middle**

The posterior surface:

It is formed by the tectum with 4 rounded elevations called colliculi (corpora quadrigemina)

2 superior colliculi: Above

2 inferior colliculi: Below

The trochlear nerves are the smallest cranial nerves and emerge from the dorsal surface.

The Contents of Crus Cerebri
- Middle 2/3: Pyramidal tract
- Medial 1/6: Frontopontine fibres
- Lateral 1/6: Temporopontine, parietopontine and occipitopontine fibres.

The connections and functions of superior colliculus

Connections:
- Afferents: From retina (visual), spinal cord (tactile), inferior colliculus (auditory), occipital cortex (modulating)
- Efferents: To retina, spinal cord (tectospinal), brain stem nuclei, tegmentum,

Function: Control reflex movements of eyes, head and neck in response to visual stimuli.

Benedikt's syndrome (paramedian midbrain syndrome)

The clinical features result because of the involvement of following structures:

Complete ipsilateral oculomotor paralysis causing abduction and depression because of sparing of lateral rectus (VI CN) and superior oblique muscle (IV CN). There is also ptosis and dilatation of ipsilateral pupil. All these are manifestations of involvement of oculomotor nerve roots.

Contralateral cerebellar dystaxia with intention tremors. This is because of involvement of superior cerebellar peduncle (dentato-thalamic fibers).

Contralateral loss of tactile sensation from extremities and trunk because of medial lemniscus involvement.

Perinaud's syndrome (dorsal midbrain syndrome)

The clinical features appear as the following structures are affected.

Absence of convergence—medial rectus paralysis

Paralysis of upwards and downwards movement—both oblique paralysis

Papillary disturbance—Edinger-Westphal nucleus involvement

Noncommunicating hydrocephalus—compression of cerebral aqueduct.

Thus, the syndrome is due to involvement of

Superior colliculus

Pretectal area

Cerebral aqueduct.

Pons

Features are

The anterior surface has:

A shallow median groove in which the basilar artery lies runs longitudinally in the mid line.

There are many thick transverse ridges (formed by transverse pontine fibers).

The abducent nerves emerge from the sulcus which separates the pons from the medulla near mid line.

B. The lateral surface

The transverse pontine fibers collect on either side to form a compact thick bundle called the middle cerebellar penduncle (or brachium pontis); which sinks into the corresponding cerebellar hemisphere.

The trigeminal nerve (V) (the largest cranial nerve) leaves the lateral part of the middle of the pons.

The pontocerebellar angle is the triangular space between the lower border of the middle cerebral peduncle, the cerebellum and the upper part of the medulla.

Two cranial nerves facial (VII) and auditory (VIII) are attached to the pons in the region of a pontocerebellar angle or the cerebellopontine angle.

C. The posterior surface: This surface forms the "upper" part of the floor of the 4th ventricle.

The cranial nerve nuclei in pons:
- Sixth nerve nucleus
- Seventh nerve nucleus
- Vestibular and cochlear nuclei
- Salivatory, lacrimatory nuclei and nucleus of spinal tract of trigeminal nerve.

Medial longitudinal bundle: Association tract, which coordinates movements of eyes, head and neck in response to stimulation of 8th cranial nerve. The nuclei of 3rd, 4th, 5th, 6th and 11th cranial nerve are interconnected by the bundle

The effect of unilateral lesion in lower part of pons: Crossed or alternate hemiplegic, i.e. paralysis of face on one side and limbs on the other side.

Pontine lesions (Stroke) result in: Pin point pupils and hyperpyrexia.

THE CEREBRUM/BRAIN

The different parts of cerebrum

The brain is divided into 3 parts:

✓ Forebrain (Prosencephalon)

✓ Midbrain (Mesencephalon)

✓ Hindbrain (Rhombencephalon)

Brain develops: From Cranial part of Neural tube. The cavity of developing brain shows three dilatations. Craniocaudally, these are prosencephalon, mesencephalon and rhombencephalon.

FOREBRAIN

The subdivisions of forebrain

- Telencephalon: made of 2 cerebral hemispheres and their cavity, i.e. lateral ventricles.
- Diencephalon: Made of thalamus, metathalamus, epithalamus and its cavity, i.e. third ventricle.

The different lobes of cerebrum

- Frontal lobe
- Parietal lobe
- Occipital lobe
- Temporal lobe

This division is done by:

Three sulci: Central, lateral, occipito-parietal.

Two imaginary lines: One from parieto-occipital sulcus to preoccipital notch and second is backward continuation of posterior ramus of lateral sulcus before it turns upwards and meets the first line.

The structural divisions of the cerebral cortex

    A. Allocortex (archipallium): Consist of piriform area and hippocampal formation, made up of 3 layers

B. **Isocortex (neopallium):** Consists of granular and agranular cortex. Made up of 6 layers.

The functional divisions of the cerebral cortex: The cortex is divided into motor and sensory areas.

The body parts are represented in the cerebral cortex

✓ The body is represented upside downwards with the legs at top and head at bottom.

✓ In motor area, angle of mouth, thumb, finger movements are represented by the larger areas.

THE FRONTAL LOBE

- The motor speech area is located in the inferior frontal gyrus. Injury to this area results in aphasia (inability to speak).
- The prefrontal area forms the remaining part of the lateral surface of the frontal lobe. Here problems are solved. This area is highly developed in humans.

PARIETAL LOBE

- It receives pain, temperature, touch and vibration from the body. The area located in the post-central gyrus is known as the primary sensory area.
- If the parietal association area is damaged the patient cannot know and identify the objects which he feels, this condition is known as agnosia.

THE TEMPORAL LOBE

- The "auditory sensory area" (or areas 41 and 42) is found in Heschl's gyrus.
- It receives the "auditory radiation" from the medial geniculate body.

THE OCCIPITAL LOBE

- The "visual sensory area" (area 17) is found in the lips of the calcarine sulcus mainly on the medial surface and receives the visual sensations.

The Important Areas

- **Brocas area:** Motor speech area (inferior frontal gyrus)
- **Motor area:** Precentral gyrus
- **Premotor area:** Anterior to motor area
- **Sensory area:** Postcentral gyrus
- **Visual area:** Occipital lobe
- **Werneckies area:** Superior temporal lobe

Main Cortical Areas of the Brain

- Area 4— Motor area (precentral gyrus)
- Area 3, 1, 2— Sensory area (post-central gyrus)

- Area 44— Brocas motor speech area (inferior frontal gyrus-posterior part)
- Area 41, 42— Auditory area (middle of superior temporal gyrus)
- Area 17— visual area (calcarine slcus)

The Limbic System

- Olfactory nerve, bulb, tract, striae and trigone
- Anterior perforated substance
- Piriform lobe
- Posterior part of parahippocampal and cingulate gyri
- Hippocampal formation
- Amygdaloid nuclei
- Septal region
- Fornix, stria terminalis, stria habenularis.

The Functions of Limbic System

It controls:

- Food habits
- Sex behavior
- Emotional behavior

The Lateral Ventricle

The communications of lateral ventricle: Each lateral ventricle communicates with the third ventricle through an interventricular foramen or foramen of monro

The different parts of the lateral ventricle

Each lateral ventricle is made up of:

1. Central part

2. Three horns: Anterior, posterior and inferior.

The constituents of white matter of cerebrum: It consists of myelinated fibres which connect various parts of cortex and other parts of the CNS.

The different types of fibres of white matter: Three types:

✓ Association fibres: Connect different cortical areas of same side.

✓ Projection fibres: Connect cerebral cortex to other part of CNS, e.g. brainstem, spinal cord by various tracts.

✓ Commissural fibres: Connect corresponding parts of two sides

The different commissures of cerebrum:

- Corpus callosum: Largest, connecting two cerebral hemispheres.
- Anterior commissure
- Posterior commissure
- Commissure of fornix
- Habenular commissure

- Hypothalamic commissure
- Commissures of cerebellum

Corpus Callosum

- It is the largest and the chief commissure. It contains fibers which connect various areas of the:
  - Two cerebral hemispheres except the right and left temporal poles.
  - Agenesis of corpus callosum is seen in certain newborns and they cannot coordinate the activity of both sides.
- Shapiro's syndrome is agenesis of corpus callosum

The different parts of corpus callosum

✓ **Genu: Anterior end connects two frontal lobes by forceps minor fibres.**

✓ **Rostrum: Connects orbital surfaces of two frontal lobes.**

✓ **Trunk.**

✓ **Splenium: Posterior end, thickest. Connects two occipital lobes by forceps major.**

DIENCEPHALON

The parts of Diencephalon

Dorsal part:

1. Thalamus

2. Metathalamus: Medial and lateral geniculate bodies

3. Epithalamus: Pineal body and Habenula

Ventral part:

1. Hypothalamus

2. Subthalamus

Thalamus:

- It is an **oval mass of grey matter and forms the dorsal part of diencephalon**. It is related laterally to internal capsule and medially two thalami are united together by inter-thalamic adhesion.
- Anteriorly it has a **tubercle and the posterior part is the pulvinar**.
- It has four surfaces, namely the superior, inferior, medial and lateral.
- Superior— It is related to lateral ventricle and forms floor of the body of lateral ventricle.
- Inferior—Its middle part lies on the subthalamus and its anterior part lies on the hypothalamus..
- Laterally—Related to internal capsule.
- Medial surface—forms part of wall of third ventricle.
- There is a thin membrane on the superior surface medially called velum interpositum.

6

Central Nervous System

The different parts and nuclei of thalamus

White matter:

1. External medullary lamina
2. Internal medullary lamina

Gray matter:

1. Paleothalamus: Anterior and medial nuclei
2. Neothalamus: Lateral and ventral nuclei
3. Intralaminar, mid line and reticular nuclei.

The efferents and afferents to the thalamus

Efferents to:

- Area 6 and 8 of cortex
- Cingulate gyrus
- Corpus striatum
- Frontal lobe in front of area 6
- Hypothalamus
- Motor area 4 and 6
- One nuclei of thalamus from another
- Other parts of cerebral cortex
- Post-central gyrus
- Pre cuneus
- Superior parietal lobule

Afferents: From

- Cerebellum
- Corpus striatum
- Frontal lobe in front of area 6
- Globus pallidus
- Hippocampus.
- Hypothalamus
- Red nucleus
- Reticular formation of brainstem
- Spinal and medial leminisci
- Trigeminal leminiscus

The functions of thalamus

- Capable of appreciating painful and thermal stimuli.
- Through RAS, participates in maintenance of state of wakefulness and alertness.
- Great sensory relay station on pathway of sensory impulses to cerebral cortex, except for sense of smell, visual and auditory impulses.
- Integration of impulses from sensory system, cerebral cortex, striatum, cerebellum, hypothalamus, reticular formation
- Control of emotions and behavior

Thalamic Syndrome

Thrombosis of arteries supplying the thalamus causes infarction leading to thalamic syndrome.

This is characterized by

- Hemianaesthesia—contralateral, followed by hyperesthesia/excruciating pain due to thalamic rebound.
- Abnormal voluntary movements, intention tremors, chorea, athetosis and ataxia.
- The other symptomatology would vary with the extent of the lesion. Thus there may be loss of stereognosis and memory.

Subthalamus

is the part of the diencephalon which lies on the tegmentum of midbrain.

The anterior part contains of part of **Red nucleus, substantia nigra, subthalamic nucleus and zona** incerta.

Zona incerta is a thin lamina of grey matter between the thalamus and subthalamic nuclei.

Meta-thalamus

- **Consists of lateral and medial geniculate body.**
- These are small collections of grey matter situated below the posterior part of the thalamus, lateral to colliculi of midbrain.
- The lateral geniculate body is the last relay station in the visual pathway. It is six layered. The afferents are from optic tract and lateral root and the efferents give rise to optic radiation fibres.
- The medial geniculate body is the last relay station on the pathway to auditory impulses. It gets afferents from Lateral lemniscus and inferior colliculi and the efferents give rise to auditory radiation.

Epithalamus

- It is a smell centre.
- Lies above the thalamus.
- Consists of **pineal body, habenular nuclei, habenular commissure and posterior commissure.**
- The habenular nuclei are relay stations on the olfactory pathway from olfactory centres in the cerebral cortex to the autonomic centres in the brainstem.
- Pineal gland occupies the caudal part of the roof of diencephalon. It is a small, conical body between the two superior colliculi. The pineal in many reptiles is represented by a double structure but the human pineal gland represents the posterior glandular part. It plays a part in the development of gonads. Melatonin and serotonin have been extracted from the gland. Pineal tumors are associated with precocious puberty.

Hypothalamus

It is called the head ganglion of the autonomic nervous system: Because it controls the various sympathetic and parasympathetic activities of the body.

The position of hypothalamus: It is present at base of brain and forms the floor and lateral wall of third ventricle. Its boundaries are

- **Anteriorly: Optic chiasma**
- **Posteriorly: Posterior perforated substance**
- **On each side: Optic tract and crus cerebri**

The functions of hypothalamus:

- **Endocrine control: By releasing or release inhibiting hormones, it regulates the functions of various endocrine glands of body.**
- **Neurosecretion: Oxytocin and ADH are secreted by hypothalamohypophyseal tract to posterior pituitary.**
- **Control of sexual behavior and reproduction through anterior pituitary.**
- **Regulation of food and water intake**
- **Temperature regulation**
- **Control of emotions and behaviour**
- **Maintains circadian rhythm of body**

Hypothalamus is Important as it Controls

- Temperature regulation through **anterior and posterior hypothalamic nuclei**
- Neuroendocrine control of hormones by release of releasing factors and inhibitory factors
- Thirst through **lateral nucleus**
- Hunger through **ventromedial nucleus**
- Sexual behavior through **anterior ventral hypothalmus**
- Defence mechanisms (fear, rage)
- Control of endocrine and circadian rhythms through **suprachiasmatic nucleus**

Hypothalmus extends from: Optic chiasma to mammillary bodies from anterior to posterior, it is related to:

- **Optic chiasma.**
- **Tuber cinereum and infundibulum.**
- **Mammillary bodies.**

Pineal Body or Pineal Gland

- It is a small conical body projecting downwards between two superior colliculi.
- Brain sand: Calcareous concretions appear in pineal body after 17 years of life and form aggregations. These are called brain sand. They appear as radio-opaque structures in X-ray.
- The clinical importance of pineal concretions: Normally the pineal concretions appear as midline structures in X-ray. They are shifted in cases of head injury.

- The Pineal gland is composed of two types of cells, pinealocytes and neuroglial cells with a rich network of blood vessels and sympathetic fibers. The vessels and the nerves enter the gland through the connective tissue septa which partly separate the lobules.
- The pineal body has far long been regarded as a vestigeal organ of no importance. Recent investigations have shown that it is an endocrine gland of great importance. It produces hormone that may have an important regulatory influence on many other endocrine organs (including the adenohypophysis, the neurohypophysis, the thyroid, the parathyroid, the adrenal cortex and medulla and the gonads). The best known hormone is melatonin.

The Third Ventricle

The recesses of third ventricle

These are the extensions of the cavity of third ventricle. These are:

- **Supraspinal**
- **Pineal**
- **Infundibular**
- **Optic**

The structures present in floor of third ventricle

- **Optic chiasma**
- **Tuber cinerium**
- **Infundibulum**
- **Mammillary bodies**
- **Posterior perforated substance**
- **Tegmenta of midbrain.**

The Fourth Ventricle

It is the space which lies between the cerebellum "behind" and the pons and the upper part of the medulla "in front".

It is a cavity of hindbrain.

It is diamond shaped when seen from above and tent shaped when seen from the side.

Situated between pons and medulla in front and cerebellum behind.

Recesses of the fourth ventricle:

- **Median dorsal recess**
- **Two lateral dorsal recesses**
- **Two lateral recesses**

The cranial nerve nuclei in floor of fourth ventricle

✓ **Hypoglossal nucleus**

✓ **Dorsal nucleus of vagus**

✓ Nucleus of tractus solitarius

✓ Inferior and medial vestibular nuclei

The floor of fourth ventricle is formed by

• Posterior surface of pons

• Posterior surface of open part of medulla.

The effect of lesion in medulla oblongata: The medulla contains the vital centres, i.e. respiratory, cardiac and vasomotor centre. The lesion in medulla will lead to the failure of vital functions especially, respiratory failure.

Basal Nuclei of Cerebrum

Basal nuclei

These are masses of gray matter, forming part of extrapyramidal system. These are:

> Corpus striatum: Having two nuclei
> 1. Caudate nucleus
> 2. Lentiform nucleus: Divided into
>   (a) Putamen: Lateral
>   (b) Globus pallidus: Medial
> Claustrum
> Amygdaloid body

Morphological Divisions of Corpus Striatum

The putamen and caudate nucleus form neostriatum and globus pallidus forms paleostriatum.

Midbrain

The sub-divisions of midbrain

• Crus cerebri

• Substantia nigra

• Tegmentum

• Tectum and its cavity, cerebral aqueduct.

Tectum: It is the posterior part of midbrain. It is made up of 4 colliculi, a pair of superior and a pair of inferior.

The Characteristic Features of Substantia Nigra

It is a lamina of grey matter, made of deeply pigmented nerve cells.

Afferents are from motor cortex and collaterals of sensory tracts.

Efferents pass to corpus striatum and tegmentum.

Parkinsonism or paralysis agitans: It is a degenerative disease affecting substantia nigra and its connections with corpus striatum. It is a misnomer since there is no paralysis.

The features are:
- Cog wheel or lead pipe rigidity
- Mask like facies/expressionless face. The lesion is confined to substantia nigra.
- Rigidity in flexors and extensors
- Stooped posture and shuffling gait.
- Tremors at rest which are alternating because of contraction of agonists and antagonists. They appear as pill rolling movements. The tremors can affect at times the entire limb and disappear during sleep and voluntary activity.

INTERNAL CAPSULE

The different parts of internal capsule
- **Anterior limb: Between caudate nucleus and lentiform nucleus**
- **Posterior limb: Between thalamus and lentiform nucleus**
- **Genu: Bend between two limbs**
- **Retrolentiform part: Behind lentiform nucleus**
- **Sublentiform part: Below lentiform nucleus.**

The clinical importance of blood supply of internal capsule:

Lateral striate artery (Charcot's artery) supplying internal capsule is the commonest site of haemorrhage in cases of hypertension and it leads to the paralysis of opposite half of body (hemiplegia), depending on which side is involved in haemorrhage.

CEREBELLUM

The lobes of cerebellum

1. Anterior lobe

2. Middle lobe

3. Flocculonodular lobe

Vermis and its parts: It joins the two cerebellar hemispheres. Parts:
- **Lingual**
- **Central lobule**
- **Culmen**
- **Declive**
- **Folium**
- **Tuber**
- **Pyramid**
- **Uvula**
- **Nodule**

Phylogenetic divisions of cerebellum:
- **Archicerebellum:** Oldest, flocculonodular lobe and lingual
- **Paleocerbellum:** Anterior lobe minus lingual, pyramid and uvula
- **Neocerebellum:** Middle lobe minus pyramid and uvula

The contents of superior cerebellar peduncle:

✓ Afferent tracts: Anterior spino-cerebellar, tecto-cerebellar

✓ Efferent tracts: Cerebello-rubral, dentate-thalamic, dentate-olivary, fastigio-reticular.

The contents of inferior cerebellar peduncle:

✓ Afferent: Posterior ponto-cerebellar, cuneo-cerebellar, olivo-cerebellar, parolivo-cerebellar, reticulo-cerebellar, vestibulo-cerebellar

✓ Efferent: cerebello-vestibular, cerebello-olivary, cerebello-reticular.

The contents of middle cerebellar peduncle:

✓ Afferent: pontocerebellar

Dandy-Walker Malformation

The Dandy-Walker malformation consists of
- **Enlarged posterior fossa**
- **High position of the tentorium**
- **Hypogenesis of the cerebellar vermis**
- **Cystic dilatation of the fourth ventricle**
- **Cerebellar hemispheres are hypoplastic**

It is due to an intrauterine outflow obstruction of the fourth ventricle. Thus the fourth ventricle grows upward between the developing cerebellar hemispheres, preventing their apposition and fusion in the midline. When the cerebellar hemispheres do not fuse, the vermis is not formed.

Features

Dandy-Walker malformation is associated with hydrocephalus in 75% of patients Corpus callosum is hypogenetic.

Polymicrogyria or gray matter heterotopia are seen in 10% of patients.

Blood Supply of Brain

The arteries supplying the brain:
- **Internal carotid arteries**
- **Vertebral arteries: At lower border of pons join to form basilar artery**

Circle of Willis: It is an arterial circle formed at the base of brain by interconnections between the main arteries supplying brain.

The arteries forming circle of Willis

✓ **Anteriorly: Anterior communicating artery**

✓ Posteriorly: Basilar artery as it divides into two posterior cerebral arteries

✓ On each side: Anterior cerebral, internal carotid, posterior communicating and posterior cerebral arteries.

Clinical Importance of Circle of Willis

• It helps in equilising pressure in arteries of two sides.

• It also helps in maintaining blood supply to different parts of brain, if the main artery of one side is obstructed

The structures forming the blood–brain barrier (BBB)

• Vessel wall

• Arachnoid layer of perivascular sheath

• Perivascular space

• Pial layer of perivascular sheath

• Neuroglia and ground substance of brain

"Areas lacking blood–brain barrier are called circumventricular organs."

Thrombosis of central branches of cerebral arteries result in infarction because they are end arteries.

The arterial supply of cerebral cortex

• Cortical branches of anterior, middle and posterior cerebral arteries

• Motor area by anterior and middle cerebral artery.

• Auditory area and speech area by middle cerebral artery.

• Visual area by posterior cerebral artery.

Contribution by internal carotid arteries with branching.

The internal carotid arteries arise from the common carotid arteries and give rise to two terminal arteries namely anterior cerebral and middle cerebral arteries. The other smaller branches are posterior communicating and anterior choroidal arteries.

Contribution by the vertebral arteries with branching.

Vertebral arteries arise from first part of subclavian arteries.

Give rise to posterior inferior cerebellar arteries, anterior spinal artery and posterior spinal arteries.

Two vertebral arteries unite at lower border of pons and form basilar artery.

The Branches of Basilar artery are:

• Anterior inferior cerebellar

• Internal auditory

• Pontine branches

• Superior cerebellar

• Posterior cerebral

The characteristics of veins supplying the cerebrum

• Vessel walls are devoid of muscle

• No valves are present

• Some open into cranial venous sinuses against direction of blood flow in sinus

6

Central Nervous System

CRANIAL NERVES

There are 12 pairs of cranial nerves:
- **Olfactory**
- **Optic**
- **Oculomotor**
- **Trochlear**
- **Trigeminal**
- **Abducent**
- **Facial**
- **Vestibulocochlear**
- **Glossopharyngeal**
- **Vagus**
- **Accessory**
- **Hypoglossal**

The cranial nerves are classified as:
- **Purely sensory: I, II and VIII**
- **Purely motor: III, IV, VI and XII**
- **Mixed: V, VII, IX, X and XI.**

Olfactory Nerve (cranial nerve I)

Is the "Nerve of Smell"

It consists of two neurons:
- **Olfactory cells (receptors)**
- **Ist order neuron: Olfactory nerve—olfactory bulb**
- **2nd order neuron: Olfactory tract divided into**
  - ✓ **Medial**
  - ✓ **Inter-mediate and—terminates in anterior perforated substance**
  - ✓ **Lateral striae—primary olfactory area**
- **The characteristic feature of olfactory nerve:** The fibers of olfactory nerve are central process of olfactory cells and not peripheral process of central ganglion cells.
- **It ends in prepyriform area and peri amygdaloid area which are the centres for smell.**

Remember:
- **Hyperosmia: It is morbid sensitiveness to smell**
- **Cacosmia: It is a condition in which a person imagines of non-existent odours.**
- **The cause of unilateral anosmia (loss of sensation of smell): Frontal lobe tumour can press upon olfactory striae.**
- **The cause of bilateral anosmia: Head injury leading to damage to both olfactory nerves.**

Optic Nerve (cranial nerve II)

Nerve of vision

Travels through optic canal along with ophthalmic artery

The characteristic features of optic nerve
- It is not a true cranial nerve but is brain tract which has developed as a lateral diverticulum of forebrain.
- It is incapable of regeneration after section because it lacks neurilemmal sheath
- Nerve is enclosed in all the three meningeal sheaths

The effects of lesions of different parts of visual pathway

Site	Effect
Retina	Scotoma (loss of corresponding field)
Optic nerve	Blindness of same side consensual
Optic chiasma	Bitemporal hemianopia.
Optic tract, lateral geniculate Body, optic radiation	Homonymous hemianopia
Visual cortex	Homonymous hemianopia. Macular sparing

Optic Nerve is Involved in:

The optic pathway

Axons of ganglion cells of retina → optic nerve → optic chiasma decussation of fibres occur → optic tract has fibres from nasal half of macula of opposite side and temporal half of macula of same side → optic radiation → terminates in lateral geniculate body!Visual cortex striate area no. 17

The Pathway of Light Reflex

Retina → optic nerve → optic chiasma → optic tract → lateral geniculate body ciliary ganglion → III cranial nerve → Edinger-Westphal nucleus of III cranial nerve → pretectal nucleus → Short ciliary nerve → constrictor pupillae muscle.

Consensual light reflex: Constriction of pupil of both eyes when the light is flashed on one eye. It is due to the connection of the pretectal nuclei of both sides with the Edinger-Westphal nucleus

The pathway for accommodation reflex

Retina → optic nerve → optic chiasma → optic tract → Superior longitudinal association tract → visual area of cortex → optic radiation → lateral geniculate body → Third nerve nucleus → ciliary ganglion → ciliary and sphincter (constrictor) papillae muscle.

Argyll Robertson pupil: It is a condition in which papillary light reflex is absent but the accommodation reflex is present. It is caused by cerebral syphilis.

Oculomotor Nerve (cranial nerve III)

Supplies the eye muscles except lateral rectus and superior oblique.

The functional components of oculomotor nerve

- General visceral efferents (parasympathetic): For constriction of pupil and accommodation
- Somatic efferent: For movements of eyeball
- General somatic afferent: For propioceptive impulses from muscles of eyeball

The position sub-divisions and structures supplied by nerves of oculomotor nucleus

Position: At level of superior colliculus in ventro-medial part of central grey matter of midbrain

Subdivisions of nucleus of third cranial nerve:

- Edinger-Westphal nucleus: For cilaris and sphincter papillae muscle
- Ventromedial nucleus: For superior rectus of both sides
- Dorsolateral nucleus: For inferior rectus of same side
- Intermediate nucleus: For inferior oblique of same side
- Ventral nucleus: For medial rectus of same side
- Caudal central nucleus: For levator palpebrae superioris of both sides.

The connections of occulomotor nucleus

To:

- Pretectal nuclei of both sides
- Pyramidal tracts of both sides
- IV, VI and VIII nerve nuclei
- Tecto-bulbar tract.

The relations of oculomotor nerve in superior orbital fissure: Nasociliary nerve lies in between and abducent nerve inferolateral to, the two rami of oculomotor nerve.

Ciliary Ganglion and What is its Position, Connections and Branches

It is a **peripheral ganglion** in course of occulomotor nerve

Position: Near apex of orbit between optic nerve and tendon of lateral rectus muscle

Connections:

1. **Motor root:** From nerve to inferior oblique
2. **Sensory root:** From nasociliary nerve
3. **Sympathetic root:** Branch from internal carotid plexus

Branches: Short ciliary nerves: 8–10 pierce sclera

Weber's syndrome: It is a midbrain lesion causing paralysis of 3rd cranial nerve of same side and Hemiplegia of opposite side.

The Effects of Infranuclear Lesion of 3rd Cranial Nerve

- **Cycloplegia** (loss of accommodation)
- **Diplopia** (double vision)
- **Lateral squint** (outward deviation of eyeball)

- **Mydraiasis** (dilatation of pupil)
- **Proptosis** (abnormal protrusion of the eyeball)
- **Ptosis** (drooping of upper eyelid)

Trochlear Nerve (IV cranial nerve)

Supplies the eye muscle Superior Oblique.
The functional components of IV cranial nerve
1. Somatic efferent: For movement of eyeball.
2. General somatic afferent: For proprioceptive impulses from superior oblique muscle.

The position of trochlear nucleus: In ventromedial part of central grey matter of mid-brain at the level of inferior colliculus.
The effect of lesion of IV cranial nerve: Diplopia occurs on looking downwards.

Trigeminal Nerve (V cranial nerve)

It is the sensory nerve of face
The three divisions of trigeminal nerve are:
- Ophthalmic nerve: Sensory
- Maxillary nerve: Sensory
- Mandibular nerve: Mixed.

The Distribution of Trigeminal Nerve

- **Motor: Muscles of mastication**
- **Sensory:**
  1. **Skin of head and face**
  2. **Mucous membrane of mouth, nose and paranasal air sinuses.**

The divisions of ophthalmic nerve and structures supplied by it
- Frontal nerve: By supratrochlear and supraorbital divisions supply upper eyelid and scalp up to lambdoid suture.
- Lacrimal nerve: To lacrimal gland and lateral part of conjunctiva and upper eye lid
- Nasociliary nerve: Eyeball, to ciliary ganglion, medial half of lower eyelid, mucosa and skin of nose and dura of anterior cranial fossa.

The divisions of maxillary nerve and its distribution
- Zygomatic nerve: Zygomaticotemporal and zygomaticofacial branches supply skin of temple and cheek.
- Superior dental: Teeth of upper jaw
- Greater and lesser palatine nerves: Mucous membrane of hard and soft palates
- Nasal branch: Mucous membrane of nose
- Sphenopalatine branch: Nasal septum
- Pharyngeal branch: Mucosa of nasopharynx

The distribution of mandibular nerve

1. Before division to anterior and posterior trunk:
   - Nerve to medial pterygoid
   - Nerve to tensor palate and tensor tympani
   - Nerve to dura mater

2. Anterior trunk:
   - Buceal nerve: Skin of cheek and mucous membrane on its inner aspect
   - Nerve to masseter, temporalis and lateral pterygoid

3. Posterior trunk:
   - Auriculotemporal nerve: Sensory to skin of temple and auricle and secretomotor fibres to parotid gland
   - Lingual nerve: Mucous membrane of floor of mouth, anterior 2/3 of tongue, sublingual and submandibular salivary gland.
   - Inferior alveolar (dental) nerve: Teeth of lower jaw and nerve to mylohyoid and anterior belly of digastrics.

The effect of complete unilateral lesion of trigeminal nerve: Unilateral anesthesia of face and anterior part of scalp, auricle and mucous membrane of nose, mouth, and anterior two-thirds of tongue, with paralysis and wasting of muscles of mastication on affected side.

Trigeminal neuralgia: It is the disease of unknown etiology in which there is sudden severe pain in the area of distribution of trigeminal nerve. Corneal reflex: is lost in damage to trigeminal nerve.

Abducent Nerve (VI cranial nerve)

Supplies the eye muscles lateral rectus

The functional components of abducent nerve
- Somatic efferent: For lateral movement of eyeball
- General somatic afferent: For proprioceptive impulses from lateral rectus muscle.

Position of VI cranial nerve nucleus: Lies at the upper part of floor of fourth ventricle beneath facial colliculus.

Effect of paralysis of abducent nerve
- **Medial squint**
- **Diplopia**

Facial Nerve (VII cranial nerve)

The functional components of facial nerve:
- Branchial afferent: Motor to muscles of facila expression and elevation of hyoid bone
- General viscerent efferent: Secretomotor to submandibular and sublingual glands, lacrimal gland and glands of nose, palate and pharynx.

- Special visceral afferent: Carries taste sensation from anterior 2/3 of tongue and palate.
- General somatic afferent: For proprioceptive impulses from muscles supplied

The branches of facial nerve and structures supplied

Within the facial canal:

- Greater petrosal nerve: Joins deep petrosal nerve, supply glands of nose, palate and pharynx and lacrimal gland. Also carries taste sensation from palate
- Nerve to stapedius muscle
- Chorda tympani: Joins lingual nerve.

Supplies:
- Secretomotor fibres to submandibular and sublingual glands
- Carries taste sensation from anterior 2/3 of tongue.

At Exit from Stylomastoid Foramen

- Muscles: Posterior auricular: Supplies auricularis posterior occipitalis and intrinsic muscles on back of auricle
- Digastric branch: To posterior belly of digastrics
- Stylohyoid branch: To stylohyoid muscle.

Terminal Branches

- Temporal branches: Supply auricularis anterior and superior intrinsic muscles on lateral side of ear, frontalis, orbicularis and corrugator supercilia
- Zygomatic branches: To orbicularis oculi
- Buccal branches: To buccal muscles
- Mandibular branch: To muscles of lower lip and chin
- Cervical branch: Supplies platysma
- Communicating branches: To trigeminal and vagus nerve.

Pes anserinus : The Branching pattern of branches of facial nerve after its exit from parotid on face is called **pes anserinus.**

Bell's palsy: It is the infranuclear lesion of facial nerve, in which the whole of face is paralysed on same side. Face becomes asymmetrical and is drawn to the normal side.

The supranuclear lesion of facial nerve, only lower part of face is paralysed: Because the lower facial muscles have a unilateral cortical representation through opposite pyramidal tract but the upper facial muscles have a bilateral representation through pyramidal tracts of both sides.

Vestibulocochlear Nerve (VIII cranial nerve)

- Dorsal and ventral cochlear nuclei, situated in relation to inferior cerebellar peduncle
- Superior, inferior, medial and lateral vestibular nuclei, situated laterally in pons and medulla

The parts of VIII cranial nerve

- Cochlear nerve: nerve of hearing
- Vestibular nerve: Nerve of equilibrium (balance)

The Auditory and Vestibular Pathways

Auditory pathway:

Receptors: Hair cells of organ of Corti

First sensory neuron: Spiral ganglion of bipolar cells (in a canal around modiolus). Central processes of ganglion forms cochlear nerve.

Second neuron: Cochlear nuclei form trapezoid body in pons and then ascend as lateral lemnisci. Fibres of lateral lemniscus terminate in inferior colliculus and medial geniculate body.

Third neuron: In medial geniculate body. From it, auditory radiations pass to auditory cortex via internal capsule

Vestibular pathway:

Receptor: Hair cells in maculae of saccule and utricle.

First neuron: Vestibular ganglion of bipolar cells central processes of ganglion forms vestibular nerve.

Second neuron: Vestibular nuclei. These send fibres to:

- Archi-cerebellum
- Motor nuclei of brain stem (of III, IV and VI nerve)
- Anterior horn cells of spinal cord.

The unilateral injury to cochlear nerve do not greatly affect auditory activity because auditory radiations to cortex are bilaterally distributed.

The effect of lesion of vestibular nerve: Vertigo, ataxia and nystagmus.

Glossopharyngeal Nerve (IX cranial nerve)

The functional components of IX cranial nerve

- Branchial afferent: Branchiomotor to stylopharyngeus
- General visceral efferent: Secretomotor to parotid
- General visceral efferent: Sensory to pharynx, tonsil and posterior 1/3 of tongue.
- Special visceral afferent: Taste sensation from posterior 1/3 of tongue
- General somatic afferent: Proprioceptive impulses from stylopharyngeus.

The nuclei of origin of ninth nerve

- **Nucleus ambiguous**
- **Nucleus of tractus solitarius**
- **Inferior salivatory nucleus**

Branches of IX Cranial Nerve

- Tympanic: To middle ear, auditory tube and lesser petrosal nerve to parotid gland

- Carotid: To carotid body and carotid sinus.
- Pharyngeal: Form pharyngeal plexus
- Muscular: To stylopharyngeus
- Tonsillar: Supply tonsil and forms a plexus.
- Lingual: Taste and general sensations from posterior 1/3 of tongue.

Vagus Nerve (X cranial nerve)

The nuclei of vagus nerve:
- **Nucleus ambiguous**
- **Nucleus of tractus solitarius**
- **Dorsal nucleus of vagus**

The ganglia on vagus and what are their connections:
- Superior ganglion: In jugular foramen connected to IX and XI nerves and superior cervical ganglion of sympathetic chain
- Inferior ganglion: Near base of skull connected to XII nerve, superior cervical ganglion and loop between C1 and C2 nerves.

The branches of vagus: The structures supplied by these

From superior ganglion:
(a) **Meningeal: Dura mater of posterior cranial fossa**
(b) **Auricular: Conchae and root of auricle posterior ½ of external auditory meatus and outer surface of tympanic membrane.**
In neck (from inferior ganglion):
(a) **Pharyngeal: It has mainly fibres of cranial accessory nerve. Forms pharyngeal plexus.**
(b) **Carotid: to carotid body.**
(c) **Superior laryngeal nerve:**
   • **External laryngeal: Inferior constrictor and cricothyroid muscle**
   • **Internal laryngeal: Densory to larynx up to vocal cord**
(d) **Right recurrent laryngeal nerve:** To muscles of larynx except cricothyroid. Sensory to larynx below vocal cord.
(e) **Cardiac: To superficial and deep cardiac plexus.** In abdomen: The two vagus nerves are distributed to stomach and celiac, hepatic and renal plexuses.

The effect of lesion of vagus nerve:

• Cadaveric position of vocal cord • Dysphagia. • Flattening of palatal arch • Hoarseness of voice • Nasal regurgitation of swallowed liquids • Nasal twang in voice

Accessory Nerve (XI cranial nerve)

Named so as it is accessory to vagus.

The roots of the accessory nerve: Two roots: Cranial and spinal roots

The roots of accessory nerve are:

- The cranial root arises from the lower part of nucleus ambiguos.
- The spinal root arises from the lateral part of anterior grey column of the cervical part, C1–5 of the spinal cord.

The spinal root enter the cranial cavity: The spinal rootlets of the accessory nerve unite to form a trunk which ascends in the vertebral canal and enters the cranial cavity through the foramen magnum.

The accessory nerve called accessory because it is accessory to the vagus nerve, hence the name. The cranial root is in fact a part of the vagus nerve

The distribution of the cranial accessory nerve: It is distributed via branches of the vagus to:

- *The muscles of the soft palate (except the tensor palate)*
- *Pharynx (except the stylopharyngeus)*
- *Intrinsic muscles of the larynx.*

The distribution of the spinal accessory nerve: It supplies the

- *Sternomastoid*
- *Trapezius*

Effects of a complete lesion of the spinal accessory nerve

There will be paralysis of the sternomastoid and trapezius muscles (lower motor neuron type of paralysis).

- *The patient will not be able to rotate his head to the healthy side (due to paralysis of sternomastoid)*
- *He will not be able to shrug the affected shoulder nor will he be able to raise the arm above the head (due to paralysis of trapezius).*

Hypoglossal Nerve (XII cranial nerve)

The "nerve of the tongue"

The distribution of the hypoglossal nerve

- Hypoglossal is the motor nerve to all muscles of the tongue except the palatoglossus.
- Branches of hypoglossal nerve containing fibres of C1 nerve.
- **Meningeal branch:** To meninges of anterior cranial fossa
- **Descending branch:** Upper root of ansa cervical
- To thyrohyoid and geniohyoid.

Damage to hypoglossal nerve on one side: *There will be ipsilateral lower motor neurone type of paralysis of muscles of the tongue. On asking the patient to protrude his tongue, It will deviate to the paralysed side called as "ipsilateral paralysis."*

Differentiating nuclear lesion from an infranuclear lesion of the hypoglossal nerve: *In addition to features of the infranuclear lesion (flaccid paralysis and wasting of muscles) there will also be fasciculation's in the muscles of the tongue on the affected side. There will be wrinkling of the mucous membrane of the tongue due to wasting of muscles and their fasciculations.*

Important Points for Revision

Important Membranes

- **Basilar** membrane — Forming floor of organ of Corti (Ear)
- **Bowman's** membrane — Anterior limiting membrane of cornea (Eye)
- **Bruch's** membrane — Pigment membrane in retina (Eye)
- **Decemet's** membrane — Posterior limiting membrane of cornea (Eye)
- **Elsching's** membrane — Astroglial membrane covering optic disc (Eye)
- **Henle's** membrane — Outer layer of cells of root sheath of hair
- **Heuser's** membrane — Exocelomic membrane
- **Huxley's** membrane — Inner layer of cells of root sheath of hair
- **Periodontal** membrane — Between cementum and socket of tooth
- **Quadrate** membrane — Extends from arytenoids cartilage to epiglottis
- **Reissner's** membrane — Forming roof of organ of Corti (Ear)
- **Schneiderian** membrane — Mucus membrane lining nasal cavities
- **Shrapnell's** membrane — Pars flaccida of the tympanic membrane
- **Thyrohyoid** membrane — Connects thyroid to hyoid bone. Pierced by internal laryngeal nerve and superior laryngeal vessels.

Important Vessels in Anatomy

- **Duodenal ulcer** is caused by bleeding of gastroduodenal artery
- **Extradural hematoma (EDH)** is caused by bleeding of middle meningeal artery
- **Gastric ulcer** is caused by bleeding of left gastric artery
- **Haemoptysis** is caused by bleeding of bronchial artery
- **Menstruation** is caused by bleeding of spiral arteries
- **Subdural hematoma** (SDH) is caused by bleeding of bridging veins
- **Tonsillar hemorrhage** is caused by bleeding of paratonsillar veins
- **Myocardial infarction** is caused by obstruction in coronary vessels
- **Wallenburg's syndrome** is caused by obstruction in posterior inferior cerebellar arteries
- **Medial medullary syndrome** is caused by obstruction in vertebral arteries
- **Superior mesenteric artery syndrome** is caused by obstruction in superior mesenteric artery

- **Leriche's syndrome** is caused by obstruction in **Aorto Iliac Vessels**.
- **Great saphenous vein** is used for **CABG** (coronary artery bypass graft)

Important Anatomical Lines

- **Hilton's line:** At level of interval between subcutaneous part of external sphincter and lower border of internal anal sphincter. Felt as a groove on digital examination.
- **Nelaton's line:** From anterior superior iliac spine to ischial tuberosity. Used for diagnosing dislocation of hip.
- **Arcuate line (fold of Douglas):** Represents posterior wall of rectus sheath, at level midway between umbilicus and pubic symphysis.
- **Pectinate line:** Circular line of attachment of anal valves.
- **Holden's line:** Lateral to pubic tubercle about 8 cms. Prevents extravasation of urine into lower limb.
- **Reid's base line:** Horizontal line between infraorbital margin and centre of external acoustic meatus.
- **Linea alba:** It is a raphe formed by interlacing fibres of aponeuroses of three muscles forming rectus sheath. It extends from xiphoid process to pubic symphysis
- **Langer's line:** Corresponds to natural orientation of collagen fibres parallel to orientation of muscle fibres (in dead).
- **Kraissel's line:** Corresponds to natural orientation of collagen fibres parallel to orientation of muscle fibres (in living).

Anatomical Canals

- **Alcock's canal:** Pudendal canal or canalis pudendalis
- **Canal of nuck:** A diverticulum of the peritoneal membrane extending into the inguinal canal, accompanying the round ligament in the female, or the testis in its descent into the scrotum in the male; usually completely obliterated in the female.
- **Dorello's canal:** An opening sometimes found in the temporal bone through which the abducens nerve and inferior petrosal sinus together enter the cavernous sinus.
- **Guyon's canal:** Canal for the ulnar nerve and vessels; defined medially by the pisiform, and posteriorly by the flexor retinaculum.
- **Haversian canals:** Central vascular channels in Haversian systems
- **Hunter's canal:** Canalis adductorius or the adductor canal
- **Palatovaginal canal:** Transmits pharyngeal branch from pterygopalatine ganglion and pharyngeal branch from maxillary artery.
- **Stilling's canal:** A minute canal running through the vitreous from the discus nervi optici to the lens.
- **Vomerovaginal canal:** Transmits pharyngeal vessels and nerves

Important Fascias in Anatomy

- **Buck's fascia:** Deep fascia of penis
- **Camper's fascia:** Superficial fatty layer of superficial fascia

- **Gerota fascia:** Fascia covering kidney
- **Denonvillier's fascia:** Fascia separating rectum from prostate
- **Fascia colli:** Investing layer of deep cervical fascia of neck
- **Fascia lata**: Deep fascia of thigh
- **Cribriform fascia:** Fascia covering saphenous opening
- **Fascia iliaca:** Forms posterior wall of femoral sheath
- **Fascia transversalis**: forms anterior wall of femoral sheath
- **Scarpa's fascia:** Deep membranous layer of superficial fascia
- **Toldt's fascia:** Anterior renal fascia
- **Waldeyer's fascia:** Fascia separating rectum from coccyx
- **Zuckerkandl fascia:** Posterior renal facia

Important Triangles in Anatomy

- **Triangle of koch:** Is bounded by Tricuspid valve, Margin of coronary sinus opening, Tendon of Todaro. It is a part of fibrous skeleton of the heart. The tendon of Todaro is a continuation of the eustachian valve of the inferior vena cava and the thebesian valve of the coronary sinus. Along with the opening of the coronary sinus and the septal cusp of the tricuspid valve it makes up the triangle of Koch. The centre of the triangle of Koch is the location of the atrioventricular node. It makes up the triangle of Koch. The centre of the triangle of Koch is the location of the atrioventricular node.
- **Triangle of auscultation:** Only part of back not covered by muscles. Respiratory sounds are best heard here. Boundaries are medial border of scapula laterally. Lateral border of trapezius medially and upper border of latissmus dorsi inferiorly.
- **Triangle of petit:** It is bounded superiorly by 12th rib, inferiorly by iliac crest and laterally by posterior border of external oblique muscle.
- **Lessers triangle** is bound by hypoglossal nerve above and two bellies of digastric on either sides.
- **Hesselbach's triangle** is bounded by lateral margin of rectus abdominis medially, inferior epigastric artery laterally and inguinal ligament inferiorly.
- **McEwans suprameatal triangle:** Triangular depression posterior to external acoustic meatus is bounded by posterosuperior margin of external acoustic meatus, supramastoid crest and a vertical line tangent to posterior border of external acoustic meatus.
- **Triangle of pain:** Lateral to triangle of doom bounded by gonadal vessels medially, iliopubic tract laterally and inferiorly by inferior edge of skin incision.
- **Trautman triangle:** Anteriorly is bounded by bony labrynth, posteriorly by sigmoid sinus and above by superior petrosal sinus.

Important Angles

- **Alpha angle:** In eye between visual axis and optical axis
- **Angle of femoral torsion**: 15°

- **Angle of humeral torsion**: 164°
- **Carrying angle:** Angle made by long axis of arm with long axis of forearm—170°
- **Cittele's angle:** Sino dural angle
- **Cerebellopontine angle:** Important site for acoustic neuromas
- **Cobb angle:** Used in scoliosis
- **Kappa angle:** (in eye) between pupillary axes
- **Lovibond's angle:** Angle between nail plate and proximal nail fold
- **Neck shaft angle of femur** in adults: 125°—More in females
- **Renal angle:** Junction of 12th rib with erector spinae muscle
- **Sternal angle:** Angle of Louis
  - Cubitus valgus is increase in carrying angle; feature of Turners syndrome.
  - Coxa vera is reduction in neck shaft angle of femur.
  - Coxa valga is increase in neck shaft angle of femur.

Important Points for Revision

Tortuous Arteries

- Facial artery
- Lingual artery
- Ophthalmic artery
- PICA (post inferior cerebellar artery)
- Splenic artery
- Uterine artery
- Vaginal artery

End Arteries

- Central artery of retina
- Central branches of cerebral artery
- Coronary artery
- Segmental branches of renal/splenic artery

Important Foramina

- Foramen of **Morgagni** refers to an opening in the diaphragm
- Foramen of **Winslow** is between greater and lesser sac
- Foramen of **Magendie, Lushka** are related to fourth ventricle
- Foramen of **Monro** is interventricular foramen (brain).
- Foramen of **Vesalius** (Emisary sphenoidal foramen)

Important Lymph Nodes

- **Epitrochlear/supratrochlear nodes** are main nodes in upper limb
- **Para-aortic lymph nodes** are enlarged in cancer testis

- **Left supraclavicular lymph nodes** are enlarged in gastric malignancy (Virchow's node)
- **Axillary nodes** are most important lymph nodes for breast cancer
- **Lymph node of lund:** Cystic lymph node of gall bladder
- **Cloquets node/Rosenmüllers node:** Nodes in femoral canal
- **Mucocutaneous lymph node syndrome:**
  - **Sister Mary Joseph node:** Seen around Umbilicus in gastrointestinal malignancies
  - **Rotter's lymph nodes** are small interpectoral lymph nodes located between the pectoralis major and pectoralis minor muscles. They receive lymphatic fluid from the muscles and the mammary gland, and deliver lymphatic fluid to the axillary lymphatic plexus.

Commonest Sites

- Commonest site of **BHP:** Periurethral zone of prostate
- Commonest site of **fertilization:** Ampulla of uterine tubes
- Commonest site of **ectopic pregnancy:** fallopian tubes
- Commonest site of **cancer prostate:** Peripheral zone of prostate
- Commonest site of **varicocele:** Left side
- Commonest position of **appendix:** Retrocecal
- Commonest site of **internal hemorrhoids:** 3, 7 and 11 o' clock.
- Commonest site of **fracture clavicle:** Lateral 1/3rd and medial 2/3rd.
- Commonest site of **sinusitis:** Maxillary sinus

Important Fractures

- Toddlers #:   Spiral # of tibia
- Smiths #:   Reverse of Colles
- Rolandos #:   (Extra articular) base of Ist metacarpal
- Potts #:   Bimalleolar ankle
- Pond #:   Depressed skull # in infants
- Monteggias #:   Proximal ulna with dislocation head of radius
- Masonneres #:   Neck of fibula
- March #:   Stress # shaft of second or third metatarsal
- Jones #:   Base of 5th metatarsal
- Jeffersons #:   Burst fracture of Atlas (C1)
- Hangmans #:   Axis
- Galezzi #:   Distal radius with dislocation of distal radio ulnar joint
- Crescent #:   Iliac bone with sacroiliac disruption
- Cottons #:   Trimalleolar #
- Cooleys #:   Fracture of distal radius
- Clay shovellers #:   Spinous process of T1

- Chauffers #:   Radius above styloid process
- Chance #:   Horizontal # through vertebrae due to sudden deceleration
- Boxers #:   Neck of fifth metacarpal
- Bennets #:   (Intra-articular) base of Ist metacarpal
- Aviators #:   Neck of talus

Important "Sites" of Injury

✓ Injury to **upper end of humerus** causes axillary nerve damage
✓ Injury **(dislocation of shoulder)** causes axillary nerve damage
✓ Injury to **mid humerus** causes radial nerve damage
✓ Injury to **lower end** (medial) of humerus causes ulnar nerve damage
✓ Injury to **supra condylar area** of humerus causes median nerve damage
✓ Injury to **upper trunk of brachial plexus** causes Erb's palsy
✓ Injury to **lower trunk of brachial plexus** causes Klumpke's palsy
✓ Injury to **neck of fibula** causes damage to common peroneal nerve
✓ **Posterior dislocation of hip** causes damage to sciatic nerve
✓ **Injury to pterion** causes damage to middle meningeal vessels
✓ **Injury to left hypochondriac region:** Splenic injury Kehr's sign positive

Multiple Choice Questions

True statement about "os Cordis" is:

A. A sesamoid bone
B. Present in lateral head of gastrocnemius
C. Present in heart
D. Present in quadriceps tendon

Ans. (C) Present in heart

Boundaries of the "Lumbar Triangle of Petit" are all except:

A. Floor: Psoas major muscle
B. Below: Crest of ilium
C. Laterally: External oblique
D. Medially: Latissimus dorsi

Ans. (A) Floor: Psoas major muscle

All are true about structures passing through smaller orifices in diaphragm except:

A. Between slips from 7th and 8th costal cartilages: musculophrenic vessels
B. Between each pair of remaining slips: One of lower five intercostal nerves and vessels
C. Behind medial lumbocostal arch: Aorta
D. Behind lateral lumbocostal arch: Subcostal nerve and vessels

Ans. (C) Behind medial lumbocostal arch: Aorta

"Benedikt's syndrome" involves:

A. Mid brain
B. Pons
C. Medulla
D. Cerebellum

Ans. (A) Mid brain

Boundary of the "Koch's triangle" is not formed by:

A. Tricuspid valve ring
B. Tendon of Todaro
C. Moderator band
D. Coronary sinus

Ans. (C) Moderator band

243

"Jacobson's nerve" is a branch of:

A. Facial

B. Vagus

C. Glossopharyngeal

D. Trigeminal

Ans. (C) Glossopharyngeal

"Dorsiflexion" of ankle is by all except:

A. Tibialis posterior

B. Extensor digitorum longus

C. Extensor hallucis longus

D. Peroneus tertius

Ans. (A) Tibialis posterior

"Plantar" flexion of ankle is by:

A. Tibialis posterior

B. Extensor digitorum longus

C. Extensor hallucis longus

D. Peroneus tertius

Ans. (A) Tibialis posterior

"Hofbauer" cells are seen in:

A. Intestine

B. Placenta

C. Adrenal gland

D. Seminiferous tubules

Ans. (B) Placenta

Most common site of "peripheral aneurysm" is:

A. Femoral artery

B. Radial artery

C. Popliteal artery

D. Brachial artery

Ans. (C) Popliteal artery

"Arnolds" nerve is name of:

A. Auriculotemporal

B. Greater auricular

C. Auricular branch of vagus

D. Nerve to stapedius

Ans. (C) Auricular branch of vagus

"Charcots's artery" is a branch of:

A. Anterior cerebral artery

B. Middle cerebral artery

C. Posterior cerebral artery

D. PICA

Ans. (B) Middle cerebral artery

"Virchow's" nodes are:

A. Pretracheal

B. Paratracheal

C. Supraclavicular

D. Posterior triangle

Ans. (C) Supraclavicular

In the cubital fossa the brachial artery lies:

A. Medial to ulnar nerve

B. Medial to radial nerve

C. Medial to biceps

D. Lateral to biceps

Ans. (C) Medial to biceps

Infections from dangerous area of face are facilitated by:

A. Veins here do not have valves
B. Difficulty to immobilize this part of the face
C. Absence of deep fascia fails to restrict infection
D. All of above

Ans. (D) All of above

Gastrulation occurs by:

A. 3 weeks
B. 8 weeks
C. 10 weeks
D. 12 weeks

Ans. (A) 3 weeks

"Columns of Bertin" are seen in:

A. Suprarenals
B. Thymus
C. Kidney
D. Palatine tonsil

Ans. (C) Kidney

Processus vaginalis is related to development of:

A. Cervix
B. Vagina
C. Testis
D. Uterine tubes

Ans. (C) Testis

"Artery of Adamkiewicz" supplies:

A. Suprarenals
B. Thymus
C. Spinal cord
D. Palatine tonsil

Ans. (C) Spinal cord

"Pterion" of skull corresponds to:

A. Middle meningeal artery
B. Bridging veins
C. Vertebral artery
D. None

Ans. (A) Middle meningeal artery

The "Rotator cuff" includes all muscles except:

A. Supraspinatus
B. Infraspinatus
C. Teres major
D. Subscapularis

Ans. (C) Teres major

True about Psoas abscess are all except:

A. Tuberculous disease gives rise to it
B. It is also called as a hot abscess
C. This abscess trickles under the psoas sheath up to the insertion of psoas major
D. May be mistaken for a femoral hernia and flexion deformity of hip it due to spasm of psoas

Ans. (B) It is also called as a hot abscess

"Bursa of Fabricus" corresponds to:

A. Spleen   B. Thymus
C. Lymph nodes   D. Palatine tonsil
Ans. (B) Thymus

Not a true statement is:

A. Left suprarenal drains into left renal vein
B. Left testicular vein drains into left renal vein
C. Left ovarian vein drains into left renal vein
D. Batesons vertebral venous plexus is valvular
Ans. (D) Batesons vertebral venous plexus is valvular

"Cords of Billroth" are seen in:

A. Liver   B. Spleen
C. Thymus   D. Lymph nodes
Ans. (B) Spleen

"Housemaid's knee" is the result of inflammation of:

A. Deep infrapatellar bursa
B. Prepatellar bursa
C. Subcutaneous infrapatellar bursa
D. Suprapatellar bursa
Ans. (B) Prepatellar bursa

Anterior spinal artery occlusion causes predominantly:

A. Motor loss   B. Sensory loss
C. Both   D. None
Ans. (A) Motor loss

"Melanocytes" in skin are developed from:

A. Ectoderm   B. Mesoderm
C. Endoderm   D. Neural crest
Ans. (D) Neural crest

Space of Mall is seen in:

A. Liver   B. Thymus
C. Spleen   D. Pituitary
Ans. (A) Liver

"Stave cells" are seen in:

A. Liver   B. Thymus
C. Spleen   D. Pituitary
Ans. (C) Spleen

Multiple Choice Questions

The root value of ilioinguinal nerve is:

A. L1   B. L1L2

C. L1L2L3   D. L3L4

Ans. (A) L1

Pain referred to the shoulder in inflammation of rotator cuff is known as:

A. Kehr's sign   B. Murphy's sign

C. Trendelenburg's sign   D. Dawbarn's sign

Ans. (D) Dawbarn's sign

Tympanic membrane is developed from:

A. Ectoderm

B. Mesoderm

C. Ectoderm + Mesoderm + Endoderm

D. Mesoderm + Endoderm

Ans. (C) Ectoderm + Mesoderm + Endoderm

Germinal epithelium of ovary is lined by:

A. Squamous epithelium   B. Columnar epithelium

C. Transitional epithelium   D. Cuboidal epithelium

Ans. (D) Cuboidal epithelium

"Moynihan's Hump" is related to

A. Coeliac trunk   B. Hepatic artery

C. Left gastric artery   D. Right gastric artery

Ans. (B) Hepatic artery

Anterior facial vein communicates with cavernous sinus through:

A. Posterior facial vein   B. Common facial vein

C. Posterior auricular vein   D. Deep facial nerve

Ans. (D) Deep facial nerve

"Space of Nuel" is seen in:

A. Heart   B. Cerebellum

C. Liver   D. Organ of Corti

Ans. (D) Organ of Corti

"Motor nerve" of tongue is:

A. Lingual nerve   B. Glossopharyngeal nerve

C. Hypoglossal nerve   D. Chorda tympani nerve

Ans. (C) Hypoglossal nerve

True about singers nodule are all except:

A. Also called as teachers' nodule
B. It is a small inflammatory growth that develops on the vocal cords of people who constantly strain their voices
C. Misuse or over use of voice leads to hyperkeratosis of the free edges of vocal cords
D. None

Ans. (D) None

"Avascular necrosis" is seen in:

A. Talus
B. Cuboid
C. Navicular
D. Calcaneum

Ans. (A) Talus

Paradidymis is embryologically developed from:

A. Metanephros
B. Mesonephros
C. Mesonephric duct
D. Mesonephric tubules

Ans. (D) Mesonephric tubules

Knee jerk tests:

A. L1, 2, 3
B. L2, 3, 4
C. L4, 5
D. L5

Ans. (B) L2, 3, 4

"Thymic hypoplasia" is due to faulty development of:

A. 2nd pharyngeal pouch
B. 3rd pharyngeal pouch
C. 4th pharyngeal pouch
D. 5th pharyngeal pouch

Ans. (B) 3rd pharyngeal pouch

"Policeman's tip" deformity refers to:

A. Erb's palsy
B. Klumpke palsy
C. Winging of scapula
D. Wrist drop

Ans. (A) Erb's palsy

Portocaval anastomosis in the form of varices are present at:

A. Bare area of liver
B. Rectum
C. Esophagus
D. All

Ans. (C) Esophagus

Pain referred to the left shoulder in the rupture of spleen is known as:

A. Kehr's sign
B. Murphy's sign
C. Fox sign
D. Dawbarn's sign

Ans. (A) Kehr's sign

Riedel's lobe pertains to:

A. Lung

B. Liver

C. Pancreas

D. Thymus

Ans. (B) Liver

Midbrain develops from:

A. Diencephalon

B. Telencephalon

C. Mesencephalon

D. Rhombencephalon

Ans. (C) Mesencephalon

The Dandy-Walker malformation consists of all except:

A. Small posterior fossa

B. High position of the tentorium

C. Hypogenesis of the cerebellar vermis

D. Cystic dilatation of the fourth ventricle

Ans. (A) Small posterior fossa

Short gastric vessels are related to:

A. Splenorenal ligament

B. Gastrosplenic ligament

C. Phrenico colic ligament

D. Falciform ligament

Ans. (B) Gastrosplenic ligament

One of the commonest area of tenderness from appendicitis is called:

A. McBurney's point

B. Murphy's point

C. Sudeck's point

D. Cullen's point

Ans. (A) McBurney's point

Opening in middle meatus are all except:

A. Opening of frontal air sinus

B. Opening of maxillary air sinus

C. Opening of middle ethmoidal air sinus

D. None

Ans. (D) None

Component of basal ganglia is:

A. Dentate nucleus

B. Emboliform nucleus

C. Globoose nucleus

D. Caudate nucleus

Ans. (D) Caudate nucleus

The total volume of CSF is about:

A. 13 ml

B. 130 ml

C. 1300 ml

D. 13000 ml

Ans. (B) 130 ml

Select the incorrect statement about patella:

A. A sesamoid bone
B. No periosteum
C. Minimizes friction
D. Develops in tendon of popliteus

Ans. (D) Develops in tendon of popliteus

Which of the following structures passes through "internal acoustic meatus":

A. Mandibular nerve
B. Maxillary nerve
C. Facial nerve
D. Middle meningeal artery

Ans. (C) Facial nerve

"Winging of the scapula" is due to injury to nerve supplying the muscle:

A. Pectoral nerve
B. Serratus anterior
C. Subscapular nerve
D. Ulnar nerve

Ans. (B) Serratus anterior

"The Reichert's cartilage" is a cartilage of:

A. 1st arch
B. 2nd arch
C. 3rd arch
D. 4th arch

Ans. (B) 2nd arch

"Main" source of blood supply to liver is:

A. Portal vein
B. Common hepatic artery
C. Left hepatic artery
D. Right hepatic artery

Ans. (A) Portal vein

Trigone of urinary bladder is derived from:

A. Ectoderm
B. Mesoderm
C. Endoderm
D. Neural crest

Ans. (B) Mesoderm

Wrist joint is an example of:

A. Hinge joint
B. Saddle joint
C. Ellipsoid joint
D. Ball and socket joint

Ans. (C) Ellipsoid joint

Which of the following muscles is NOT supplied by hypoglossal nerve?

A. Hypoglossus
B. Styloglossus
C. Palatoglossus
D. Genioglossus

Ans. (C) Palatoglossus

Nerve in relation to "neck of fibula" is:

A. Saphenous nerve

B. Common peroneal nerve

C. Tibial nerve

D. Obturator nerve

Ans. (B) Common peroneal nerve

"Safety muscle" of tongue is:

A. Mylohyoid

B. Geniohyoid

C. Stylohyoid

D. Genioglossus

Ans. (D) Genioglossus

Mesothelium is developed from:

A. Ectoderm

B. Mesoderm

C. Ectoderm + Mesoderm + Endoderm

D. Mesoderm + Endoderm

Ans. (B) Mesoderm

"Left gastric artery" is a branch of:

A. Common hepatic artery

B. Splenic artery

C. Celiac trunk

D. Gastroduodenal artery

Ans. (C) Celiac trunk

Lymphatic drainage of testis is predominantly to:

A. Inguinal lymph node

B. External iliac lymph node

C. Internal iliac lymph node

D. Pre and para-aortic lymph nodes

Ans. (D) Pre and para-aortic lymph nodes

Ovula Nabothi are seen in relation to:

A. Spleen

B. Ovary

C. Cervix

D. Testis

Ans. (C) Cervix

"Erb's paralysis" occurs due to injury at which level?

A. C5–C6

B. C6–C7

C. C7–C8

D. C8–T1

Ans. (A) C5–C6

The histological layer absent in esophagus is:

A. Mucosa

B. Submucosa

C. Muscular layer

D. Serosa

Ans. (D) Serosa

Multiple Choice Questions

The lateral rectus muscle of eye is supplied by:

A. 3rd cranial nerve   B. 4th cranial nerve
C. 5th cranial nerve   D. 6th cranial nerve
Ans. (D) 6th cranial nerve

Which among the following does not open into coronary sinus?

A. Great cardiac vein   B. Middle cardiac vein
C. Small cardiac vein   D. Anterior cardiac vein
Ans. (D) Anterior cardiac vein

Elastic cartilage is present in:

A. Trachea   B. Intervertebral disc
C. Menisci   D. Epiglottis
Ans. (D) Epiglottis

Auriculotemporal nerve is a direct branch of:

A. Mandibular nerve   B. Maxillary nerve
C. Ophthalmic nerve   D. Trigeminal ganglion
Ans. (A) Mandibular nerve

True about the arterial supply of pancreas are all except:

A. Pancreatic branches of splenic artery
B. Superior pancreaticoduodenal artery, a branch of coeliac trunk
C. Inferior pancreaticoduodenal artery, a branch of superior mesenteric artery
D. Arteria cauda pancreatica: a branch of superior mesenteric artery
Ans. (D) Arteria cauda pancreatica: a branch of superior mesenteric artery

"Foramen of Morgagni" refers to an opening in:

A. The brain   B. The lesser omentum
C. The skull   D. The diaphragm
Ans. (D) The diaphragm

Facial artery is a branch of:

A. External carotid artery   B. Thyrocervical trunk
C. Costocervical trunk   D. Internal carotid artery
Ans. (A) External carotid artery

"Pes anserinus" is seen in relation to:

A. Abducent nerve   B. Oculomotor nerve
C. Glossopharyngeal nerve   D. Facial nerve
Ans. (D) Facial nerve

Hassall's corpuscles are a histological feature of:

A. Spleen
B. Thymus
C. Lymph nodes
D. Palatine tonsil

Ans. (B) Thymus

Which cranial nerve is associated with meninges covering it?

A. Optic nerve
B. Trigeminal nerve
C. Trochlear nerve
D. Abducent nerve

Ans. (A) Optic nerve

Fracture of surgical neck of humerus leads to loss of abduction movement of the corresponding shoulder joint due to injury of:

A. Radial nerve
B. Musculocutaneous nerve
C. Axillary nerve
D. Median nerve

Ans. (C) Axillary nerve

Contents of rectus sheath are all except:

A. Pyramidalis
B. Superior epigastric artery
C. Inferior epigastric vein
D. Rectus femoris

Ans. (D) Rectus femoris

Nerves: lower 5-intercostal nerves, subcostal nerve
Not a corresponding match of cranial nerves is:

A. Glossopharyngeal IX
B. Vagus X
C. Accessory VII
D. Hypoglossal XII

Ans. (C) Accessory VII

Structure opening in left atrium of heart is:

A. Coronary sinus
B. Superior vena cava
C. Inferior vena cava
D. Pulmonary veins

Ans. (D) Pulmonary veins

Accessory nerve supplies:

A. Sternomastoid
B. Buccinator
C. Platysma
D. Stapedius

Ans. (A) Sternomastoid

Superior orbital fissure transmits all cranial nerves except:

A. III
B. IV
C. VI
D. VII

Ans. (D) VII

Glisson's capsule is seen in:

A. Liver

B. Thymus

C. Kidney

D. Adrenal

Ans. (A) Liver

Chromaffin cells are seen in:

A. Liver

B. Thymus

C. Kidney

D. Adrenal

Ans. (D) Adrenal

Injury to median nerve causes:

A. Saturday night palsy

B. Erb's palsy

C. Elbow drop

D. Ape thumb deformity

Ans. (D) Ape thumb deformity

Lateral ligament of ankle joint consists of all except:

A. Anterior talofibular ligament

B. Posterior talofibular ligament

C. Calcaneofibular ligament

D. Tibiocalcaneal ligament

Ans. (D) Tibiocalcaneal ligament

Parkinsonism effects mainly:

A. Cerebellum

B. Substantia nigra

C. Nucleus basalis

D. Frontal lobe

Ans. (B) Substantia nigra

The structure passing through optic canal is:

A. Mandibular nerve

B. Maxillary nerve

C. Middle meningeal artery

D. Optic nerve

Ans. (D) Optic nerve

The Dandy-Walker malformation consists of all except:

A. Small posterior cranial fossa

B. High position of the tentorium

C. Hypogenesis of the cerebellar vermis

D. Cystic dilatation of the fourth ventricle

Ans. (A) Small posterior cranial fossa

"Hip joint" is an example of:

A. Hinge joint

B. Ellipsoid joint

C. Saddle joint

D. Ball and socket joint

Ans. (D) Ball and socket joint

"Mandibular" nerve supplies:

A. Posterior belly of digastric
B. Buccinator
C. Masseter
D. Stapedius

Ans. (C) Masseter

Taste sensations from the anterior 2/3 of tongue are carried by nerve:

A. Chorda tympani
B. Glossopharyngeal
C. Lingual
D. Vagus

Ans. (A) Chorda tympani

The epithelial lining of the trachea is composed of:

A. Pseudostratified columnar nonciliated cells, goblet cells and basal cells
B. Pseudostratified columnar ciliated cells, goblet cells and basal cells
C. Stratified columnar nonciliated cells, goblet cells and basal cells
D. Stratified noncolumnar ciliated cells, goblet cells and basal cells

Ans. (B) Pseudostratified columnar ciliated cells, goblet cells and basal cells

Elbow is an example of:

A. Hinge joint
B. Ellipsoid joint
C. Saddle joint
D. Ball and socket joint

Ans. (A) Hinge joint

Lymphatic drainage of ovaries is predominantly to the nodes:

A. Deep inguinal
B. Superficial inguinal
C. Para-aortic
D. Common iliac

Ans. (C) Para-aortic

Left testicular vein drains into:

A. Left splenic vein
B. Left renal vein
C. Inferior vena cava
D. Right renal vein

Ans (B) Left renal vein

Intervertebral disc is made up of:

A. Fibrocartilage
B. Elastic cartilage
C. Hyaline cartilage
D. None

Ans. (A) Fibrocartilage

Space of Disse is seen in:

A. Liver
B. Thymus
C. Spleen
D. Pituitary

Ans. (A) Liver

The axis of rotation of gut is in relation to:

A. Common hepatic artery

B. Splenic artery

C. Celiac trunk

D. Superior mesenteric artery

Ans. (D) Superior mesenteric artery

Discus proligerus is seen in relation to:

A. Spleen

B. Ovary

C. Lymph nodes

D. Testis

Ans. (B) Ovary

Paramesonephric duct forms which of the following structure?

A. Ureter

B. Uterus

C. Urethra

D. Uvula

Ans. (B) Uterus

Teres minor is supplied by nerve:

A. Thoracodorsal

B. Axillary

C. Dorsal scapular

D. Lower subscapular

Ans. (B) Axillary

Stapedius is supplied by:

A. Abducent nerve

B. Oculomotor nerve

C. Glossopharyngeal nerve

D. Facial nerve

Ans. (D) Facial nerve

All of the following are contents of broad ligament except:

A. Fallopian tube

B. Round ligament

C. Ovarian ligament

D. Ovary

Ans. (D) Ovary

The nerve passing between two heads of gastrocnemius is:

A. Saphenous nerve

B. Sural nerve

C. Femoral nerve

D. Obturator nerve

Ans. (B) Sural nerve

Heart failure cells are seen in:

A. Heart

B. Lung

C. Liver

D. Veins

Ans. (B) Lung

"Vessel" seen in substance of cavernous sinus is:

A. External carotid artery

B. Thyrocervical trunk

C. Costocervical trunk

D. Internal carotid artery

Ans. (D) Internal carotid artery

Pseudoganglion is usually seen in nerve to:

A. Infraspinatus   B. Teres major
C. Teres minor   D. Long head of triceps

Ans. (C) Teres minor

Sharipos syndrome is agenesis of:

A. Corpus callosum
B. Anterior commissure
C. Posterior commissure
D. Hippocampal commissure

Ans. (A) Corpus callosum

NOT a branch of cerebral part of ICA is:

A. Ophthalmic   B. Anterior cerebral
C. Middle cerebral   D. Anterior communicating

Ans. (D) Anterior communicating

Hyperacusis is due to involvement of:

A. Auriculotemporal   B. Greater auricular
C. Auricular branch of vagus   D. Nerve to stapedius

Ans. (D) Nerve to stapedius

Iliolumbar artery is a branch of:

A. Anterior division of internal iliac artery
B. Posterior division of internal iliac artery
C. Anterior division of external iliac artery
D. Posterior division of external iliac artery

Ans. (B) Posterior division of internal iliac artery

Sural nerve passes between which muscle?

A. Semimembranosus   B. Semitendinosus
C. Biceps femoris   D. Gastrocnemius

Ans. (D) Gastrocnemius

All structures open in right atrium of heart except:

A. Coronary sinus   B. Superior vena cava
C. Inferior vena cava   D. Pulmonary veins

Ans. (D) Pulmonary veins

Defective cilia are seen in:

A. Cystic fibrosis syndrome   B. Ehlers-Danlos syndrome
C. Mounier-Kuhn syndrome   D. Kartagener's syndrome

Ans. (D) Kartagener's syndrome

The base of the mesentery attaches to the posterior abdominal wall:

A. To the right of the third lumbar vertebra and passes obliquely to the left and inferiorly to the right sacroiliac joint

B. To the left of the third lumbar vertebra and passes obliquely to the left and inferiorly to the right sacroiliac joint

C. To the right of the second lumbar vertebra and passes obliquely to the left and inferiorly to the right sacroiliac joint

D. To the left of the second lumbar vertebra and passes obliquely to the right and inferiorly to the right sacroiliac joint

Ans. (D) To the left of the second lumbar vertebra and passes obliquely to the right and inferiorly to the right sacroiliac joint

Axillary sheath is derived from:

A. Clavipectoral fascia
B. Prevertebral fascia
C. Pretracheal fascia
D. None

Ans. (B) Prevertebral fascia

Gag reflex is absent in injury to the following nerve:

A. Facial (VII)
B. Glossopharyngeal (IX)
C. Hypoglossal (XII)
D. Spinal accessory (XI)

Ans. (B) Glossopharyngeal (IX)

Allantois is related to:

A. Liver
B. Pancreas
C. Kidney
D. Urinary bladder

Ans. (B) Urinary bladder

Facial nerve supplies all muscles except:

A. Sternomastoid
B. Buccinator
C. Platysma
D. Stapedius

Ans. (A) Sternomastoid

Local spread of cancer of esophagus is rapid due to absence of:

A. Mucosa
B. Submucosa
C. Muscular layer
D. Serosa

Ans. (D) Serosa

Central artery of retina is branch of:

A. External carotid artery
B. Internal carotid artery
C. Ophthalmic artery
D. Basilar artery

Ans. (C) Ophthalmic artery

Embryologically the diaphragm is developed from all except:

A. Ventral and dorsal mesenteries of esophagus
B. Septum transversum
C. Pleuroperitoneal membrane
D. Endoderm of body wall

Ans. (D) Endoderm of body wall

Not true about optic nerve is:

A. It is a tract of CNS
B. Formed by axons of bipolar neurons
C. The optic nerve is not covered with meninges
D. It is crossed by ophthalmic artery

Ans. (C) The optic nerve is not covered with meninges

Hirschsprung's disease is due to faulty migration of cells from:

A. Ectoderm
B. Mesoderm
C. Endoderm
D. Neural crest

Ans. (D) Neural crest

Fabella is seen in which of the following muscle?

A. Semimembranosus
B. Semitendinosus
C. Medial head of gastrocnemius
D. Lateral head of gastrocnemius

Ans. (D) Lateral head of gastrocnemius

Schmidt-Lanterman clefts are seen in relation to:

A. Cardiac muscle
B. Skeletal muscle
C. Smooth muscle
D. Neurons

Ans. (B) Skeletal muscle and **(D)** Neurons

Cords of Billroth are seen in:

A. Liver
B. Spleen
C. Thymus
D. Lymph nodes

Ans. (B) Spleen

The posterior end of thalamus attaches:

A. Lateral geniculate body
B. Medial geniculate body
C. Both
D. None

Ans. (C) Both

Intervertebral disc is made up of:

A. Fibrocartilage
B. Elastic cartilage
C. Hyaline cartilage
D. None

Ans. (A) Fibrocartilage

Ophthalmic artery accompanies which nerve?

A. Optic
B. Oculomotor
C. Maxillary
D. Mandibular

Ans. (A) Optic

Prepyriform area is concerned with which modality?

A. Visual
B. Auditory
C. Gustatory
D. Olfactory

Ans. (D) Olfactory

True about splenic artery is/are:

A. Arises from celiac trunk
B. Gives short gastric arteries
C. Tortuous
D. All of the above

Ans. (D) All of the above

Trendelenburg's sign is positive due to injury in which of the following nerve?

A. Superior gluteal nerve
B. Inferior gluteal nerve
C. Femoral nerve
D. Pudendal nerve

Ans. (A) Superior gluteal nerve

Nerve related to surgical neck of humerus is:

A. Thoracodorsal
B. Axillary
C. Dorsal scapular
D. Lower subscapular

Ans. (B) Axillary

Tailors muscle is:

A. Sartorius
B. Gluteus maximus
C. Iliopsoas
D. Pectineus

Ans. (A) Sartorius

One of the commonest area of colonic ischemia is called:

A. McBurney's point
B. Murphy's point
C. Sudeck's point
D. Cullen's point

Ans. (C) Sudeck's point

Radial nerve originates from:

A. Posterior cord of brachial plexus
B. Medial cord of brachial plexus
C. Lateral cord of brachial plexus
D. Erb's point

Ans. (A) Posterior cord of brachial plexus

Coracoid process is a_____type of epiphysis.

A. Pressure
B. Traction
C. Atavistic
D. Aberrant

Ans. (C) Atavistic

Length of inguinal canal is:

A. Less than 5 cm
B. 15–20 cm
C. 25–30 cm
D. 40–45 cm

Ans. (A) Less than 5 cm

Connective tissue is developed predominantly from:

A. Ectoderm
B. Mesoderm
C. Ectoderm + Mesoderm + Endoderm
D. Mesoderm + Endoderm

Ans. (B) Mesoderm

First carpometacarpal joint is an example of:

A. Hinge joint
B. Ellipsoid joint
C. Saddle joint
D. Ball and socket joint

Ans. (C) Saddle joint

Lymphatic drainage of glans penis is to the nodes:

A. Deep inguinal
B. Superficial inguinal
C. Para-aortic
D. Common iliac

Ans. (A) Deep inguinal

Quinsy is the name given to:

A. Peritonsillar abscess
B. Retropharyngeal abscess
C. Parapharyngeal abscess
D. Sublingual abscess

Ans. (A) Peritonsillar abscess

The SA node is usually supplied by branch from the:

A. Left coronary artery
B. Right coronary artery
C. Ascending aorta
D. Descending aorta

Ans. (B) Right coronary artery

Amacrine cells are seen in:

A. Lens
B. Organ of Corti
C. Cervix
D. Retina

Ans. (D) Retina

Thymus gland develops from:

A. 2nd pharyngeal pouch
B. 3rd pharyngeal pouch
C. 4th pharyngeal pouch
D. 5th pharyngeal pouch

Ans. (B) 3rd pharyngeal pouch

Content of Hunter's canal are all of the following except:

A. Femoral nerve
B. Femoral artery
C. Saphenous nerve
D. Nerve to vastus medialis

Ans. (A) Femoral nerve

In humans the notochord:

A. Completely disappers
B. Persists as vertebral body
C. Persists as the intervertebral disc
D. Persists as nucleus pulposus

Ans. (D) Persists as nucleus pulposus

Müllerian duct forms which of the following structure?

A. Ureter
B. Uterus
C. Urethra
D. Uvula

Ans. (B) Uterus

Features of Horner's syndrome are all except:

A. Ptosis
B. Miosis
C. Enophthalmos
D. Hydrosis

Ans. (D) Hydrosis

Endothelium of blood vessels is lined by:

A. Squamous epithelium
B. Columnar epithelium
C. Transitional epithelium
D. Cuboidal epithelium

Ans. (A) Squamous epithelium

Wolffian duct is:

A. Metanephros
B. Mesonephros
C. Mesonephric duct
D. Mesonephric tubules

Ans. (C) Mesonephric duct

Pulmonary sequestration is supplied by:

A. Pulmonary artery
B. Bronchial artery
C. Intercostal artery
D. Systemic artery

Ans. (D) Systemic artery

Occulsion of which of the following arteries can result in Wallenberg syndrome?

A. Vertebral artery
B. Medial cerebral artery
C. Posterior cerebral artery
D. Posterior inferior cerebellar artery

Ans. (D) Posterior inferior cerebellar artery

Broad ligament contains all except:

A. Round ligament of the uterus   B. Ligament of the ovary
C. Uterine vessels   D. Internal iliac vessels

Ans. (D) Internal iliac vessels

Broad ligament contains all except:

A. External iliac vessels   B. Ovarian vessels
C. Epoophoron   D. Paraoophoron

Ans. (A) External iliac vessels

Stomach bed is formed by all except:

A. Diaphragm   B. Right suprarenal
C. Pancreas   D. Splenic artery

Ans. (B) Right suprarenal

Incorrect statement about arterial supply of suprarenal is:

A. Superior suprarenal artery: Branch of inferior phernic
B. Middle suprarenal artery: Branch of abdominal aorta
C. Inferior suprarenal artery: Branch of renal artery
D. None

Ans. (D) None

Portocaval anastomosis is present at all sites except:

A. Bare area of liver   B. Rectum
C. Esophagus   D. Spleen

Ans. (D) Spleen

Ape-hand deformity is due to injury of:

A. Ulnar nerve   B. Median nerve
C. Radial nerve   D. Postinterosseus nerve

Ans. (B) Median nerve

Which one is a tortuous artery?

A. Vertebral artery   B. Ovarian artery
C. Vaginal artery   D. Uterine artery

Ans. (D) Uterine artery

Nasolacrimal duct opens into which meatus?

A. Inferior
B. Superior
C. Middle
D. All

Ans. (A) Inferior meatus

Vital point is found in:

A. Cerebellum
B. Medulla oblongata
C. Hypothalamus
D. Thalamus

Ans. (B) Medulla oblongata

Urothelium is the name given to:

A. Squamous epithelium
B. Columnar epithelium
C. Transitional epithelium
D. Cuboidal epithelium

Ans. (C) Transitional epithelium

Superior thyroid artery is a branch of:

A. External carotid artery
B. Thyrocervical trunk
C. Costocervical trunk
D. Internal carotid artery

Ans. (A) External carotid artery

Opening of jaw is done by:

A. Medial pterygoid
B. Temporalis
C. Lateral pterygoid
D. Masseter

Ans. (C) Lateral pterygoid

Platysma is supplied by the following nerve:

A. Mandibular nerve
B. Maxillary nerve
C. Facial nerve
D. Cervical plexus

Ans. (C) Facial nerve

Myelination of CNS is done by:

A. Schwann cells
B. Microglia
C. Oligodendrocytes
D. Astrocytes

Ans. (C) Oligodendrocytes

The muscles producing movement of plantar flexion at ankle joint is:

A. Extensor digitorum longus
B. Extensor hallucis longus
C. Peroneus tertius
D. Tibialis posterior

Ans. (D) Tibialis posterior

The structures passing through inguinal canal are all except:

A. Ilioinguinal nerve in both sexes
B. Round ligament of uterus in females
C. Spermatic cord in males
D. None
Ans. (D) None

Skin around umbilicus is supplied by which dermatome?

A. T9
B. T10
C. T11
D. T12
Ans. (B) T10

"Facial angle" is a rough index of the degree of development of:

A. Mandible
B. Nose
C. Brain
D. Eyes
Ans. (C) Brain

Hyperpyrexia and pin point pupils are seen in lesion of:

A. Mid brain
B. Pons
C. Medulla
D. Cerebellum
Ans. (B) Pons

Sustentacular cells are seen in:

A. Spleen
B. Ovary
C. Lymph nodes
D. Testis
Ans. (D) Testis

The nerve of "third pharyngeal arch" is:

A. Abducent nerve
B. Oculomotor nerve
C. Glossopharyngeal nerve
D. Facial nerve
Ans. (C) Glossopharyngeal nerve

Ear pinna is made up of:

A. Fibrocartilage
B. Elastic cartilage
C. Hyaline cartilage
D. None
Ans. (B) Elastic cartilage

Nerve present in the substance of parotid gland is:

A. Facial
B. Vagus
C. Glossopharyngeal
D. Trigeminal
Ans. (A) Facial

Caroticotympanic artery is a branch of:

A. Vertebral artery

C. Labyrinthine artery

B. Basilar artery

D. Internal carotid artery

Ans. (D) Internal carotid artery

Serratus anterior is supplied by which nerve?

A. Thoracodorsal

C. Axillary

B. Long thoracic

D. Radial

Ans. (B) Long thoracic

All structure passes through aortic opening except:

A. Aorta

C. Thoracic duct

B. Azygous vein

D. Left recurrent laryngeal nerve

Ans. (D) Left recurrent laryngeal nerve

Vessel seen in anatomical snuff box is:

A. Ulnar artery

C. Anterior interosseous artery

B. Radial artery

D. Brachial artery

Ans. (B) Radial artery

Injury to which nerve causes foot drop?

A. Femoral nerve

C. Tibial nerve

B. Common peroneal nerve

D. Obturator nerve

Ans. (B) Common peroneal nerve

Main source of blood supply to liver is by:

A. Hepatic artery

C. Left gastric artery

B. Hepatic vein

D. Portal vein

Ans. (D) Portal vein

Breast is developed predominantly from:

A. Ectoderm

C. Ectoderm + Endoderm

B. Mesoderm

D. Mesoderm + Endoderm

Ans. (A) Ectoderm

Deep fascia of neck is:

A. Colles fascia

C. Campers fascia

B. Fascia colli

D. Waldeyers fascia

Ans. (B) Fascia colli

Nerve innervation of tensor palati is:

A. Facial nerve

C. Maxillary nerve

B. Ophthalmic nerve

D. Mandibular nerve

Ans. (D) Mandibular nerve

Uterus develops from:

A. Metanephros

B. Mesonephros

C. Mesonephric duct

D. Paramesonephric duct

Ans. (D) Paramesonephric duct

Lateral branches of abdominal aorta are all except:

A. Testicular or ovarian

B. Renal

C. Middle suprarenal

D. Inferior mesenteric

Ans. (D) Inferior mesenteric

Crypts are a histological feature of:

A. Spleen

B. Thymus

C. Lymph nodes

D. Palatine tonsil

Ans. (D) Palatine tonsil

The loss of opposition movement of the thumb is due to injury to the nerve:

A. Anterior interosseous nerve

B. Median nerve

C. Radial nerve

D. Ulnar nerve

Ans. (B) Median nerve

The structure present in the centre of cavernous sinus is:

A. Maxillary nerve

B. Trochlear nerve

C. Oculomotor nerve

D. Abducent nerve

Ans. (D) Abducent nerve

Cells of Merkel are seen in relation to:

A. Cardiac muscle

B. Skeletal muscle

C. Smooth muscle

D. Skin

Ans. (D) Skin

Stylopharyngeus is supplied by cranial nerve:

A. Abducent nerve

B. Oculomotor nerve

C. Glossopharyngeal nerve

D. Facial nerve

Ans. (C) Glossopharyngeal nerve

Nails are derived from:

A. Ectoderm

B. Mesoderm

C. Endoderm

D. Neural crest

Ans. (A) Ectoderm

Length of trachea is:

A. 5–10 cm

B. 10–15 cm

C. 15–20 cm

D. 20–25 cm

Ans. (B) 10–15 cm

Lateral boundary of cubital fossa is formed by:

A. Brachioradialis
B. Pronator teres
C. Brachialis
D. Biceps

Ans. (A) Brachioradialis

Ito cells are a histological feature of:

A. Spleen
B. Prostate
C. Pituitary
D. Liver

Ans. (D) Liver

Miner's knee is the result of inflammation of:

A. Deep infrapatellar bursa
B. Prepatellar bursa
C. Subcutaneous infrapatellar bursa
D. Suprapatellar bursa

Ans. (B) Prepatellar bursa

Motor supply of diaphragm is by following nerve:

A. Phrenic nerve
B. Accessory phrenic nerve
C. Cranial accessory nerve
D. Spinal accessory nerve

Ans. (A) Phrenic nerve

Inferior rectal artery is a branch of:

A. Aorta artery
B. External iliac artery
C. Internal iliac artery
D. Pudendal artery

Ans. (D) Pudendal artery

Which among the following opens into coronary sinus?

A. Great cardiac vein
B. Middle cardiac vein
C. Small cardiac vein
D. All of above

Ans. (D) All of above

Paramesonephric duct forms which of the following structure?

A. Uterine tubes
B. Uterus
C. Appendix of testis
D. All of the above

Ans. (D) All of the above

The Meckel's cartilage is a cartilage of:

A. 1st arch
B. 2nd arch
C. 3rd arch
D. 4th arch

Ans. (A) 1st arch

Duct of Wirsung pertain to:

A. Lung
B. Liver
C. Pancreas
D. Thymus

Ans. (C) Pancreas

The root value of saphenous nerve is:

A. L1
B. L1 L2
C. L1 L2 L3
D. L3 L4

Ans. (D) L3 L4

The chief abductor of vocal is:

A. Posterior cricothyroid
B. Posterior cricoarytenoid
C. Cricohyoid
D. Mylohyoid

Ans. (B) Posterior cricoarytenoid

Oral diaphragm is:

A. Mylohyoid
B. Geniohyoid
C. Stylohyoid
D. Genioglossus

Ans. (A) Mylohyoid

The artery of mid gut is:

A. Common hepatic artery
B. Splenic artery
C. Celiac trunk
D. Superior mesentric artery

Ans. (D) Superior mesentric artery

Opening in middle meatus are all except:

A. Opening of frontal air sinus
B. Opening of maxillary air sinus
C. Opening of middle ethmoidal air sinus
D. Opening of posterior ethmoidal air sinus

Ans. (D) Opening of posterior ethmoidal air sinus

Gluteus medius is supplied by:

A. Superior gluteal nerve
B. Inferior gluteal nerve
C. Femoral nerve
D. Pudendal nerve

Ans. (A) Superior gluteal nerve

True about appendices epiploicae is:

A. Helps in active peristalsis
B. Present in alimentary canal along with mesentery
C. Present in small intestine
D. Present in rectum

Ans. (B) Present in alimentary canal along with mesentery

Multiple Choice Questions

The following provides maximum support to uterus:

A. Broad ligament
B. Mackenrodt's ligament
C. Round ligament
D. Vesicouterine fold

Ans. (B) Mackenrodt's ligament

Lesser petrosal nerve is a branch of:

A. Facial
B. Vagus
C. Glossopharyngeal
D. Trigeminal

Ans. (C) Glossopharyngeal

Feeding centre lies in:

A. Cerebral cortex
B. Hypothalamus
C. Midbrain
D. Pons

Ans. (B) Hypothalamus

Most common position of appendix is:

A. Splenic
B. Retrocaecal
C. Pelvic
D. Paracolic

Ans. (B) Retrocaecal

'Chassaignac's tubercle' is:

A. Erb's point
B. Carotid tubercle on C6 vertebra
C. Found on first rib
D. Medial condyle of humerus

Ans. (B) Carotid tubercle on C6 vertebra

Valves of Kerckring are seen in:

A. Appendix
B. Small intestine
C. Cecum
D. Sigmoid colon

Ans. (B) Small intestine

Main action of popliteus muscle is:

A. Unlocking of knee joint
B. Locking of knee joint
C. Extension of knee joint
D. Medial rotation of knee joint

Ans. (A) Unlocking of knee joint

Brunner's glands are located in the:

A. Duodenum
B. Jejunum
C. Ileum
D. All

Ans. (A) Duodenum

Artery of hind gut is:

A. Coeliac trunk

B. Superior mesenteric artery

C. Inferior mesenteric artery

D. Ileocolic artery

Ans. (C) Inferior mesenteric artery

Collecting ducts of kidney are developed from:

A. Mesonephros

B. Metanephros

C. Ureteric bud

D. Pronephros

Ans. (C) Ureteric bud

Intention tremor is seen in lesion of:

A. Cerebellum

B. Medulla oblongata

C. Hypothalamus

D. Thalamus

Ans. (A) Cerebellum

Trapezius is supplied by:

A. Glossopharyngeal nerve

B. Vagus nerve

C. Cranial accessory nerve

D. None

Ans. (D) None

The number of pleural recesses is:

A. 2

B. 3

C. 4

D. 5

Ans. (A) 2

Motor nerve supply to face is by:

A. Abducent nerve

B. Oculomotor nerve

C. Glossopharyngeal nerve

D. Facial nerve

Ans. (D) Facial nerve

Tail of pancreas is related to:

A. Splenorenal ligament

B. Gastrosplenic ligament

C. Phrenicocolic ligament

D. Falciform ligament

Ans. (A) Splenorenal ligament

The boundaries of Hesselbach's triangle are all except:

A. Medially: Lateral border of rectus abdominis

B. Laterally: Superior epigastric artery

C. It is divided into two unequal portions by obliterated umbilical artery

D. Inferiorly: Medial half of inguinal ligament

Ans. (B) Laterally: Superior epigastric artery

Stave cells are seen in:

A. Spleen
B. Kidney
C. Liver
D. Duodenum

Ans. (A) Spleen

Structure passing between pronator teres is:

A. Ulnar nerve
B. Median nerve
C. Radial nerve
D. Post interosseus nerve

Ans. (B) Median nerve

All are true about the boundaries of the popliteal fossa except:

A. Superolaterally: Biceps brachii tendon
B. Superomedially: Semimembranosus and semitendinosus
C. Inferomedially: Medial head of gastrocnemius
D. Inferolaterally: Lateral head of gastrocnemius and plantaris

Ans. (A) Superolaterally: Biceps brachii tendon

Tonsil is lined by:

A. Stratified squamous keratinized epithelium
B. Stratified squamous nonkeratinized epithelium
C. Columnar epithelium
D. Cuboidal epithelium

Ans. (B) Stratified squamous nonkeratinized epithelium

Middle meningeal artery passes through:

A. Foramen lacerum
B. Foramen spinosum
C. Foramen rotundum
D. Foramen ovale

Ans. (B) Foramen spinosum

Walking on a slippery floor the lady fell onto her outstretched right hand. After sometime she felt tenderness in the area of anatomical snuff box. The bone she would have most likely fractured is:

A. Capitate
B. Hamate
C. Lunate
D. Scaphoid

Ans. (D) Scaphoid

All of the following statements are true regarding internal jugular vein except:

A. In the jugular foramen it lies posterior to 9th, 10th and 11th cranial nerves
B. It joins the subclavian vein behind the sternal end of clavicle
C. It forms a content of carotid sheath
D. It receives the external jugular vein

Ans. (D) It receives the external jugular vein

The apex of lung:

A. Is covered by clavipectoral fascia

B. Is notched by subclavian artery

C. Is related to intermediate 1/3 of clavicle

D. Rises 1.0 cm above the first rib

Ans. (B) Is notched by subclavian artery

The spinal cord:

A. Terminates at the upper border of L3 in adult

B. Is uniform in width throughout its length except at the conus medullaris

C. Gives rise to a component of 11th cranial nerve

D. Lacks a subarachnoid space

Ans. (C) Gives rise to a component of 11th cranial nerve

A patient diagnosed as having cervical rib may feel pain along the:

A. Medial side of forearm

B. Medial side of forearm and hand

C. Lateral side of forearm

D. Lateral side of forearm and hand

Ans. (B) Medial side of forearm and hand

The embryological cause of extrophy of bladder is:

A. Defective migration of mesoderm

B. Early amniotic rupture

C. Dorsal body wall defect

D. Imperforate anus

Ans. (A) Defective migration of mesoderm

Calcitonin secreting parafollicular cells are derived from endodermal pouch:

A. 2nd   B. 3rd

C. 4th   D. 5th

Ans. (D) 5th

The structures passing through lesser sciatic foramen are all except:

A. Tendon of obturator externus   B. Internal pudendal vessels

C. Pudendal nerve   D. Nerve to obturator internus

Ans. (A) Tendon of obturator externus

Brodmann areas classify:

A. Cerebral cortex   B. Thalamus

C. Mid brain   D. Pons

Ans. (A) Cerebral cortex

Gubernaculum is related to development of:

A. Cervix
B. Vagina
C. Testis
D. Uterine tubes

Ans. (C) Testis

Klumpke's paralysis occurs due to injury at which level?

A. C5–C6
B. C6–C7
C. C7–C8
D. C8–T1

Ans. (D) C8–T1

Wrist drop is due to injury of:

A. Ulnar nerve
B. Median nerve
C. Radial nerve
D. Post interosseus nerve

Ans. (C) Radial nerve

All open in to coronary sinus except:

A. Great cardiac vein
B. Middle cardiac vein
C. Small cardiac vein
D. Oblique vein of the right atrium

Ans. (D) Oblique vein of the right atrium

The contents of the adductor canal are all except:

A. Femoral artery
B. Femoral vein
C. Descending genicular branch of the femoral artery
D. Saphenous vein

Ans. (D) Saphenous vein

Superior parathyroid glands develops from:

A. 2nd pharyngeal pouch
B. 3rd pharyngeal pouch
C. 4th pharyngeal pouch
D. 5th pharyngeal pouch

Ans. (C) 4th pharyngeal pouch

Posterior spinal artery occlusion causes predominantly:

A. Motor loss
B. Sensory loss
C. Both
D. None

Ans. (B) Sensory loss

Internal carotid artery lies in close relation to:

A. Foramen lacerum
B. Foramen spinosum
C. Foramen rotundum
D. Foramen ovale

Ans. (A) Foramen lacerum

The pharyngeal/branchial arch which disappears is the?

A. 1st arch
B. 2nd arch
C. 3rd arch
D. 5th arch

Ans. (D) 5th arch

The pyramidalis is supplied by:

A. The terminal branches of the subcostal nerve
B. The terminal branches of the iliohypogastric nerve
C. The terminal branches of the ilioinguinal nerve
D. The terminal branches of the genitofemoral nerve

Ans. (A) The terminal branches of the subcostal nerve

APUD system refers to:

A. Chief cells
B. Parietal cells
C. Argentaffin cells
D. Goblet cells

Ans. (C) Argentaffin cells

Fertilization occurs in:

A. Uterus
B. Ovary
C. Abdomen
D. Fallopian tube

Ans. (D) Fallopian tube

Smallest muscle in human body is:

A. Stapedius
B. Pectoralis minor
C. Lumbrical
D. Erector pilorum

Ans. (D) Erector pilorum

Which of the following structures passes through foramen rotundum?

A. Mandibular nerve
B. Maxillary nerve
C. Facial nerve
D. Middle meningeal artery

Ans. (B) Maxillary nerve

Corpora arenacea are a histological feature of:

A. Spleen
B. Thymus
C. Pituitary
D. Pineal

Ans. (D) Pineal

Foramen of Morgagni refers to an opening in:

A. The brain
B. The lesser omentum
C. The skull
D. The diaphragm

Ans. (D) The diaphragm

Sinus of Morgagni refers to an opening in:

A. The brain   B. The lesser omentum
C. The base of skull   D. The diaphragm
Ans. (C) The base of skull

Glands of Krause are a histological feature of:

A. Les of eye   B. Skin
C. Conjuctiva of eye   D. Adrenal medulla
Ans. (C) Conjuctiva of eye

All are correct about arterial supply of stomach except:

A. Left gastric artery: Branch of coeliac trunk
B. Left gastroepiploic artery: Branch of left gastric
C. Right gastric artery: Branch of common hepatic
D. Right gastroepiploic artery: Branch of gastroduodenal
Ans. (B) Left gastroepiploic artery: Branch of left gastric

The branches of inferior mesenteric artery are all except:

A. Left colic   B. Sigmoid
C. Superior rectal artery   D. Ileocolic
Ans. (D) Ileocolic

Not a correct statement is:

A. Flexion of trunk: Rectus abdominis
B. Lateral flexion: Oblique muscles
C. Pyramidalis relaxes linea alba
D. Cremaster can elevate testes
Ans. (C) Pyramidalis relaxes linea alba

Strongest flexor of the hip is:

A. Sartorius   B. Gluteus maximus
C. Iliopsoas   D. Pectineus
Ans. (D) Iliopsoas

Urinary bladder is lined by:

A. Squamous epithelium   B. Columnar epithelium
C. Transitional epithelium   D. Cuboidal epithelium
Ans. (C) Transitional epithelium

Epididymis is derived from:

A. Paramesonephric duct   B. Wolffian duct
C. Nephric duct   D. None
Ans. (B) Wolffian duct

Multiple Choice Questions

Nystagmus and scanning speech are seen in lesion of:

A. Cerebellum
B. Medulla oblongata
C. Hypothalamus
D. Thalamus

Ans. (A) Cerebellum

Stapedius muscle is supplied by which cranial nerve?

A. 5th nerve
B. 6th nerve
C. 7th nerve
D. 8th nerve

Ans. (C) 7th nerve

Which one of the following muscle is superficial?

A. Platysma
B. Palmaris brevis
C. Dartos
D. All of above

Ans. (D) All of above

Bilateral chemosis and proptosis is a presenting feature following infection of the nasal vestibule. Most likely cause is:

A. Lateral sinus thrombosis
B. Cavernous sinus thrombosis
C. Optic apex syndrome
D. Frontal lobe abscess

Ans. (B) Cavernous sinus thrombosis

Limbus fossa ovalis is seen in:

A. Right atrium
B. Right ventricle
C. Left atrium
D. All of above

Ans. (A) Right atrium

Cochlear division is a part of which cranial nerve?

A. 5th nerve
B. 6th nerve
C. 7th nerve
D. 8th nerve

Ans. (D) 8th nerve

Jugular foramen transmits all cranial nerves except:

A. IX
B. X
C. XI
D. XII

Ans. (D) XII

Thyroid follicles are lined by:

A. Squamous epithelium
B. Columnar epithelium
C. Transitional epithelium
D. Cuboidal epithelium

Ans. (D) Cuboidal epithelium

Implantation in humans occurs in:

A. Uterus   B. Ovary
C. Abdomen   D. Fallopian tube

Ans. (A) Uterus

All of the following are branches of internal iliac artery except:

A. Superior vesical artery   B. Uterine artery
C. Inferior vesical artery   D. Ovarian artery

Ans. (D) Ovarian artery

Medial ligament of ankle joint consists of a part of:

A. Anterior talofibular ligament
B. Posterior talofibular ligament
C. Calcaneofibular ligament ·
D. Tibiocalcaneal ligament

Ans. (D) Tibiocalcaneal ligament

Broca's area is localized in:

A. Superior temporal gyrus   B. Parietal lobe
C. Inferior frontal gyrus   D. Angular gyrus

Ans. (C) Inferior frontal gyrus

A pituitary tumor most often causes:

A. Bitemporal hemianopia
B. Binasal hemianopia
C. Unilateral hemianopia
D. Superior quadrant unilateral hemianopia

Ans. (A) Bitemporal hemianopia

Which of the following bone ossifies in membrane?

A. Humerus   B. Clavicle
C. Femur   D. Radius

Ans. (B) Clavicle

Sensory nerve supply for face is:

A. VI cranial nerve   B. VII cranial nerve
C. V cranial nerve   D. III cranial nerve

Ans. (C) V cranial nerve

All are cerebellar nuclei except:

A. Dentate nucleus   B. Emboliform nucleus
C. Globoose nucleus   D. Lentiform nucleus

Ans. (D) Lentiform nucleus

All are neural crest derivatives except:

A. Mesothelial cells
B. Adrenal medulla
C. Melanoblast
D. Odontoblasts

Ans. (A) Mesothelial cells

Which of the following is known as 'the police man of the abdomen'?

A. Peritoneal cavity
B. Lesser sac
C. Greater omentum
D. Appendices epiploicae

Ans. (D) Appendices epiploicae

Anterior interventricular artery is a branch of:

A. Right coronary artery
B. Left coronary artery
C. Circumflex artery
D. Left anterior descending artery

Ans. (B) Left coronary artery

The tonsillar artery is a branch of the:

A. Facial artery
B. Lingual artery
C. Maxillary artery
D. Superior thyroid artery

Ans. (A) Facial artery

Ovary develops from:

A. Metanephros
B. Mesonephros
C. Mesonephric duct
D. None

Ans. (D) None

Greater petrosal nerve is a branch of:

A. Facial
B. Vagus
C. Glossopharyngeal
D. Trigeminal

Ans. (A) Facial

Testis is covered by all except:

A. Tunica vaginalis
B. Tunica albuginea
C. Tunica vasculosa
D. None

Ans. (D) None

Not a branch of lumbar plexus is:

A. Femoral nerve (L2, 3, 4)
B. Genitofemoral nerve (L1, L2)
C. Iliohypogastric nerve (L1)
D. None

Ans. (D) None

Denonvilliers' fascia is:

A. Fascia of perenium
B. Fascia of penis
C. Renal fascia
D. Rectoprostatic fascia

Ans. (D) Rectoprostatic fascia

Primitive streak forms:

A. Ectoderm
B. Endoderm
C. Mesoderm
D. None

Ans. (C) Mesoderm

Alcock's canal is related to:

A. Superior gluteal nerve
B. Inferior gluteal nerve
C. Femoral nerve
D. Pudendal nerve

Ans. (A) Superior gluteal nerve

Latest concept of number of bronchopulmonary segments in right and left lungs are:

A. 10 and 10
B. 10 and 9
C. 10 and 8
D. 10 and 7

Ans. (A) 10 and 10

Müllerian duct is also known as:

A. Metanephros
B. Mesonephros
C. Mesonephric duct
D. Paramesonephric duct

Ans. (D) Paramesonephric duct

Length of thoracic duct is:

A. 5–10 cm
B. 10–15 cm
C. 15–20 cm
D. 40–45 cm

Ans. (D) 40–45 cm

Splenic artery is a branch of:

A. Coeliac trunk
B. Hepatic artery
C. Left gastric artery
D. Right gastric artery

Ans. (A) Coeliac trunk

Ligament of Treitz is related to:

A. Spleen
B. Small intestine
C. Cecum
D. Sigmoid colon

Ans. (B) Small intestine

Most common site of ectopic implantation is:

A. Uterus

B. Ovary

C. Abdomen

D. Fallopian tube

Ans. (D) Fallopian tube

The malleus is a derivative of:

A. 1st arch

B. 2nd arch

C. 3rd arch

D. 4th arch

Ans. (A) 1st arch

Volkmann's canals are seen in:

A. Liver

B. Spleen

C. Bone

D. Lymph nodes

Ans. (C) Bone

Descemet's membrane is seen in:

A. Liver

B. Spleen

C. Bone

D. Eye

Ans. (D) Eye

Not a feature of oxyntic cells is:

A. They are highly basophilic

B. Intrinsic factor of Castle is secreted by parietal cells

C. They secrete HCL

D. Also called parietal cells

Ans. (A) They are highly basophilic

Not a component of Waldeyer's ring is:

A. Pharyngeal tonsils

B. Palatine tonsils

C. Lingual tonsils

D. Peyer's patches

Ans. (D) Peyer's patches

Müllerian duct forms which of the following structure?

A. Ureter

B. Uterine tube

C. Urethra

D. Uvula

Ans. (B) Uterine tube

Content of carotid sheath is:

A. Vertebral artery

B. Basilar artery

C. Labyrinthine artery

D. Internal carotid artery

Ans. (D) Internal carotid artery

About the positions of testis during its descent in foetal life, all are correct except:

A. 3rd month: Reaches iliac fossa
B. 7th month: Traverses inguinal canal
C. 4th month: Reaches superficial inguinal ring
D. 9th month: Descends into scrotum

Ans. (C) 4th month: Reaches superficial inguinal ring

The ligaments attached and specific to liver are all except:

A. Falciform ligament
B. Coronary ligament
C. Right triangular ligament
D. None

Ans. (B) Coronary ligament

Meckel's ganglion is related to which cranial nerve:

A. Facial
B. Vagus
C. Glossopharyngeal
D. Trigeminal

Ans. (D) Trigeminal

Female genital tract develops from:

A. Metanephros
B. Mesonephros
C. Mesonephric duct
D. Paramesonephric duct

Ans. (D) Paramesonephric duct

Length of ductus deferens is:

A. 5–10 cm
B. 10–15 cm
C. 15–20 cm
D. 40–45 cm

Ans. (D) 40–45 cm

Kidney is surrounded by a special layer of fascia called:

A. Waldeyer's fascia
B. Fascia colli
C. Denonvilliers' fascia
D. Gerota's fascia

Ans. (D) Gerota's fascia

A man while trying to save his head from muggers got injured on his forearm. He went to a nearby clinic where the examining physician found that he could not adduct his thumb. The nerve affected in this case would be:

A. Anterior interosseus
B. Median
C. Radial
D. Ulnar

Ans. (D) Ulnar

A person was operated for the removal of a tumor of the right parotid gland. After the surgery he could not close his right eye properly and there was loss of expression on the right side of face. The affected nerve would be the branches of the following nerve:

A. Chorda tympani

B. Facial

C. Mandibular

D. Maxillary

Ans. (B) Facial

The tendon of one of the following muscles strengthens and stabilizes the knee joint on the lateral side:

A. Soleus

B. Sartorius

C. Gracilis

D. Biceps femoris

Ans. (D) Biceps femoris

Injury to common peroneal nerve results in foot drop because of the paralysis of the following group of muscles of leg:

A. Deep flexors

B. Extensors

C. Peroneus longus and brevis

D. Superficial flexors

Ans. (B) Extensors

While giving intramuscular injection into deltoid muscle, the intern needs to be careful in not damaging the following nerve:

A. Radial

B. Musculocutaneous

C. Median

D. Long thoracic

Ans. (A) Radial

True about portal vein are all except:

A. Formed by splenic vein and superior mesenteric vein

B. Receive blood from GI tract

C. Lies behind the neck of pancreas

D. Lies anterior to epiploic foramen

Ans. (D) Lies anterior to epiploic foramen

Temperature control is by:

A. Cerebral cortex

B. Hypothalamus

C. Midbrain

D. Pons

Ans. (B) Hypothalamus

After trauma, pseudocysts are common in relation to:

A. Liver

B. Pancreas

C. Kidney

D. Urinary bladder

Ans. (B) Pancreas

The branches of arch of aorta are all except:

A. Brachiocephalic artery, divides into right common carotid and right subclavian artery

B. Left common carotid

C. Thyroidea ima

D. None

Ans. (D) None

The contents of femoral triangle are all except:

A. Femoral vein

B. Femoral sheath

C. Femoral nerve

D. Genital branch of genitofemoral nerve

Ans. (D) Genital branch of genitofemoral nerve

Cells of Hensen are seen in:

A. Heart

B. Cerebellum

C. Liver

D. Organ of Corti

Ans. (D) Organ of Corti

Musculocutaneous nerve supplies:

A. Brachialis

B. Biceps brachi

C. Coracobrachialis

D. All of the above

Ans. (D) All of the above

A patient can approximate both shoulders in absence of:

A. Scapula

B. Clavicle

C. Humerus

D. None

Ans. (B) Clavicle

Heister valve is seen in:

A. Liver

B. Gall bladder

C. Ureter

D. Pancreas

Ans. (B) Gall bladder

The nerve of Wrisberg is a branch of:

A. Recurrent laryngeal nerve

B. Mandibular nerve

C. Facial nerve

D. Maxillary nerve

Ans. (C) Facial nerve

Hypoglossal canal transmits cranial nerve:

A. IX   B. X
C. XI   D. XII

Ans. (C) XI

Heubner's artery is a branch of:

A. Anterior cerebral artery   B. Middle cerebral artery
C. Posterior cerebral artery   D. PICA

Ans. (A) Anterior cerebral artery

Visual cortex is supplied by:

A. Anterior cerebral artery   B. Middle cerebral artery
C. Posterior cerebral artery   D. PICA

Ans. (C) Posterior cerebral artery

Cells of claudius are seen in:

A. Heart   B. Cerebellum
C. Liver   D. Organ of Corti

Ans. (D) Organ of Corti

Payer's patches are most commonly located in the:

A. Duodenum   B. Jejunum
C. Ileum   D. All

Ans. (C) Ileum

Saturday night palsy is caused due to:

A. Radial nerve injury in spiral groove
B. Radial nerve injury in hand
C. Ulnar nerve injury in spiral groove
D. Ulnar nerve injury in hand

Ans. (A) Radial nerve injury in spiral groove

Occlusion of which of the following arteries can result in lateral medullary syndrome?

A. Vertebral artery
B. Middle cerebral artery
C. Posterior cerebral artery
D. Posterior inferior cerebellar artery

Ans. (D) Posterior inferior cerebellar artery

Space of Disse are a histological feature of:

A. Spleen   B. Prostate
C. Pituitary   D. Liver

Ans. (D) Liver

Ureter develops from:

A. Metanephros
B. Mesonephros
C. Mesonephric duct
D. Paramesonephric duct

Ans. (C) Mesonephric duct

Brunner's glands are present in which of the following?

A. Duodenum
B. Jejunum
C. Colon
D. Stomach

Ans. (A) Duodenum

Umbilicus is supplied by which spinal segment:

A. T4
B. T6
C. T8
D. T10

Ans. (D) T10

Clitoris develops from:

A. Genital tubercle
B. Genital ridge
C. Wolffian duct
D. Müllerian duct

Ans. (A) Genital tubercle

Which of the following cells are responsible for myelination in central nervous system?

A. Astrocytes
B. Ependymocytes
C. Microglial cells
D. Oligodendrocytes

Ans. (D) Oligodendrocytes

Mechanism preventing inguinal hernia development are all except:

A. Obliquity of inguinal canal
B. Shutter mechanism of the arched fibers of the internal oblique and transversus abdominis
C. Sphincter action of transversus abdominis and internal oblique muscles at deep inguinal ring
D. Ball valve action of pyramidalis muscle

Ans. (D) Ball valve action of pyramidalis muscle

Tibial collateral ligament represents degenerated tendon of:

A. Sartorius
B. Gracilis
C. Soleus
D. Adductor magnus

Ans. (D) Adductor magnus

Most common position of appendix is:

A. Pelvic
B. Preileal
C. Postileal
D. Retrocecal

Ans. (D) Retrocecal

Podocytes are seen in:

A. Liver
B. Kidney
C. Ear
D. Eye

Ans. (B) Kidney

Descmet's membrane is seen in:

A. Sclera
B. Iris
C. Cornea
D. Choroid

Ans. (C) Cornea

Following structure passes through deep inguinal ring except:

A. Spermatic cord
B. Internal spermatic fascia
C. Round ligament
D. Ilioinguinal nerve

Ans. (D) Ilioinguinal nerve

Lymphatic drainage of uterus is to:

A. Internal iliac nodes
B. Para-aortic
C. Superficial-inguinal
D. Deep inguinal nerve

Ans. (A) Internal iliac nodes

Auditory cortex lies in:

A. Parietal lobe
B. Temporal lobe
C. Frontal lobe
D. Occipital lobe

Ans. (B) Temporal lobe

Waiter's tip deformity is:

A. Erb's paralysis
B. Klumpke's paralysis
C. Sprengel deformity
D. Colles' fracture

Ans. (A) Erb's paralysis

Lesser petrosal nerve passes through:

A. Foramen lacerum
B. Foramen spinosum
C. Foramen rotundum
D. Foramen ovale

Ans. (D) Foramen ovale

Axillary nerve damage may result in difficulty of:

A. Abduction
B. Adduction
C. Flexion
D. Lateral rotation

Ans. (A) Abduction

Epithelial lining of GIT is developed predominantly from:

A. Ectoderm
B. Mesoderm
C. Endoderm
D. Mesoderm + Endoderm

Ans. (C) Endoderm

Corpora amylacea are a histological feature of:

A. Spleen
B. Prostate
C. Pituitary
D. Pineal

Ans. (B) Prostate

The branches of lumbar plexus are all having correct root values except:

A. Femoral nerve (L2, 3, 4)
B. Genitofemoral nerve (L1, 2)
C. Iliohypogastric nerve (L1)
D. Iloinguinal nerve (L3)

Ans. (D) Iloinguinal nerve (L3)

Nerve injured in posterior dislocation of hip is:

A. Saphenous nerve
B. Common peroneal nerve
C. Sciatic nerve
D. Obturator nerve

Ans. (C) Sciatic nerve

Claw hand is caused by:

A. Median nerve palsy
B. Ulnar nerve palsy
C. Radial nerve palsy
D. Anterior interosseous nerve

Ans. (B) Ulnar nerve palsy

Structure not present in the substance of parotid gland is:

A. Facial nerve
B. Retromandibular vein
C. External carotid artery
D. Internal carotid artery

Ans. (D) Internal carotid artery

Jugular foramen transmits all cranial nerves except:

A. IX
B. X
C. XI
D. XII

Ans. (D) XII

Fabella is seen in which of the following muscle?

A. Semimembranous
B. Semitendinosus
C. Biceps femoris
D. Gastrocnemius

Ans. (D) Gastrocnemius

Nerve innervation of tensor tympani is:

A. Facial nerve
B. Ophthalmic nerve
C. Maxillary nerve
D. Mandibular nerve

Ans. (D) Mandibular nerve

Ligament of Treitz is made up of:

A. Striated muscle fibres in upper part
B. Elastic fibres in middle part
C. Smooth muscle fibres in lower part
D. All of above

Ans. (D) All of above

Flexors of knee joints are all except:

A. Gracilis
B. Semimembranosus
C. Quadriceps femoris
D. Gastrocnemius

Ans. (C) Quadriceps femoris

Cystic artery is commonly a branch of:

A. Coeliac trunk
B. Common hepatic artery
C. Left hepatic artery
D. Right hepatic artery

Ans. (D) Right hepatic artery

Taste sensations from the posterior 1/3 of tongue are carried by nerve:

A. Chorda tympani
B. Glossopharyngeal
C. Lingual
D. Vagus

Ans. (B) Glossopharyngeal

Ultimobranchial body is derived from endodermal pouch:

A. 2nd
B. 3rd
C. 4th
D. 5th

Ans. (D) 5th

Nerve of Ist pharyngeal arch is:

A. Facial nerve
B. Ophthalmic nerve
C. Maxillary nerve
D. Mandibular nerve

Ans. (D) Mandibular nerve

The structure which is not a component of basal ganglia is:

A. Caudate nucleus
B. Putamen
C. Globus pallidus
D. Thalamus

Ans. (D) Thalamus

Uterus basically develops from:

A. Metanephros
B. Mesonephros
C. Mesonephric duct
D. Paramesonephric duct

Ans. (D) Paramesonephric duct

The auditory bone incus is a derivative of:

A. 1st arch
B. 2nd arch
C. 3rd arch
D. 4th arch

Ans. (A) 1st arch

"Window artery" is:

A. Right coronary artery
B. Left anterior descending coronary artery
C. Left coronary artery
D. None

Ans. (B) Left anterior descending coronary artery

Fallopian tube is lined by:

A. Squamous epithelium
B. Columnar epithelium
C. Transitional epithelium
D. Cuboidal epithelium

Ans. (B) Columnar epithelium

Branches from anterior division internal iliac artery are except:

A. Superior vesical
B. Inferior vesical
C. Iliolumbar
D. Middle rectal

Ans. (C) Iliolumbar

Among the following subcutaneous muscle is:

A. Buccinator
B. Anterior belly of digastric
C. Platysma
D. Stapedius

Ans. (C) Platysma

The most common dislocation of hip joint is:

A. Anterior
B. Posterior
C. Medial
D. Lateral

Ans. (B) Posterior

Visual cortex lies in:

A. Parietal lobe
B. Temporal lobe
C. Frontal lobe
D. Occipital lobe

Ans. (D) Occipital lobe

The posterior surface of neck of pancreas is closely related to:

A. Pylorus of stomach
B. Aorta
C. Common iliac vein
D. Portal vein

Ans. (D) Portal vein

All are true except:

A. Hepatic artery is a branch of superior mesenteric artery
B. Cystic artery usually arise from right hepatic artery
C. Left gastric artery is a branch of celiac trunk
D. Celiac artery is a branch of aorta

Ans. (A) Hepatic artery is a branch of superior mesenteric artery

The embryological first pharyngeal arch ligament is the:

A. Sphenomandibular ligament
B. Stylohyoid ligament
C. Stylomandibular ligament
D. Styloid ligament

Ans. (A) Sphenomandibular ligament

Valves of Gerlach guards the orifice of:

A. Appendix
B. Small intestine
C. Cecum
D. Sigmoid colon

Ans. (A) Appendix

"Inferior" parathyroid glands develops from:

A. 2nd pharyngeal pouch
B. 3rd pharyngeal pouch
C. 4th pharyngeal pouch
D. 5th pharyngeal pouch

Ans. (B) 3rd pharyngeal pouch

Tanycytes are special cells seen in:

A. Intestine
B. Placenta
C. Adrenal gland
D. Brain

Ans. (D) Brain

Branches from posterior division of internal iliac artery are except:

A. Superior gluteal
B. Superior vesical
C. Ilio lumbar
D. Lateral sacral

Ans. (B) Superior vesical

Rexed's lamina classify:

A. Cerebral cortex
B. Thalamus
C. Mid brain
D. Spinal cord

Ans. (D) Spinal cord

Gall bladder is lined by:

A. Squamous epithelium
B. Columnar epithelium
C. Transitional epithelium
D. Cuboidal epithelium

Ans. (B) Columnar epithelium

Intervertebral disc is made up of:

A. Fibrocartilage

B. Elastic cartilage

C. Hyaline cartilage

D. None

Ans. (A) Fibrocartilage

"Winging of scapula" occurs due to injury to which nerve:

A. Thoracodorsal

B. Long thoracic

C. Axillary

D. Radial

Ans. (B) Long thoracic

Deep petrosal nerve is a branch of plexus around:

A. Common carotid artery

B. Internal carotid artery

C. External carotid artery

D. Middle meningeal artery

Ans. (B) Internal carotid artery

External petrosal nerve is a branch of plexus around:

A. Common carotid artery

B. Internal carotid artery

C. External carotid artery

D. Middle meningeal artery

Ans. (D) Middle meningeal artery

Adrenal medulla is developed predominantly from:

A. Ectoderm

B. Mesoderm

C. Endoderm

D. Neural crest

Ans. (D) Neural crest

The supports of uterus are strong except:

A. Pelvic diaphragm

B. Perineal body

C. Uterovesical fold

D. Urogenital diaphragm

Ans. (C) Uterovesical fold

Cremasteric muscle is supplied by which of the following nerve?

A. Illiohypogastric

B. Illioinguinal

C. Femoral

D. Genitofemoral

Ans. (D) Genitofemoral

"Herrings bodies" are a histological feature of:

A. Spleen

B. Pineal

C. Pituitary

D. Adrenal medulla

Ans. (C) Pituitary

Multiple Choice Questions

First carpometacarpal joint is a type of:

A. Saddle joint   B. Ball and socket joint

C. Secondary cartilaginous joint   D. Hinge joint

Ans. (A) Saddle joint

"Nucleus pulposus" is an embryological remnant of:

A. Notochord   B. Spinal cord

C. Mesoderm   D. Ectoderm

Ans. (A) Notochord

Not true about arterial supply of stomach is:

A. Right gastroepiploic artery: Branch of gastroduodenal

B. Right gastric artery: Branch of common hepatic

C. Left gastroepiploic artery: Branch of splenic

D. Left gastric artery: Branch of inferior mesenteric artery

Ans. (D) Left gastric artery: Branch of inferior mesenteric artery

Internal auditory meatus transmits cranial nerve:

A. IX, X   B. X, XI

C. VII, VIII   D. XII, X

Ans. (C) VII, VIII

Duct of Santorini pertains to:

A. Lung   B. Liver

C. Pancreas   D. Thymus

Ans. (C) Pancreas

"Anterior spinal artery" is a branch of:

A. Vertebral artery   B. Basilar artery

C. Labyrinthine artery   D. Internal carotid artery

Ans. (A) Vertebral artery

The structure lying in the lienorenal ligament are all except:

A. Body of pancreas

B. Splenic vessels

C. Pancreaticosplenic lymph nodes

D. Lymphatics

Ans. (A) Body of pancreas

Which one of the following muscle is not subcutaneous?

A. Platysma   B. Palmaris longus

C. Dartos   D. Facial muscles

Ans. (B) Palmaris longus

Anterior spinal artery occlusion predominantly causes:

A. Motor loss
B. Sensory loss
C. Both
D. None

Ans. (A) Motor loss

Structures passes through foramen ovale are all except:

A. Mandibular nerve
B. Greater petrosal nerve
C. Accessory meningeal artery
D. Emissary vein

Ans. (B) Greater petrosal nerve

The structures passing through foramen spinosum are all except:

A. Middle meningeal artery
B. Meningeal branch of mandibular nerve
C. Posterior trunk of middle meningeal vein
D. None

Ans. (D) None

Human intestinal glands contains:

A. Paneth cells
B. Neuroendocrine cells
C. Stem cells
D. All of the above

Ans. (D) All of the above

Length of anal canal is:

A. 3–4 cm
B. 4–5 cm
C. 15–20 cm
D. 40–45 cm

Ans. (A) 3–4 cm

Which of the following arteries supplies blood to trigeminal ganglion?

A. Basilar artery
B. Anterior cerebral artery
C. Posterior communicating artery
D. Cavernous part of internal carotid artery

Ans. (D) Cavernous part of internal carotid artery

Not a corresponding match of cranial nerves is:

A. Olfactory I
B. Optic II
C. Oculomotor III
D. Trochlear V

Ans. (D) Trochlear V

Which muscle has double nerve supply?

A. Brachioradialis
B. Biceps brachi
C. Coracobrachialis
D. Brachialis

Ans. (D) Brachialis

"Dorsalis pedis artery" is the continuation of:

A. Anterior tibial artery
B. Posterior tibial artery
C. Popliteal artery
D. Femoral artery

Ans. (A) Anterior tibial artery

Secretomotor nerve fibers to the parotid gland are supplied by which of the following nerve?

A. Facial
B. Vagus
C. Glossopharyngeal
D. Trigeminal

Ans. (C) Glossopharyngeal

"Femoral sheath" contains all of the following except:

A. Femoral artery
B. Femoral vein
C. Femoral nerve
D. Lymph node

Ans. (C) Femoral nerve

"Lens" of the eye develops from which of the following?

A. Endoderm
B. Mesoderm
C. Surface ectoderm
D. Neuroectoderm

Ans. (C) Surface ectoderm

Maxillary sinus opens into which meatus?

A. Inferior
B. Superior
C. Middle
D. All

Ans. (C) Middle meatus

The ligaments attached and specific to liver are all except:

A. Falciform ligament
B. Coronary ligament
C. Right triangular ligament
D. None

Ans. (D) None

The skin over the "angle of mandible" is supplied by which nerve?

A. Great auricular nerve
B. Facial
C. Auriculotemporal
D. Mandibular

Ans. (A) Great auricular nerve

"Horner's syndrome" is characterized by all of the following except:

A. Miosis
B. Enophthalmos
C. Ptosis
D. Cycloplegia

Ans. (D) Cycloplegia

Not a part of male urethra is:

A. Spongy   B. prostatic
C. Membranous   D. Fleshy

Ans. (D) Fleshy

"Pointing index" is seen in injury to:

A. Median nerve
B. Radial nerve
C. Ulnar nerve
D. Posterior interosseous nerve

Ans. (A) Median nerve

SVC opens into:

A. Right atrium   B. Right ventricle
C. Posterior wall of left atrium   D. All of above

Ans. (A) Right atrium

Ovary develops from:

A. Genital tubercle   B. Mesonephros
C. Mesonephric duct   D. Genital ridge

Ans (D) Genital ridge

The tortuous "uterine artery" is branch of:

A. Internal iliac artery
B. External iliac artery
C. Abdominal aorta
D. Inferior mesenteric artery

Ans. (A) Internal iliac artery

Injury to radial nerve causes:

A. Saturday night palsy   B. Crutch palsy
C. Wrist drop   D. All of the above

Ans. (D) All of the above

Branchial cysts are in relation to upper and lower thirds of:

A. Platysma   B. Sternocleidomastoid
C. Stylopharyngeus   D. Stylohyoid

Ans. (B) Sternocleidomastoid

The nerve of Wrisberg is a branch of:

A. Recurrent laryngeal nerve   B. Mandibular nerve
C. Facial nerve   D. Maxillary nerve

Ans. (C) Facial nerve

Root value of the "Obturator nerve" is from:

A. Ventral division of L2 L3 L4   B. Dorsal division of L2 L3 L4
C. Ventral rami of L1 L2   D. Dorsal rami of L1 L2
Ans. (A) Ventral division of L2 L3 L4

"Clavipectoral fascia" is pierced by all of the following except:

A. Lateral pectoral nerve   B. Medial pectoral nerve
C. Cephalic vein   D. Thoracoacromial artery
Ans. (B) Medial pectoral nerve

"Couinaud's segments" are in relation to:

A. Liver   B. Pancreas
C. Kidney   D. Urinary bladder
Ans. (A) Liver

The most common site of tubal pregnancy is:

A. Ampulla   B. Interstitial portion
C. Isthmus of tube   D. Fimbrial portion
Ans. (A) Ampulla

Sever's disease is osteochondritis of:

A. Capitate   B. Lunate
C. Trapezium   D. Calcaneum
Ans. (D) Calcaneum

Which muscle is not supplied by "12th cranial nerve"?

A. Hyoglossus   B. Genioglossus
C. Palatoglossus   D. Styloglossus
Ans. (C) Palatoglossus

"Moderator band" in heart lies in:

A. RA   B. RV
C. LA   D. LV
Ans. (B) RV

"Oblique popliteal ligament" is actually a part of:

A. Semimembranosus   B. Semitendinosus
C. Sartorius   D. Biceps femoris
Ans. (A) Semimembranosus

Which of the following is not a tributary of portal vein?

A. Splenic vein   B. Superior mesenteric vein
C. Hepatic vein   D. Rt. gastric vein
Ans. (C) Hepatic vein

Ligamentum teres contains:

A. Lt. umbilical vein
B. Rt. umbilical vein
C. Lt. umbilical artery
D. Rt. umbilical artery
Ans. (A) Lt. umbilical vein

Spermatic cord does not contain:

A. Testicular artery
B. Femoral branch of genitofemoral nerve
C. Ductus deferens
D. Pampiniform plexus
Ans. (B) Femoral branch of genitofemoral nerve

"Extradural hemorrhage" occurs due to rupture of:

A. Middle meningeal artery
B. Bridging veins
C. Vertebral artery
D. None
Ans. (A) Middle meningeal artery

All of the following are tributaries of coronary sinus except:

A. Middle cardiac vein
B. Small cardiac vein
C. Anterior cardiac vein
D. Great cardiac vein
Ans. (C) Anterior cardiac vein

Vessel lying in stem of "lateral sulcus" of cerebrum is:

A. Middle cerebral artery
B. Anterior cerebral artery
C. Posterior cerebral artery
D. None
Ans. (A) Middle cerebral artery

Appendicular artery is a branch of:

A. Coeliac trunk
B. Superior mesenteric artery
C. Inferior mesenteric artery
D. Ileocolic artery
Ans. (D) Ileocolic artery

Not a true statement is:

A. Short saphenous vein accompanies femoral nerve
B. Great saphenous vein accompanies saphenous nerve
C. Superior thyroid vessels accompany external laryngeal nerve
D. Superior laryngeal vessels accompany internal laryngeal nerve
Ans. (A) Short saphenous vein accompanies femoral nerve

"CSF-rhinorrhoea" is commonest in fracture to:

A. Temporal bone
B. Cribriform plate
C. Nasal bones
D. Temporosphenoid
Ans. (B) Cribriform plate

Most common congenital abnormality of the larynx is:

A. Laryngomalacia
B. Laryngeal web
C. Subglottic stenosis
D. Subglottic haemangioma

Ans. (A) Laryngomalacia

Not a true statement is:

A. In adults spinal cord ends at lower border of L4 vertebra
B. In newborn spinal cord may extend up to L3
C. Cauda equina extends from lumbar vertebra to coccyx
D. In embryonic period cord extends up to coccyx

Ans. (A) In adults spinal cord ends at lower border of L4 vertebra

Structure seen in "anatomical snuff box" is:

A. Ulnar artery
B. Radial nerve
C. Anterior interosseous artery
D. Cephalic vein

Ans. (D) Cephalic vein

"Clergyman's knee" is the result of inflammation of:

A. Deep infrapatellar bursa
B. Prepatellar bursa
C. Subcutaneous infrapatellar bursa
D. Suprapatellar bursa

Ans. (C) Subcutaneous infrapatellar bursa

Kidney is embryologically developed from:

A. Metanephros
B. Mesonephros
C. Mesonephric duct
D. Paramesonephric duct

Ans. (A) Metanephros

Injury to "axillary nerve" causes:

A. Loss of abduction of shoulder
B. Rounded contour of shoulder is lost
C. Sensory loss over lower half of deltoid
D. All of the above

Ans. (D) All of the above

All are true about the positions of testis during its descent in foetal life except:

A. 3rd month: Reaches iliac fossa
B. 4th month: Traverses inguinal canal
C. 8th month: Reaches superficial inguinal ring
D. 9th month: Descends into scrotum

Ans. (B) 4th month: Traverses inguinal canal

"Heubner's artery" is a branch of:

A. Anterior cerebral artery
C. Posterior cerebral artery

B. Middle cerebral artery
D. PICA

Ans. (A) Anterior cerebral artery

All are muscles of anterior abdominal wall except:

A. Internal oblique
C. Rectus abdominis

B. Transversus abdominis
D. None

Ans. (D) None

The cell types present in glands of stomach are all except

A. Serous cells
C. Oxyntic cells

B. Zymogen cells
D. Mucous neck cells

Ans. (A) Serous cells

Nerve supply of tensor tympani muscle is:

A. Recurrent laryngeal nerve
C. Facial nerve

B. Mandibular nerve
D. Maxillary nerve

Ans. (B) Mandibular nerve

"Charcot's artery" is a branch of:

A. Anterior cerebral artery
B. Middle cerebral artery
C. Posterior cerebral artery
D. PICA

Ans. (B) Middle cerebral artery

"Aldermans nerve" is name of:

A. Auriculotemporal
C. Auricular branch of vagus

B. Greater auricular
D. Nerve to stapedius

Ans. (C) Auricular branch of vagus

Length of fallopian tube is:

A. 5–10 cm
C. 25–30 cm

B. 15–20 cm
D. 40–45 cm

Ans. (A) 5–10 cm

Hip joint is supplied by all except:

A. Femoral nerve through nerve to rectus femoris
B. Anterior division of obturator nerve
C. Nerve to quadrates femoris
D. Inferior gluteal nerve

Ans. (D) Inferior gluteal nerve

The extensions of inguinal ligament are all except:

A. Reflected part of inguinal ligament
B. Pectineal part of inguinal ligament
C. Ligament of Cooper
D. None

Ans (D) None

Not a true statement is:

A. Structure passing between two heads of gastrocnemius: Sural nerve
B. Structure passing between two heads of lateral pterygoid: Maxillary artery
C. Structure passing between pronator teres: Median nerve
D. Structure passing between two planes of fibres of supinator: Anterior interosseous nerve

Ans. (D) Structure passing between two planes of fibres of supinator: Anterior interosseous nerve

True about "the muscle of Müller" are all except:

A. It is a thin layer of smooth muscle that bridges the inferior orbital fissure
B. It is supplied by sympathetic nerves
C. Its contraction produces a slight forward protrusion of the eyeball
D. Its palsy may thus lead to exophthalmos

Ans. (D) Its palsy may thus lead to exophthalmos

"Uterus and vagina" develops from:

A. Müllerian ducts
B. Wolffian ducts
C. Mesonephros
D. Metanephros

Ans. (A) Müllerian ducts

Geniculate bodies are present at the end of:

A. Cerebral cortex
B. Thalamus
C. Midbrain
D. Pons

Ans. (B) Thalamus

"Glissons" capsule is seen in:

A. Liver
B. Spleen
C. Bone
D. Eye

Ans. (A) Liver

Lymph node of Lund pertains to:

A. Liver
B. Gall bladder
C. Ureter
D. Pancreas

Ans. (B) Gall bladder

Not true about dimensions of duodenum is:

A. First (superior) part, 06 inches long
B. Second (descending) part, 03 inches long
C. Third (horizontal or inferior) part, 04 inches long
D. Fourth (ascending) part, 01 inch long

Ans. (A) First (superior) part, 06 inches long

The cranial nerve nuclei in floor of fourth ventricle are all except:

A. Hypoglossal nucleus
B. Dorsal nucleus of vagus
C. Nucleus of tractus solitarius
D. Fastigial nucleus

Ans. (D) Fastigial nucleus

Appendix of epididymis is embryologically developed from:

A. Metanephros
B. Mesonephros
C. Mesonephric duct
D. Ureteric bud

Ans. (C) Mesonephric duct

Pancreas is a J-shaped organ. Uncinate process is a part of:

A. Head
B. Neck
C. Body
D. Tail

Ans. (A) Head

Paired cranial venous sinuses are all except:

A. Cavernous
B. Superior petrosal
C. Inferior petrosal
D. None

Ans. (D) None

Pseudocysts are common to:

A. Lung
B. Liver
C. Pancreas
D. Thymus

Ans. (C) Pancreas

Structures in lateral wall of cavernous sinus are all except:

A. Maxillary nerve
B. Oculomotor nerve
C. Ophthalmic nerve
D. None

Ans. (D) None

Myelination of CNS is done by:

A. Schwann cells
B. Microglia
C. Oligodendrocytes
D. Astrocytes

Ans. (C) Oligodendrocytes

All are branches of internal thoracic artery except:

A. Mediastinal
B. Superior epigastric
C. Musculophrenic
D. None

Ans. (D) None

Flexor of knee joint are all except:

A. Semitendinosus
B. Sartorius
C. Biceps femoris
D. Quadriceps femoris

Ans. (D) Quadriceps femoris

Holden's line is seen in relation to:

A. Pelvis
B. Thigh
C. Skull
D. Anal canal

Ans. (B) Thigh

Reissner's membrane is seen in:

A. Liver
B. Kidney
C. Ear
D. Eye

Ans. (C) Ear

Lobule is seen in .... as a characteristic feature:

A. Liver
B. Thymus
C. Spleen
D. Pituitary

Ans. (B) Thymus

Dust cells are seen in:

A. Liver
B. Lung
C. Heart
D. Pituitary

Ans. (C) Heart

The muscles producing movement of dorsiflexion at ankle joint are all except:

A. Extensor digitorum longus
B. Extensor hallucis longus
C. Peroneus tertius
D. Tibialis posterior

Ans. (D) Tibialis posterior

The root value of femoral branch of genitofemoral nerve is:

A. L1
B. L1, L2
C. L1, L2, L3
D. L3, L4

Ans. (B) L1, L2

"Avascular necrosis" is seen in:

A. Scaphoid   B. Cuboid
C. Navicular   D. Lunate

Ans. (A) Scaphoid

Kienböck's disease is osteochondritis of:

A. Scaphoid   B. Cuboid
C. Navicular   D. Lunate

Ans. (D) Lunate

The right free margin of lesser omentum contains all except:

A. Hepatic artery   B. Portal vein
C. Bile duct   D. Hepatic vein

Ans. (D) Hepatic vein

Midbrain develops from:

A. Diencephalon   B. Telencephalon
C. Mesencephalon   D. Rhombencephalon

Ans. (C) Mesencephalon

"CSF-otorrhea" is commonest in fracture to:

A. Temporal bone   B. Cribriform plate
C. Nasal bones   D. Mastoid

Ans. (D) Mastoid

Paramesonephric duct/Müllerian duct forms which of the following structure?

A. Ureter   B. Uterine tube
C. Urethra   D. Uvula

Ans. (B) Uterine tube

Area 17 of visual cortex is supplied mainly by:

A. Middle cerebral artery
B. Anterior cerebral artery
C. Posterior cerebral artery
D. None

Ans. (C) Posterior cerebral artery

All arise from anterior surface of aorta except:

A. Coeliac trunk
B. Superior mesenteric artery
C. Inferior mesenteric artery
D. Ileocolic artery

Ans. (D) Ileocolic artery

Artery of midgut is:

A. Coeliac trunk
B. Superior mesenteric artery
C. Inferior mesenteric artery
D. None

Ans. (B) Superior mesenteric artery

Vessel present closest to foramen lacerum is:

A. Thyrocervical trunk
B. Internal carotid artery
C. External carotid artery
D. Costocervical trunk

Ans. (B) Internal carotid artery

Vessel present inside the trabeculated cavernous sinus is:

A. Thyrocervical trunk
B. Internal carotid artery
C. External carotid artery
D. Costocervical trunk

Ans. (B) Internal carotid artery

Accessory spleen can be found at all sites, except:

A. Hilum of spleen itself
B. Tail of pancreas
C. Greater omentum
D. All of the above

Ans. (D) All of the above

Not a true statement about anatomical landmarks is:

A. Xiphoid process at the level of 9th thoracic vertebra
B. Subcostal plane passes through 3rd lumbar vertebra
C. Pubic symphysis lies at the level of coccyx
D. Highest point of iliac crest at the level of 1st lumbar vertebra

Ans. (D) Highest point of iliac crest at the level of 1st lumbar vertebra

Nerve supply to knee joint is by:

A. Femoral nerve
B. Obturator nerve
C. Tibial nerve
D. All of the above

Ans. (D) All of the above

Cranial nerve which is secretomotor to GIT is:

A. Facial nerve
B. Glossopharyngeal nerve
C. Vagus nerve
D. Cranial accessory nerve

Ans. (C) Vagus nerve

Thickest nerve in body is:

A. Sciatic
B. Pudendal
C. Inferior rectal
D. Obturator

Ans. (A) Sciatic

Milk line is seen in relation to:

A. Pelvis
B. Thigh
C. Skull
D. Breast

Ans. (D) Breast

Not a component of anserine bursa is:

A. Sartorius
B. Gracilis
C. Semitendinosus
D. Semimembranosus

Ans. (D) Semimembranosus

Wry neck is due to central irritation of:

A. Facial nerve
B. Glossopharyngeal nerve
C. Vagus nerve
D. Cranial accessory nerve

Ans. (D) Cranial accessory nerve

Bell's palsy effects:

A. Facial nerve
B. Glossopharyngeal nerve
C. Vagus nerve
D. Cranial accessory nerve

Ans. (A) Facial nerve

Meralgia parasthetica is due to compression of:

A. Saphenous nerve
B. Deep peroneal nerve
C. Tibial nerve
D. Lateral cutaneous nerve of thigh

Ans. (D) Lateral cutaneous nerve of thigh

Sharpey's fibres are seen in relation to:

A. Adipose tissue
B. Kidney
C. Ear
D. Bone

Ans. (D) Bone

Squamo-columnar junction is seen in relation to:

A. Uterus
B. Lung
C. Cervix
D. Anal canal

Ans. (C) Cervix

Mesothelium is lined by:

A. Squamous epithelium
B. Columnar epithelium
C. Transitional epithelium
D. Cuboidal epithelium

Ans. (A) Squamous epithelium

Direct branch of aorta is:

A. Superior vesical artery
C. Inferior vesical artery
B. Uterine artery
D. Ovarian artery

Ans. (D) Ovarian artery

Guyon's canal is associated with:

A. Erb's paralysis
B. Ulnar nerve compression
C. Median nerve compression
D. Carpal tunnel syndrome

Ans. (B) Ulnar nerve compression

Inferior thyroid artery is a branch of:

A. Thyrocervical trunk
B. External carotid artery
C. Intercostal artery
D. Subclavian artery

Ans. (A) Thyrocervical trunk

The structures transmitted by inferior orbital fissure are all except:

A. Emissary vein
B. Supraorbital vessels
C. Maxillary nerve
D. Orbital branches of pterygopalatine ganglion

Ans. (B) Supraorbital vessels

Collecting part of kidney is embryologically developed from:

A. Metanephros
C. Mesonephric duct
B. Mesonephros
D. Ureteric bud

Ans. (D) Ureteric bud

The structures transmitted by foramen transversarium are all except:

A. Vertebral artery
B. Vertebral vein
C. Branch from inferior cervical ganglion
D. None

Ans. (D) None

Reid's base line is seen in relation to:

A. Pelvis
C. Skull
B. Thigh
D. Anal canal

Ans. (C) Skull

Carpal tunnel syndrome is associated with:

A. Erb's paralysis
B. Ulnar nerve compression
C. Median nerve compression
D. Carpal fracture
Ans. (C) Median nerve compression

Sudden death as a result of cardiac arrest can be due to irritation of:

A. Facial nerve
B. Glossopharyngeal nerve
C. Vagus nerve
D. Cranial accessory nerve
Ans (C) Vagus nerve

Which of the following structures passes through foramen rotundum:

A. Mandibular nerve
B. Maxillary nerve
C. Facial nerve
D. Middle meningeal artery
Ans. (B) Maxillary nerve

The four pulmonary veins which carry oxygenated blood open into:

A. Right atrium
B. Right ventricle
C. Left atrium
D. All of the above
Ans. (C) Left atrium

The tortuous splenic artery arises from:

A. Coeliac trunk
B. Superior mesenteric artery
C. Inferior mesenteric artery
D. Aorta
Ans. (A) Coeliac trunk

SA node is seen in:

A. Right atrium
B. Right ventricle
C. Left atrium
D. All of the above
Ans. (A) Right atrium

Panninculosis carnosus in lower animals represents:

A. Platysma
B. Palmaris longus
C. Dartos
D. Facial muscles
Ans. (D) Facial muscles

Posterior pituitary bodies are:

A. Herring bodies
B. Brain sand
C. Councilmann bodies
D. Amyloid bodies
Ans. (A) Herring bodies

Nerve accompanying vestibulocochlear nerve in some part of its course is:

A. Facial nerve
B. Glossopharyngeal nerve
C. Vagus nerve
D. Cranial accessory nerve
Ans. (A) Facial nerve

"Figure of 8 bandage" is applied in fracture of:

A. Scapula

B. Clavicle

C. Humerus

D. None

Ans. (B) Clavicle

All of the following structures pass through optic foramen except:

A. Optic nerve

B. Ophthalmic artery

C. Ophthalmic nerve

D. Dural matter

Ans. (C) Ophthalmic nerve

Control of gait is by:

A. Vermis of cerebellum

B. Medulla oblongata

C. Hypothalamus

D. Thalamus

Ans. (A) Vermis of cerebellum

Caterpillar turn is related to:

A. Coeliac trunk

B. Hepatic artery

C. Left gastric artery

D. Right gastric artery

Ans. (B) Hepatic artery

The constituents of spermatic cord is/are:

A. Vas deferens

B. Pampiniform plexus

C. Artery of vas

D. All of the above

Ans. (D) All of the above

Which nerve escapes entrapment syndrome?

A. Radial

B. Ulnar

C. Median

D. None

Ans. (D) None

Delphic nodes are:

A. Pretracheal

B. Paratracheal

C. Supraclavicular

D. Posterior triangle

Ans. (A) Pretracheal

Muscles used in normal walk during stance and swing:

A. Iliopsoas

B. Tibialis anterior

C. Gastrocnemius

D. Popliteus

Ans. (C) Gastrocnemius

Temporomandibular joint is a:

A. Saddle shaped joint

B. Ball and socket joint

C. Condyloid joint

D. Plane joint

Ans (C) Condyloid joint

The first bone to ossify in body is:

A. Lower end of femur   B. Clavicle

C. Upper end of humerus   D. Upper end of tibia

Ans. (B) Clavicle

Nucleus brain common to IX, X and VII cranial nerves is:

A. Nucleus of tractus solitarius   B. Nucleus ambiguous

C. Dentate nucleus   D. Red nucleus

Ans. (A) Nucleus of tractus solitarius

Nucleus IIIrd cranial nerve is:

A. Nucleus of tractus solitarius   B. Nucleus ambiguous

C. Dentate nucleus   D. Edinger-Westphal nucleus

Ans. (D) Edinger-Westphal nucleus

The structures lying at level of L1 vertebra are all except:

A. Duodenojejunal flexure   B. Hilum of kidneys

C. Pancreas   D. Cardiac end of stomach

Ans. (D) Cardiac end of stomach

Not true about dimensions of duodenum is:

A. First (superior) part, 02 inches long

B. Second (descending) part 03 inches long

C. Third (horizontal or inferior) part, 04 inches long

D. Fourth (ascending) part, 06 inches long.

Ans. (D) Fourth (ascending) part, 06 inches long

Cleidocranial dysostosis mainly effects in:

A. Lower end of femur   B. Clavicle

C. Upper end of humerus   D. Upper end of tibia

Ans. (B) Clavicle

The following structures do not have lymphatics, except:

A. Bone marrow   B. Bronchi

C. Cervix   D. Epidermis

Ans. (A) Bone marrow

The parafollicular cells (C cells) of the thyroid gland develop from which pharyngeal pouch?

A. Second   B. Third

C. Fourth   D. Fifth

Ans. (D) Fifth

Multiple Choice Questions

The following glands contain the myoepithelial cells, except:

A. Mammary glands   B. Salivary glands
C. Sebaceous glands   D. Sweat glands

Ans. (C) Sebaceous glands

The fenestrated capillaries are present in the following structures, except:

A. Lungs   B. Kidneys
C. Intestine   D. Endocrine glands

Ans. (A) Lungs

The carotid sheath surrounds the following structures, except:

A. Common and internal carotid arteries
B. Internal jugular vein
C. Sympathetic trunk
D. Vagus nerve

Ans. (C) Sympathetic trunk

Crescents of Giannuzzi or Demilunes are present in the following:

A. Lungs   B. Kidneys
C. Intestine   D. Salivary glands

Ans. (D) Salivary glands

Injury to radial nerve causes:

A. Saturday night palsy   B. Erb's palsy
C. Elbow drop   D. All of the above

Ans. (A) Saturday night palsy

Freiberg's disease is osteochondritis of:

A. Capitate   B. Lunate
C. Trapezium   D. Metatarsal

Ans. (D) Metatarsal

The contents of hypoglossal canal are all except:

A. Hypoglossal nerve
B. Meningeal branch of ascending pharyngeal artery.
C. Emissary vein
D. None

Ans. (D) None

The effects of infranuclear lesion of 3rd cranial nerve are all except:

A. Cycloplegia   B. Diplopia
C. Medial squint   D. Mydraiasis

Ans. (C) Medial squint

Vena cordis minimi open into:

A. Right atrium
C. Posterior wall of left atrium

B. Right ventricle
D. All of the above

Ans. (D) All of the above

Lesion of vagus nerve leads to all except:

A. Nasal regurgitation of swallowed liquids
B. Nasal twang in voice
C. Hoarseness of voice
D. Arching of palate

Ans. (D) Arching of palate

The nuclei of origin of ninth nerve are all except:

A. Nucleus ambiguous
B. Nucleus of tractus solitarius
C. Inferior salivatory nucleus
D. Nucleus of Clarke

Ans. (D) Nucleus of Clarke

The folds of dura mater are all except:

A. Falx cerebri
C. Ligamentum denticulatum

B. Tentorium cerebelli
D. Diaphragma sellae

Ans. (C) Ligamentum denticulatum

Which of the following have lesser number of dendrites:

A. Astrocytes
C. Microglial

B. Oligodendrocytes
D. Schwann cells

Ans. (B) Oligodendrocytes

Lens develops from which of the following?

A. Endoderm
C. Surface ectoderm

B. Mesoderm
D. Neuroectoderm

Ans. (C) Surface ectoderm

Connective tissue cells develop from which of the following?

A. Endoderm
C. Surface ectoderm

B. Mesoderm
D. Neuroectoderm

Ans. (B) Mesoderm

Presence of Hassall's corpuscles with absence of germinal centers is a feature of:

A. Thymus
C. Tonsils

B. Lymph node
D. Peyer's patches

Ans. (A) Thymus

The prostate is supplied by branches from vessels except:

A. Inferior vesical
B. Middle rectal
C. Penile
D. Internal pudendal

Ans. (C) Penile

Dentate nucleus is present in:

A. Midbrain
B. Pons
C. Medulla
D. Cerebellum

Ans. (D) Cerebellum

Cardiac arrest can be due to:

A. Glossopharyngeal
B. Vagus
C. Facial
D. Trigeminal

Ans. (B) Vagus

Spermatic cord contains all of the following except:

A. Testicular artery
B. Loose areolar tissue
C. Artery to vas
D. None

Ans. (D) None

All are true about umbilicus except:

A. It is the site for umbilical hernia
B. It is a site for vicarious menstruations
C. It is the site for cherry red tumor or raspberry tumor
D. Laproscopic ports are never applied through umbilicus

Ans. (D) Laproscopic ports are never applied through umbilicus

Deep inguinal ring is the defect in:

A. External oblique
B. Transverse abdominis
C. Internal oblique
D. Fascia transversalis

Ans. (D) Fascia transversalis

Abdominal aorta divides at the level of:

A. L1
B. L2
C. L4
D. S3

Ans. (C) L4

Structure opening in left atrium of heart is:

A. Coronary sinus
B. Superior vena cava
C. Inferior vena cava
D. Pulmonary veins

Ans. (D) Pulmonary veins

Accessory nerve supplies:

A. Sternomastoid
B. Buccinator
C. Platysma
D. Stapedius

Ans. (A) Sternomastoid

Superior orbital fissure transmits all cranial nerves except:

A. III
B. IV
C. VI
D. VII

Ans. (D) VII

Embryologically the nerve of the second pharyngeal arch is:

A. Recurrent laryngeal nerve
B. Mandibular nerve
C. Facial nerve
D. Maxillary nerve

Ans. (C) Facial nerve

Injury to median nerve causes:

A. Saturday night palsy
B. Erb's palsy
C. Elbow drop
D. Ape thumb deformity

Ans. (D) Ape thumb deformity

"Hip joint" is an example of:

A. Hinge joint
B. Ellipsoid joint
C. Saddle joint
D. Ball and socket joint

Ans. (D) Ball and socket joint

"Mandibular" nerve supplies:

A. Posterior belly of digastric
B. Buccinator
C. Masseter
D. Stapedius

Ans. (C) Masseter

Taste sensations from the anterior 2/3 of tongue are carried by nerve:

A. Chorda tympani
B. Glossopharyngeal
C. Lingual
D. Vagus

Ans. (A) Chorda tympani

The epithelial lining of the trachea is composed of:

A. Pseudostratified columnar nonciliated cells, goblet cells and basal cells
B. Pseudostratified columnar ciliated cells, goblet cells and basal cells
C. Stratified columnar nonciliated cells, goblet cells and basal cells
D. Stratified noncolumnar ciliated cells, goblet cells and basal cells

Ans. (B) Pseudostratified columnar ciliated cells, goblet cells and basal cells

Elbow is an example of:

A. Hinge joint
B. Ellipsoid joint
C. Saddle joint
D. Ball and socket joint

Ans. (A) Hinge joint

Lymphatic drainage of ovaries is predominantly to the nodes:

A. Deep inguinal
B. Superficial inguinal
C. Para-aortic
D. Common iliac

Ans. (C) Para-aortic

Left testicular vein drains into:

A. Left splenic vein
B. Left renal vein
C. Inferior vena cava
D. Right renal vein

Ans. (B) Left renal vein

The axis of rotation of gut is in relation to:

A. Common hepatic artery
B. Splenic artery
C. Celiac trunk
D. Superior mesenteric artery

Ans. (D) Superior mesenteric artery

Not a component of Guy ropes is:

A. Sartorius
B. Gracilis
C. Semitendinosus
D. Semimembranosus

Ans. (D) Semimembranosus

Discus proligerous is seen in relation to:

A. Spleen
B. Ovary
C. Lymph nodes
D. Testis

Ans. (B) Ovary

Teres minor is supplied by nerve:

A. Thoracodorsal
B. Axillary
C. Dorsal scapular
D. Lower subscapular

Ans. (B) Axillary

Stapedius is supplied by:

A. Abducent nerve
B. Oculomotor nerve
C. Glossopharyngeal nerve
D. Facial nerve

Ans. (D) Facial nerve

All of the following are contents of broad ligament except:

A. Fallopian tube
B. Round ligament
C. Ovarian ligament
D. Ovary

Ans. (D) Ovary

Multiple Choice Questions

The nerve passing between two heads of gastrocnemius is:

A. Saphenous nerve   B. Sural nerve

C. Femoral nerve   D. Obturator nerve

Ans. (B) Sural nerve

Heart failure cells are seen in:

A. Heart   B. Lung

C. Liver   D. Veins

Ans. (B) Lung

"Vessel" seen in substance of cavernous sinus is:

A. External carotid artery

B. Thyrocervical trunk

C. Costocervical trunk

D. Internal carotid artery

Ans. (D) Internal carotid artery

Pseudoganglion is usually seen in nerve to:

A. Infraspinatus   B. Teres major

C. Teres minor   D. Long head of triceps

Ans. (C) Teres minor

All are branches of posterior cord of brachial plexus, except:

A. Thoracodorsal nerve   B. Upper subscapular nerve

C. Suprascapular nerve   D. Axillary nerve

Ans. (C) Suprascapular nerve

Most prominent spinous process is of which vertebra?

A. C6   B. C7

C. L1   D. T12

Ans. (B) C7

The branches of hepatic artery are all except:

A. Gastroduodenal artery

B. Hepatic artery proper

C. Infraduodenal artery

D. Right gastric artery

Ans. (C) Infraduodenal artery

Angle of mandible is supplied by which nerve?

A. Great auricular nerve   B. Facial

C. Auriculotemporal   D. Mandibular

Ans. (A) Great auricular nerve

True about arterial supply of adrenal/suprarenal gland is all except:

A. Superior suprarenal artery: Branch of inferior phrenic
B. Middle suprarenal artery: Branch of abdominal aorta
C. Inferior suprarenal artery: Branch of renal artery.
D. None
Ans. (D) None

Circumvallate papillae of tongue are supplied by which nerve?

A. Glossopharyngeal   B. Facial
C. Lingual   D. Chorda tympani
Ans. (A) Glossopharyngeal

Sensory nerve supply to posterior 1/3 of tongue is by which nerve?

A. Glossopharyngeal   B. Facial
C. Lingual   D. Chorda tympani
Ans. (A) Glossopharyngeal

Length of external auditory canal is:

A. 20 mm   B. 22 mm
C. 24 mm   D. 15 mm
Ans. (C) 24 mm

Signet ring shaped cells are:

A. Plasma cells   B. Adipose cells
C. Pigment cells   D. Osteoclasts
Ans. (B) Adipose cells

"Rexed's laminae" are seen in:

A. Liver   B. Spinal cord
C. Brain   D. Lymph nodes
Ans. (B) Spinal cord

Maxillary sinus opens into which meatus?

A. Inferior   B. Superior
C. Middle   D. All
Ans. (C) Middle

Urachus is the remnant of:

A. Umbilical cord   B. Umbilicus
C. VID   D. Allantois
Ans. (D) Allantois

Hyperaccusis is due to involvement of:

A. Auriculotemporal
B. Greater auricular
C. Auricular branch of vagus
D. Nerve to stapedius

Ans. (D) Nerve to stapedius

Richert's cartilage develops from:

A. I branchial arch
B. II branchial arch
C. III branchial arch
D. IV branchial arch

Ans. (B) II branchial arch

Bile duct opens into:

A. First part of duodenum
B. Second part of the duodenum
C. Third part of duodenum
D. None

Ans. (B) Second part of the duodenum

Iliolumbar artery is a branch of:

A. Anterior division of internal iliac artery
B. Posterior division of internal iliac artery
C. Anterior division of external iliac artery
D. Posterior division of external iliac artery

Ans. (B) Posterior division of internal iliac artery

Sural nerve passes between which muscle?

A. Semimembranosus
B. Semitendinosus
C. Biceps femoris
D. Gastrocnemius

Ans. (D) Gastrocnemius

All structures open in right atrium of heart except:

A. Coronary sinus
B. Superior vena cava
C. Inferior vena cava
D. Pulmonary veins

Ans. (D) Pulmonary veins

Defective cilia are seen in:

A. Cystic fibrosis syndrome
B. Ehlers-Danlos syndrome
C. Mounier-Kuhn syndrome
D. Kartagener's syndrome

Ans. (D) Kartagener's syndrome

Visceral surface of spleen has impressions for all except:

A. Renal impression: For right kidney
B. Pancreatic impression: For tail of pancreas
C. Gastric impression: For fundus of stomach
D. Colic impression: For splenic flexure of colon

Ans. (A) Renal impression: For right kidney

The components of chromaffin system are all except:

A. Small masses of cells among ganglia of sympathetic chain
B. Paraganglia
C. Para-aortic bodies
D. Adrenal cortex

Ans. (D) Adrenal cortex

Trigone of bladder is embryologically developed from:

A. Metanephros
B. Mesonephros
C. Mesonephric duct
D. Ureteric bud

Ans. (C) Mesonephric duct

Axillary sheath is derived from:

A. Clavipectoral fascia
B. Prevertebral fascia
C. Pretracheal fascia
D. None

Ans. (B) Prevertebral fascia

Gag reflex is absent in injury to the following nerve:

A. Facial (VII)
B. Glossopharyngeal (IX)
C. Hypoglossal (XII)
D. Spinal accessory (XI)

Ans. (B) Glossopharyngeal (IX)

Allantois is related to:

A. Liver
B. Pancreas
C. Kidney
D. Urinary bladder

Ans. (D) Urinary bladder

Paramesonephric duct in males remains as:

A. Prostatic utricle
B. Prostatic urethra
C. Colliculus seminalis
D. Ejaculatory duct

Ans. (A) Prostatic utricle

Human intestinal glands contains:

A. Paneth cells
B. Neuroendocrine cells
C. Stem cells
D. All of the above

Ans. (D) All of the above

Carpometacarpal joint of thumb is_____ type of joint.

A. Ball and socket
B. Hinge
C. Plane
D. Saddle

Ans. (D) Saddle

The abductor of vocal cord is:

A. Posterior cricoarytenoid
B. Lateral cricoarytenoid
C. Thyroarytenoid
D. Cricoarytenoid

Ans. (A) Posterior cricoarytenoid

Length of portal vein is:

A. 5–10 cm
C. 25–30 cm

B. 15–20 cm
D. 40–45 cm

Ans. (A) 5–10 cm

Porters tip deformity occurs due to involvement of _____ of brachial plexus.

A. Upper trunk
C. Medial cord

B. Middle trunk
D. Lateral trunk

Ans. (A) Upper trunk

Lymphatics of testis/ovaries drain into_____ lymph nodes:

A. Internal iliac
C. Superficial inguinal

B. Para-aortic
D. Coeliac

Ans. (B) Para-aortic

Meckel's cartilage develops from:

A. I branchial arch
C. III branchial arch

B. II branchial arch
D. IV branchial arch

Ans. (A) I branchial arch

Portal vein is formed by:

A. Junction of superior mesenteric vein and inferior mesenteric vein
B. Junction of splenic vein and inferior mesenteric vein
C. Junction of splenic vein and superior mesenteric vein
D. Continuation of superior mesenteric vein

Ans. (C) Junction of splenic vein and superior mesenteric vein

Left gonadal vein drains into:

A. Left splenic vein
C. Inferior vena cava

B. Left renal vein
D. Right renal vein

Ans. (B) Left renal vein

The structure which is not a component of basal ganglia:

A. Caudate nucleus
C. Globus pallidus

B. Putamen
D. Thalamus

Ans. (D) Thalamus

Peritoneal folds related to stomach are all except:

A. Lesser omentum

B. Greater omentum

C. Gastrosplenic ligament

D. Leinorenal ligament

Ans. (D) Leinorenal ligament

Foramen cecum is an important landmark for development of:

A. Superior parathyroids

B. Inferior parathyroids

C. Tonsils

D. Thyroid

Ans. (D) Thyroid

Which of the following develops from the third pharyngeal pouch?

A. Superior parathyroids

B. Inferior parathyroids

C. Tonsils

D. Thyroid

Ans. (B) Inferior parathyroids

Which of the following muscle has double nerve supply?

A. Brachioradialis

B. Biceps brachii

C. Coracobrachialis

D. Brachialis

Ans. (D) Brachialis

Dorsalis pedis artery is the continuation of:

A. Anterior tibial artery

B. Posterior tibial artery

C. Popliteal artery

D. Lateral tarsal artery

Ans. (A) Anterior tibial artery

Intention tremor is due to damage to:

A. Basal ganglia

B. Brain stem

C. Thalamus

D. Cerebellum

Ans. (D) Cerebellum

Pectinate line is seen in relation to:

A. Pelvis

B. Thigh

C. Skull

D. Anal canal

Ans. (D) Anal canal

The Stensen's duct opens in the oral cavity opposite to the level of:

A. Crown of upper second molar tooth

B. Crown of lower second molar tooth

C. Crown of upper second molar tooth

D. Crown of lower second molar tooth

Ans. (A) Crown of upper second molar tooth

Nerve supply of tensor palati muscle is:

A. Recurrent laryngeal nerve   B. Mandibular nerve
C. Facial nerve   D. Maxillary nerve
Ans. (B) Mandibular nerve

Main mechanical support to the uterus is provided by:

A. Broad ligament of uterus
B. Utero-vesical ligament
C. Transverse cervical ligament
D. Round ligament of uterus
Ans. (C) Transverse cervical ligament

Temporary foot drop is due to compression of:

A. Saphenous nerve   B. Deep peroneal nerve
C. Tibial nerve   D. Obturator nerve
Ans. (B) Deep peroneal nerve

Structure passing through the Dorello's canal is:

A. Branch of mandibular nerve
B. Middle meningeal artery
C. Maxillary artery
D. Abducens nerve
Ans. (D) Abducens nerve

Umbilical cord contains:

A. 1 vein and 2 arteries   B. 2 veins and 2 arteries
C. 1 artery and 2 veins   D. 1 vein and 1 artery
Ans. (A) 1 vein and 2 arteries

Axillary nerve damage may result in difficulty in:

A. Abduction   B. Extension
C. Flexion   D. Lateral rotation
Ans. (A) Abduction

Length of spinal cord in adults is:

A. 5–10 cm   B. 15–20 cm
C. 25–30 cm   D. 40–45 cm
Ans. (D) 40–45 cm

Scavenging in CNS is done by:

A. Schwann cells   B. Microglia
C. Oligodendrocytes   D. Astrocytes
Ans. (B) Microglia

Lymphatic drainage of testis is:

A. Inguinal lymph node
B. External iliac lymph node
C. Internal iliac lymph node
D. Pre and para-aortic lymph nodes

Ans. (D) Pre and para-aortic lymph nodes

Left ovarian veins drain into:

A. Portal vein
B. Inferior vena cava
C. Left renal vein
D. Inferior mesenteric vein

Ans. (C) Left renal vein

Sensory nerve supply to some muscles of face is from:

A. Recurrent laryngeal nerve   B. Abducent nerve
C. Facial nerve   D. Maxillary nerve

Ans. (D) Maxillary nerve

Left gastric artery is a branch of:

A. Common hepatic artery   B. Splenic artery
C. Celiac trunk   D. Gastroduodenal artery

Ans. (C) Celiac trunk

Schultz line is seen in relation to:

A. Pelvis   B. Thigh
C. Skull   D. Breast

Ans. (D) Breast

Descemet's membrane is seen in:

A. Liver   B. Kidney
C. Ear   D. Eye

Ans. (D) Eye

Bowman's membrane is seen in:

A. Liver   B. Kidney
C. Ear   D. Eye

Ans. (D) Eye

Arteriae pancreatica magna is a branch of:

A. Common hepatic artery   B. Splenic artery
C. Celiac trunk   D. Gastroduodenal artery

Ans. (B) Splenic artery

Cystic artery is usually a branch of:

A. Common hepatic artery

C. Gastroduodenal artery

B. Left hepatic artery

D. None

Ans. (D) None

The deltoid is supplied by:

A. Ulnar nerve

C. Axillary nerve

B. Median nerve

D. Radial nerve

Ans. (C) Axillary nerve

The carpal tunnel syndrome is due to:

A. Axillary nerve

C. Radial nerve

B. Median nerve

D. Ulnar nerve

Ans. (B) Median nerve

Hypertrophy of .... in leprosy behind medial epicondyle of humerus is due to:

A. Axillary nerve

C. Radial nerve

B. Median nerve

D. Ulnar nerve

Ans. (D) Ulnar nerve

Stapes is derived from branchial arch:

A. 2nd

C. 4th

B. 3rd

D. 5th

Ans. (A) 2nd

The structures lying in the gastrosplenic ligament are all except:

A. Left gastroepiploic vessels

B. Short gastric vessels

C. Right gastric artery

D. Lymphatics

Ans. (C) Right gastric artery

The pharyngeal arch which does not persist is:

A. 2nd

C. 4th

B. 3rd

D. 5th

Ans. (D) 5th

Osgood-Schlatter disease is osteochondritis of:

A. Capitate

C. Trapezium

B. Tibial tubercle

D. Metatarsal

Ans. (B) Tibial tubercle

Two vertebral arteries join to form:

A. Anterior-cerebral artery
C. Posterior-cerebellar artery

B. Basilar artery
D. Posterior-communicating artery

Ans. (B) Basilar artery

Muscles of tongue develop from:

A. Lingual swelling
C. Tuberculum impar

B. Occipital somites
D. Hypobranchial prominence

Ans. (B) Occipital somites

Left anterior descending is usually a branch of:

A. Right coronary
C. Both

B. Left coronary
D. None

Ans. (B) Left coronary

Trachea is lined by:

A. Squamous epithelium
B. Stratified columnar
C. Transitional
D. Pseudostratified ciliated columnar

Ans. (D) Pseudostratified ciliated columnar

Superior thyroid artery is a branch of:

A. Thyrocervical trunk
C. Intercostal artery

B. External carotid artery
D. Subclavian artery

Ans. (B) External carotid artery

Rotator cuff is formed by all except:

A. Infraspinatus
C. Teres major

B. Supraspinatus
D. Teres minor

Ans. (D) Teres major

Peripheral heart is:

A. Sartorius
C. Soleus

B. Gracilis
D. Semimembranosus

Ans. (C) Soleus

Saturday night palsy caused due to:

A. Radial nerve injury in hand
B. Radial nerve injury in spiral groove
C. Ulnar nerve injury in hand
D. Ulnar nerve injury in spiral groove

Ans. (B) Radial nerve injury in spiral groove

All are branches of femoral artery:

A. Superficial circumflex iliac
B. Superficial epigastric
C. Superficial external pudendal
D. Superficial internal pudendal
Ans. **(D)** Superficial internal pudendal

Columns of Bertin are seen in:

A. Suprarenals
C. Kidney
B. Thymus
D. Palatine tonsil
Ans. **(C)** Kidneys

"Cords of Billroth" are seen in:

A. Liver
C. Thymus
B. Spleen
D. Lymph nodes
Ans. **(B)** Spleen

Corpora arenacea are seen in:

A. Liver
C. Pancreas
B. Pineal
D. Pituitary
Ans. **(B)** Pineal

Urinary bladder is lined by:

A. Squamous epithelium
B. Stratified columnar epithelium
C. Transitional epithelium
D. Pseudostratified ciliated columnar epithelium
Ans. **(C)** Transitional epithelium

Light pathway involves:

A. Lateral geniculate body
C. Olivary nucleus
B. Medial geniculate body
D. Trapezoid body
Ans. **(A)** Lateral geniculate body

Crescents are a histological feature of:

A. Sweat gland
C. Salivary glands
B. Sebaceous glands
D. Pancreas
Ans. **(C)** Salivary glands

Which nerve is basically considered a tract with meninges covering it?

A. Optic
C. Facial
B. Oculomotor
D. Mandibular
Ans. **(A)** Optic nerve

Porter's tip deformity is seen in:

A. Erb's paralysis
C. Sprengel deformity
B. Klumpke's paralysis
D. Colles' fracture

Ans. (A) Erb's paralysis

Horner's syndrome accompanies:

A. Erb's paralysis
C. Sprengel deformity
B. Klumpke' s paralysis
D. Colles' fracture

Ans. (B) Klumpke's paralysis

Scapula is involved in:

A. Erb's paralysis
C. Sprengel deformity
B. Klumpke's paralysis
D. Colles' fracture

Ans. (C) Sprengel deformity

Demilunes are a histological feature of:

A. Pancreas
C. Sebaceous glands
B. Salivary glands
D. Sweat gland

Ans. (B) Salivary glands

Musculocutaneous nerve does not supply:

A. Brachialis
C. Coracobrachialis
B. Biceps femoris
D. None

Ans. (B) Biceps femoris

The fate of the notochord is that it:

A. Completely disappers
B. Persists as vertebral body
C. Persists as the intervertebral disc as a whole
D. Persists as nucleus pulposus

Ans. (D) Persists as nucleus pulposus

Nerve of Bell is:

A. Saphenous nerve
B. Sural nerve
C. Long thoracic nerve
D. Intercostobrachial nerve

Ans. (C) Long thoracic nerve

Vessel present inside carotid sheath is:

A. External carotid artery
C. Costocervical trunk
B. Thyrocervical trunk
D. Internal carotid artery

Ans. (D) Internal carotid artery

In carotico cavernous fistula vessel involved is:

A. Thyrocervical trunk   B. Internal carotid artery
C. External carotid artery   D. Costocervical trunk
Ans. (B) Internal carotid artery

The nerve of second pharyngeal arch is:

A. Recurrent laryngeal nerve   B. Mandibular nerve
C. Facial nerve   D. Maxillary nerve
Ans. (C) Facial nerve

Coronary sinus opens into:

A. Right atrium   B. Right ventricle
C. Posterior wall of left atrium   D. All of the above
Ans. (A) Right atrium

Hypoglossal nucleus lies in:

A. Lower pons   B. Medulla
C. Pons   D. Midbrain
Ans. (B) Medulla

Tonsil is lined by:

A. Stratified squamous keratinized epithelium
B. Stratified squamous non keratinized epithelium
C. Columnar epithelium
D. Cuboidal epithelium
Ans. (B) Stratified squamous nonkeratinized epithelium

Epididymis is embryologically developed from:

A. Metanephros   B. Mesonephros
C. Mesonephric duct   D. Ureteric bud
Ans. (C) Mesonephric duct

Germinal epithelium is:

A. Stratified squamous keratinized epithelium
B. Stratified squamous non keratinized epithelium
C. Columnar epithelium
D. Cuboidal epithelium
Ans. (D) Cuboidal epithelium

Pineal gland contains:

A. Herring bodies   B. Brain sand
C. Councilman's bodies   D. Amyloid bodies
Ans. (B) Brain sand

Central artery of retina is branch of:

A. External carotid artery

B. Internal carotid artery

C. Ophthalmic artery

D. Basilar artery

Ans. (C) Ophthalmic artery

Allantoic diverticulum is a prolongation of:

A. Primitive streak

B. Yolk sac

C. Embryo proper

D. Trophoblast

Ans. (B) Yolk sac

The embryological first pharyngeal arches remains as:

A. Styloid ligament

B. Stylomandibular ligament

C. Stylonoid ligament

D. Sphenomandibular ligament

Ans. (D) Sphenomandibular ligament

Pars cystica forms:

A. Thoracic duct

B. Gartner's duct

C. Cystic duct

D. Hepatic duct

Ans. (C) Cystic duct

Pin point pupils and hyperpyrexia are seen in lesions of:

A. Midbrain

B. Pons

C. Medulla

D. Cerebellum

Ans. (B) Pons

Safety muscle of tongue is:

A. Styloglossus

B. Stylopharyngeus

C. Palatoglossus

D. Genioglossus

Ans. (D) Genioglossus

Muscle of tongue not supplied by hypoglossal nerve is:

A. Styloglossus

B. Stylopharyngeus

C. Palatoglossus

D. Genioglossus

Ans. (B) Stylopharyngeus

Mid shaft fracture humerus causes:

A. Axillary nerve palsy

B. Median nerve palsy

C. Radial nerve palsy

D. Ulnar nerve palsy

Ans. (C) Radial nerve palsy

Rule of 2 applies to:

A. Ligament of Treitz

B. Meckel's diverticulum

C. Appendicis epiploicae

D. Sacculations

Ans. (B) Meckel's diverticulum

The vagina is a muscular tube lined with:

A. Non stratified squamous epithelium that is histologically similar to the mucosa of the cervix and vulva

B. Stratified squamous epithelium that is histologically similar to the mucosa of the cervix and vulva

C. Stratified cuboidal epithelium that is not histologically similar to the mucosa of the cervix and vulva

D. Stratified cuboidal epithelium that is histologically similar to the mucosa of the cervix and vulva

Ans (B) Stratified squamous epithelium that is histologically similar to the mucosa of the cervix and vulva

Adrenal cortex arises from:

A. Mesonephros

B. Mesoderm

C. Endoderm

D. Ectoderm

Ans. (B) Mesoderm

Tonsillar artery is a branch of:

A. Superficial temporal artery

B. Maxillary artery

C. Lingual artery

D. Facial artery

Ans. (D) Facial artery

Epidural hematoma is due to:

A. Subdural veins

B. Ophthalmic artery

C. Occipital artery

D. Middle meningeal artery

Ans. (D) Middle meningeal artery

Deep cervical fascia of neck is:

A. Colles' fascia

B. Fascia colli

C. Camper's fascia

D. Waldeyer's fascia

Ans. (B) Fascia colli

True about long thoracic nerve is:

A. Known as nerve of Bell

B. Supplies serratus anterior

C. Paralysis results in 'winged scapula'

D. All of the above

Ans. (D) All of the above

Oral diaphragm is formed by:

A. Hypoglossus

B. Mylohyoid

C. Geniohyoid

D. Genioglossus

Ans. (B) Mylohyoid

Frey syndrome involves:

A. Flushing and sweating of the skin
B. Presence of cutaneous hyperaesthesia
C. Auriculotemporal nerve
D. All of the above

Ans. (D) All of the above

Over head abduction of shoulder is by:

A. Trapezius
B. Latissimus dorsi
C. Deltoid
D. Supraspinatus

Ans. (A) Trapezius

Superior epigastric vessels lie in:

A. Fascia transversalis
B. Rectus sheath
C. External oblique aponeurosis
D. Pelvic fascia

Ans. (B) Rectus sheath

Ligament of Treitz is related to:

A. Suprarenal gland
B. Stomach
C. Duodenum
D. Liver

Ans. (C) Duodenum

Chromaffin tissue is:

A. Suprarenal gland
B. Stomach
C. Duodenum
D. Liver

Ans. (A) Suprarenal gland

Traube's space is related to:

A. Oesophagus
B. Right kidney
C. Stomach
D. Right lobe of liver

Ans. Stomach

Couinaud's segments are related to:

A. Spleen
B. Kidneys
C. Liver
D. Thymus

Ans. (B) Kidneys

In anterior cord syndrome true is/are:

A. Loss of motor function below the level of lesion
B. Loss of pain and temperature sensation below the level of lesion
C. Relative preservation of vibration and position sense
D. All of the above

Ans. (D) All of the above

Fabella is present in:

A. Sartorius   B. Gracilis
C. Soleus   D. Gastrocnemius

Ans. (D) Gastrocnemius

Axillary nerve may be injured in:

A. Crutch paralysis
B. Dislocation of shoulder
C. Fracture of surgical neck of humerus
D. All of the above

Ans. (D) All of the above

When the patient is asked to place his hands on the wall in front and asked to push, the medial border of the scapula on the affected side stands out. It is because of damage to:

A. Posterior interosseous nerve   B. Suprascapular nerve
C. Radial nerve   D. Long thoracic nerve

Ans. (D) Long thoracic nerve

Perthe's disease is osteochondritis of:

A. Capitate   B. Tibial tubercle
C. Humeral head   D. Femoral head

Ans. (D) Femoral head

Triangle of auscultation is bounded by all except:

A. Trapezius   B. Latissimus dorsi
C. Medial border of scapula   D. Rhomboidius minor

Ans. (D) Rhomboidius minor

Features of mediastinal syndrome are all except:

A. Superior vena cava—engorgement of veins in upper half of body
B. Trachea-dyspnea
C. Left recurrent laryngeal nerve—hoarseness of voice
D. Vagus nerve—paralysis of diaphragm on the affected side

Ans. (D) Vagus nerve—paralysis of diaphragm on the affected side

All are true for Frey syndrome, except:

A. This syndrome is a sequel anastomosis of auriculotemporal nerve to great auricular nerve
B. It is characterized by unilateral facial flushing
C. Hyperesthesia over the cutaneous distributions of auriculotemporal nerve
D. None of above

Ans. (D) None of above

All are true about Arnold-Chiari syndrome except:

A. This is the most common congenital anomaly involving cerebellum
B. The vermis of cerebellum herniates into the vertebral canal through foramen magnum
C. This anomaly results in hydrocephalus
D. This is rarely associated with spina bifida

Ans. (D) This is rarely associated with spina bifida

In cauda equina syndrome all are true except:

A. Sensory loss along the distribution of affected spinal nerves
B. Lower motor neuron paralysis
C. Bladder and bowel involvement is seen
D. None

Ans. (D) None

Frankfurts plane is seen in relation to:

A. Pelvis
B. Thigh
C. Skull
D. Breast

Ans. (C) Skull

Weber's syndrome involves:

A. Midbrain
B. Pons
C. Medulla
D. Cerebellum

Ans. (A) Midbrain

The Hilum of the right lung is arched by:

A. Vagus nerve
B. Thoracic duct
C. Azygous vein
D. Esophagus

Ans. (C) Azygous vein

Nuclei of cerebellum are all except:

A. Nucleus globosus
B. Nucleus emboliformis
C. Nucleus dentate
D. Nucleus caudatus

Ans. (D) Nucleus caudatus

Nerve accompanying cranial nerve VIII is:

A. Recurrent laryngeal nerve
B. Abducent nerve
C. Facial nerve
D. Maxillary nerve

Ans. (C) Facial nerve

Kienböck's disease is osteochondritis of:

A. Capitate
B. Lunate
C. Trapezium
D. Scaphoid

Ans. (B) Lunate

All of the following muscles are supplied by pharyngeal plexus except:

A. Cricopharyngeus

B. Paltoglossus

C. Salpingopharyngeus

D. Stylopharyngeus

Ans. (D) Stylopharyngeus

Peg cells are seen in:

A. Liver

B. Intestine

C. Uterine tube

D. Uterus

Ans. (C) Uterine tube

The number of bronchopulmonary segments in each lung is:

A. 8

B. 9

C. 10

D. 11

Ans. (C) 10

Anterior cardiac vein open into:

A. Right atrium

B. Right ventricle

C. Posterior wall of left atrium

D. Anterior wall of left ventricle

Ans. (B) Right ventricle

Howships lacunae are seen around:

A. Plasma cells

B. Adipose cells

C. Pigment cells

D. Osteoclasts

Ans. (D) Osteoclasts

Fallopian tube is lined by:

A. Squamous epithelium

B. Columnar epithelium

C. Transitional epithelium

D. Cuboidal epithelium

Ans. (B) Columnar epithelium

"Hassall's corpuscles" are seen in:

A. Liver

B. Spleen

C. Thymus

D. Lymph nodes

Ans. (C) Thymus

Not related to the development of tongue is:

A. Lingual swelling

B. First pharyngeal arch

C. Tuberculum impar

D. Hypobranchial prominence

Ans. (B) First pharyngeal arch

The muscle attached to root of spine of scapula is:

A. Teres minor

B. Teres major

C. Rhomboidius minor

D. Rhomboidius major

Ans. (C) Rhomboidius minor

The bone which undergoes avascular necrosis after a fall on outstretched hand is:

A. Trapezium
B. Lunate
C. Scaphoid
D. Trapezoid

Ans. (C) Scaphoid

The joint formed in glenohumeral articulation is:

A. Ellipsoid
B. Hinge
C. Ball and socket
D. Saddle

Ans. (C) Ball and socket

The structures in relation to spiral groove of humerus is:

A. Axillary nerve
B. Radial nerve
C. Ulnar nerve
D. Musculocutaneous nerve

Ans. (B) Radial nerve

The nerve lies behind the medial epicondyle of humerus. The most likely nerve is:

A. Ulnar nerve
B. Radial nerve
C. Musculocutaneous nerve
D. Axillary nerve

Ans. (A) Ulnar nerve

Patella is classified as:

A. Long bone
B. Short bone
C. Undifferentiated bone
D. Sesamoid bone

Ans. (D) Sesamoid bone

The damage to the nerve passing in relation to the neck of fibula. Palsy of this nerve would result in:

A. Meralgia parasthetica
B. Foot drop
C. Sciatica
D. None of the above

Ans. (B) Foot drop

The arrangement of branches of facial nerve is called as:

A. Pes cavus
B. Ansa subclavian
C. Pes anserinus
D. None of the above

Ans. (D) None of the above

Follicles are seen in:

A. Ovary
B. Thyroid
C. None
D. Both

Ans. (D) Both

Multiple Choice Questions

Sertoli cells are seen in:

A. Epididymis
B. Uterine tube
C. Uterus
D. Testis

Ans. (D) Testis

Corpora amylacea are seen in:

A. Prostate
B. Pineal
C. Pancreas
D. Pituitary

Ans. (A) Prostate

Palsy of axillary nerve would lead to:

A. Paralysis of pectoralis major
B. Paralysis of pectoralis minor
C. Paralysis of deltoid
D. Paralysis of serratus anterior

Ans. (C) Paralysis of deltoid

All are true about menisci except:

A. The tear in the medial meniscus may be in the longitudinal direction (bucket handle tear) or transverse
B. The medial meniscus is firmly adherent to the deep part of tibial collateral ligament
C. Medial meniscus is more prone to injury than lateral meniscus
D. Injury to the lateral meniscus is less common because the meniscus is relatively fixed

Ans. (D) Injury to the lateral meniscus is less common because the meniscus is relatively fixed.

Examphalos is:

A. The persistence of physiological hernia of foregut loop outside the abdominal cavity
B. The persistence of physiological hernia of midgut loop outside the abdominal cavity
C. The persistence of physiological hernia of hindgut loop outside the abdominal cavity
D. None of the above

Ans. (B) The persistence of physiological hernia of midgut loop outside the abdominal cavity

The gall bladder is supplied by:

A. Cystic artery which is usually a branch of right hepatic artery
B. Cystic artery which is usually a branch of left hepatic artery
C. Cystic artery which is usually a branch of common hepatic artery
D. Cystic artery which is usually a branch of celiac artery

Ans. (A) Cystic artery which is usually a branch of right hepatic artery

Suprapubic incision is called as:

A. Lanz incision
B. Pfannensteil
C. Kocher
D. McBurney

Ans. (B) Pfannensteil

The vessel shown supplying this part of stomach and denoted by arrow is:

A. Left gastroepiploic artery
B. Right gastroepiploic artery
C. Right gastric artery
D. Left gastric artery

Ans. (A) Left gastroepiploic artery

All are true except:

A. Radial artery is used for arterial blood gas estimation
B. Brachial artery is used for BP measurement
C. Axillary artery has no branch
D. Radial artery is a branch of brachial artery

Ans. (C) Axillary artery has no branch

Teres minor is supplied by:

A. Radial nerve
B. Axillary nerve
C. Ulnar nerve
D. Musculocutaneous nerve

Ans. (B) Axillary nerve

White pulp is seen in:

A. Tonsil
B. Spleen
C. Thymus
D. Lymph nodes

Ans. (B) Spleen

"Kupffer cells" are seen in:

A. Liver
B. Spleen
C. Thymus
D. Lymph nodes

Ans. (A) Liver

Parafollicular cells are is seen in:

A. Parathyroid
B. Parotid
C. Thyroid
D. Pituitary

Ans. (C) Thyroid

The nerve which causes wrist drop is:

A. Axillary
B. Radial
C. Ulnar
D. None

Ans. (B) Radial

Cavernous sinus is:

A. An air sinus

B. A lymphatic sinus

C. An arterial sinus

D. A venous sinus

Ans. (D) A venous sinus

The sites where blood–brain barrier it is absent are called:

A. Ventricular organs

B. Circumventricular organs

C. Intraventricular organs

D. Nonventricular organs

Ans. (B) Circumventricular organs

Nissl granules in a neuron represent:

A. Golgi body

B. Fat

C. Mitochondria

D. ER

Ans. (D) ER

Most cerebral aneurysms are present:

A. In anterior circulation

B. In posterior circulation

C. Outside circle of Willis

D. Along basilar artery

Ans. (A) In anterior circulation

Suprapleural membrane is called:

A. Waldeyer's fascia

B. Colles' fascia

C. Deep cervical fascia

D. Sibson's fascia

Ans. (D) Sibson's fascia

Dorsiflexion of foot is by all muscles except:

A. Tibialis anterior

B. Peroneus tertius

C. Extensor hallucis longus

D. Soleus

Ans. (D) Soleus

The evertors of foot are:

A. Perroneus brevis

B. Peroneus longus

C. Peroneus tertius

D. All of the above

Ans. (D) All of the above

Anatomically the ureter is constricted at:

A. Two places

B. Three places

C. Five places

D. Six places

Ans. (B) Three places

True statement about femoral hernia is:

A. It is more common in males
B. It is more common in females
C. Occurs with equal frequency in both
D. Never occurs in females

Ans. (B) It is more common in females

White line is also known as:

A. Schwalbe's line
B. Rosenmüller's line
C. Reid's line
D. Hilton's line

Ans. (D) Hilton's line

"Level 1" lymph nodes draining breast are represented by:

A. Lymph nodes below pectoralis minor
B. Lymph nodes above pectoralis minor
C. Lymph nodes behind pectoralis minor
D. Lymph nodes below pectoralis major

Ans. (A) Lymph nodes below pectoralis minor

Pathway for "Light Reflex" is by:

A. Afferent: Optic nerve   Efferent: Oculomotor nerve
B. Afferent: Ophthalmic nerve   Efferent: Facial nerve
C. Afferent: Optic nerve   Efferent: Facial nerve
D. Afferent: Ophthamic nerve   Efferent: Oculomotor nerve

Ans (A) Afferent: Optic nerve   Efferent: Oculomotor nerve

Dorsalis pedis artery is a continuation of:

A. Anterior tibial artery
B. Posterior tibial artery
C. Peroneal artery
D. Fibular artery

Ans. (A) Anterior tibial artery

"Lacis" cells are:

A. Glial cells of cerebellum
B. Stellate cells in liver
C. Extraglomerular mesangial cells
D. Secretory cells in mucosa of uterine tube

Ans. (C) Extraglomerular mesangial cells

The "Encapsulated" mechanoreceptors include:

A. Pacinian corpuscles
B. Meissner's corpuscles
C. Ruffini's corpuscles
D. Merkel's disc

Ans. (D) Merkel's disc

Salient features of histology of gall bladder distinguishing it from intestines are all except:

A. Tallest columnar

B. Highly folded irregular and branched mucosa

C. No villi

D. Plenty of goblet cells

Ans. (D) Plenty of goblet cells

Ear pinna is made up of:

A. Fibrocartilage

B. Elastic cartilage

C. Hyaline cartilage

D. None

Ans. (B) Elastic cartilage

Tunica albuginea lines:

A. Epididymis

B. Uterine tube

C. Uterus

D. Testis

Ans. (D) Testis

Crypts are a feature of:

A. Tonsil

B. Spleen

C. Thymus

D. Lymph nodes

Ans. (A) Tonsil

All except following are features of large intestine:

A. Appendicis epiploicae

B. Sacculations

C. Taenia coli

D. Brunner's glands

Ans. (D) Brunner's glands

Cranial accessory nerve supplies:

A. Sternocleidomastoid

B. Trapezius

C. Lattisimus dorsi

D. Muscles of pharynx

Ans. (D) Muscles of pharynx

"Corpora arenacea" are present in:

A. Pituitary gland

B. Pineal gland

C. Prostate

D. Thymus

Ans. (B) Pineal gland

Area likely involved in schizophrenia is:

A. The locus ceruleus

B. The basal nucleus of Meynert

C. The caudate nucleus

D. The ventral tegmental area

Ans. (D) The ventral tegmental area

Left-sided hemiplegia and sensory deficits mainly of the face and arms and left visual field neglect with inability to gaze to the left and neglect of the left side is caused by thrombosis of:

A. Left middle cerebral artery

B. Right middle cerebral artery

C. Left anterior cerebral artery

D. Right anterior cerebral artery

Ans. (B) Right middle cerebral artery

"Satiety centre" is represented by which nucleus of hypothalamus?

A. Ventromedial nucleus

B. Lateral nucleus

C. Septal nucleus

D. Periventricular nucleus

Ans. (A) Ventromedial nucleus

The "Superior para thyroids" develop from:

A. The first pharyngeal pouch

B. The third pharyngeal pouch

C. The fourth pharyngeal pouch

D. The fifth pharyngeal pouch

Ans. (C) The fourth pharyngeal pouch

Main extensor of hip joint is:

A. Psoas major

B. Gluteus maximus

C. Pectineus

D. Gracilis

Ans. (B) Gluteus maximus

Herniation of "cerebellar tonsils" is a feature of:

A. Arnold-Chiari malformation

B. Dandy-Walker malformation

C. Holoprosencephaly

D. Lissencephaly

Ans. (A) Arnold-Chiari malformation